EARTHLY GOODS

Also by Christopher Joyce

Witnesses from the Grave: The Stories Bones Tell
(with Eric Stover)

EARTHLY GOODS

Medicine-Hunting in the Rainforest

by Christopher Joyce

Little, Brown and Company

Boston   New York   Toronto   London

First Edition

"The Force That Through the Green Fuse Drives the Flower" by Dylan Thomas from *Poems of Dylan Thomas*. Copyright 1939 by New Directions Publishing Corp. Reprinted by permission of New Directions Publishing Corp.

Library of Congress Cataloging-in-Publication Data

Joyce, Christopher.
    Earthly goods : medicine-hunting in the rainforest / by Christopher Joyce.—1st ed.
        p.   cm.
    Includes bibliographical references and index.
    ISBN 0-316-47408-8
    1. Materia medica, Vegetable. 2. Medicinal plants. 3. Rain forest plants. 4. Pharmacognosy.   I. Title.
    RS164.J69   1994   615'.32'0913—dc20   93-49736

            10 9 8 7 6 5 4 3 2 1

                    RRD-VA

Published simultaneously in Canada by Little, Brown & Company (Canada) Limited

Printed in the United States of America

To my father

The force that through the green fuse drives the flower
Drives my green age; that blasts the roots of trees
Is my destroyer.
And I am dumb to tell the crooked rose
My youth is bent by the same wintry fever.

The force that drives the water through the rocks
Drives my red blood; that dries the mouthing streams
Turns mine to wax.
And I am dumb to mouth unto my veins
How at the mountain spring the same mouth sucks.

The hand that whirls the water in the pool
Stirs the quicksand; that ropes the blowing wind
Hauls my shroud sail.
And I am dumb to tell the hanging man
How of my clay is made the hangman's lime.

The lips of time leech to the fountain head;
Love drips and gathers, but the fallen blood
Shall calm her sores.
And I am dumb to tell a weather's wind
How time has ticked a heaven round the stars.

And I am dumb to tell the lover's tomb
How at my sheet goes the same crooked worm.

—Dylan Thomas, ''The Force That Through the
    Green Fuse Drives the Flower''

Contents

Acknowledgments

Dragging a writer along on a botanical expedition into the rainforest is a dubious undertaking, and I would like to thank Brad Bennett of Florida International University and the New York Botanical Garden for taking the risk. Thanks go also to Costa Rica's National Institute of Biodiversity and Merck & Company for permitting me to accompany their scientists into the field; and to Michael Balick, Rosita Arvigo, and Gregory Shropshire for accommodating me in Belize. Also, the hospitality of Patricia Terrack and the people of San Miguel in Ecuador was second to none. Closer to home, I am most grateful that Michael Boyd and his colleagues at the National Cancer Institute opened their doors wide to me. I thank Walt Reid and Doug Fuller for their advice and encouragement, and writer Margaret Krieg, whose book *Green Medicine*, published in 1964, was an inspiration.

The loving and wise editorial hand of my wife, Melissa Hendricks, deftly polished what I crudely set down, and computer wizard Steve Rubin transmuted it into black and white. As always, literary agent Kristine Dahl steered me in the right direction, and William Phillips and Catherine Crawford at Little, Brown and Company delivered me safe and sound to my destination.

Introduction

A tall, shirtless white man stands in a clearing cut from a towering
rainforest in southeastern Colombia. His gray trousers hang loosely
around his thin waist, his cheeks are dark with stubble, and his fair hair
is cut close as fuzz on a peach. Carefully, he inserts the end of an
eight-inch-long bone tube into his left nostril. The other end of the tube
is held by a Yukuna Indian, a brown, compact man who, with a faint
suggestion of a smile, puts his end of the tube to his lips. Inside the tube
is a fine, rust-colored powder. It is called *lukux-rí*, a narcotic ground
from the dried leaves of a plant cultivated by the Yukuna. The Indian
takes a deep breath. . . .

The snuff is tobacco, among the mildest of the narcotic plants of
South American Indian cultures. The snuff has many names in the
western Amazon — *yema*, *ali*, and *mulu* are common ones in Colombia.
Indigenous people take it for recreation, as a medicine, and during
religious ceremonies. The Yukuna and the white man in the village
clearing are preparing themselves for a *Kai-ya-ree* dance, a three-day
ritual reenactment of the evolution of the Yukuna, during which the
celebrants will inhale bucketsful of the snuff. Like many tropical plant

drugs, it is said by its users to contain spirits that will put them in touch with the divinities that rule heaven and earth. The white man with the tube in his nose, however, is of the opinion that the magic comes from about a dozen pyridine alkaloids, including anabasine, nornicotine, and nicotine. After all, he is a Harvard man. He is Richard Evans Schultes, the world's foremost hunter of medicinal and hallucinogenic plants.

My first sight of Schultes was with the Yukuna snuff tube stuck into his nose, in a photograph in an old book on plant medicines. He was described as an ethnobotanist, someone who studies how different cultures, especially aboriginal peoples, use plants. *Lukux-rí* was among the more benign of many potent medicinal and hallucinogenic plants Schultes sampled during the thirteen years, from 1941 to 1954, he spent in South America. Most of it he spent in the Amazon, that luxuriously forested basin that stretches like an aerial sea from the Brazilian Atlantic to the Andes in the west, and south to the heart of the South American continent. When Schultes came back to Harvard, he brought twenty-four thousand plant specimens with him, including two thousand used by traditional healers. The collection is still being studied, and Schultes believes there might yet be undiscovered new medicines within it.

Searching for new medicines in the plant kingdom has been a cyclical science in the twentieth century. A chance discovery would encourage new exploration, but soon people would weary of plant-hunting's physical demands and unpredictable payoffs. Eventually, drugmakers turned away from nature, believing that it had already yielded its useful novelties. For all his charm, his Latin, his Harvard breeding, Schultes and his ilk were eccentrics, they said, people who lived in huts, slept in hammocks, and took hallucinogenic drugs with half-naked Indians.

Schultes's students took him more seriously, however. For three decades, he sent them into the rainforests to learn for themselves, and many returned with tales of powerful plants. Then, in the mid-1980s, two things happened. First, while drugmakers improved their understanding of how diseases work, they also started to run short of ideas for new chemical compounds to treat them. Second, the world started to grasp that tropical forests were shrinking like parchment put to flame. The chance to see if Schultes and his fellow tropical botanists were right could pass by in our lifetimes. Soon, an unlikely brigade formed to snatch at the flames for clues to the rest of nature's pharmacopoeia.

These people are ethnobotanists and anthropologists, many trained by Schultes himself, who follow the shamans and healers who live in the forests. They are also ecologists and conservationists who read the rainforest's intricate codex in a rolled leaf, a rotting tree limb, or a spider's web. They are cancer researchers in multimillion-dollar labs and northwestern loggers peeling bark from yew trees. And they are businesses that see profits in rainforest products. Together, they are part of a radical experiment. Its goal is twofold: to change the way people search for and test potential new medicines while at the same time preserving the world's great forests by showing how much more valuable they are standing than cut. This book describes that experiment and the people who are caught up in it.

There is a deeper connection between these plant-hunters and tropical forests, however, than simply the desire to turn green to gold. Many sense a deep-seated, almost ineffable connection, a spiritual umbilicus, with the natural world. It is a connection, they fear, that we are cutting at our peril.

The indigenous peoples of the Amazon have long believed that humans are connected to their creator through the elemental cord of the branch, the stem, or the vine. In his book *Plants of the Gods*, written with Albert Hofmann, Schultes relates the myth of *yopo*, an hallucinogenic snuff. "In the beginning, the Sun created various beings to serve as intermediaries between Him and Earth. He created hallucinogenic snuff powder in his navel, but the Daughter of the Sun found it. Thus it became available to man — a vegetal product acquired directly from the gods." So also came the Indians' food, their houses, their medicine — from root and bark, flesh and feather, earth and river.

Reflect for a moment on our species' history. During our evolution from knuckle-walkers to mall-builders, we spent most of our time as hunter-gatherers living in and from nature. Whether it was savannah, rainforest, tropical island, alpine meadow, or northern steppe, the land sustained us. Even now, we deliberately seek out environments that remind us of our ancestral home in nature. Our paintings, our vacation spots, our parks, even our landscaped gardens reflect our species' innate attachment to nature, our "biophilia." Likewise, our innate phobias about darkness, snakes, or enclosed spaces without avenues of escape point to a flip side, a biophobia. In both cases, says Harvard biologist Edward O. Wilson, who has tried to locate the source of these affinities and phobias, we appear to have a built-in preference for learning certain ways of choosing and manipulating our environments, ways that favor survival.

No environment has been richer, more varied in life — more bio-diverse — than the rainforests. These forests have been and probably still are the deep, sweet wells from which flow not only the means of life but new forms of life as well. So if we raze them now, dust off our hands, and walk away, what are the consequences?

One consequence will be the extinction of nature's best-endowed library of chemical invention, a library far larger than anything humans have ever created. That explains the seriousness with which biologists and ecologists take this renaissance in plant-hunting. Moreover, as the forests go, so go the cultures — the Witoto, the Yukuna, the Tubeos, the Tukanos, the Gwananos — that, like living time capsules, have survived in a sort of suspended animation within them. Schultes and his disciples have paged through the rainforests' volumes with these people. "You must remember," Schultes says, "when you go into the forest, the Indians are the professors and you are the student." This book is written in that spirit.

Part

1

Return to the Native

1

Paradise Revisited

The eye prefers to view landscapes from back to front, from the horizon to the foreground. A view of the rainforest that rolls down the slopes of the Ecuadorean Andes, for example, begins as a gray suggestion of mountains behind a milky haze. From there on in, the land itself is hidden: no jut of scarp, bowl of brown earth, or rocky outcrop to signal the work of geology. Shapes are vague and repetitive, and no geometry arrests the eye, no real contrasts except variegations in greenness that are almost too subtle to catch for someone raised amid pasture or prairie. Here it seems as if the carbonaceous essence of the Earth has oozed to the surface and been twisted into vermiculite shapes and packed like fibers in a felt carpet.

For millions of years, rainforests such as this girdled the globe, more or less following the imaginary line of the equator. These huge forests expanded and contracted according to the rules of nature, controlled by climate, geology, and geography. Within them teemed hundreds of thousands, perhaps millions of species of animals and plants, including humans, who like their fellow forest creatures drew everything they needed from the forest itself, and in such a way that what marks they made were quickly subsumed within the body of the vegetation that is master of the land.

The great forests of Africa, Asia, and Central and South America that began assembling themselves about one hundred million years ago have for the most part become archipelagos now. Human colonization over the past five hundred years, with its demand for wood, pasture, and farmland, has cut away half of them. Yet when combined, the islands of rainforest that remain still occupy about eight million square kilometers, about the area of the continental United States, or 6 percent of the Earth's land surface. And although their reach has been greatly curtailed, these forests still reign as undisputed champions of life. Home to as many as half the planet's species, they are Earth's incubators, magnificent not so much for their appearance but for what they represent: a part of the planet that still belongs to the plant, the insect, the serpent, and the bird. They are as much an idea as a place, a world created out of the collective unconscious of all that is *non*human, a presence that has thrived in total indifference to humanity. These forests make us feel small.

Experiencing a moist tropical lowland forest, the kind usually associated with the image of "jungle," is disconcerting at first. Inside it, there is too much for the eye to behold, and the parts appear to be even greater than the sum. Within a near-uniformity of greenness, the chaos of shape and shadow is unlike any other earthly scene. It is overwhelmingly *vegetable* — 99 percent of the forest's biomass consists of plants. One's gaze roves, unable to fasten on a single object. No two shapes are quite the same, yet all are kin: leaves as hearts and ovals and pointy-tipped lances, feathery leaves in parallel rows like a rib cage, recumbent leaves that hug the ground in rosettes or circle upright stems in whorls, leaves like elephant ears turned upward to find shafts of sunlight. Branches swoop and twist, linear only in the way spaghetti is.

For all its anarchy of shape, the forest interior is a curiously static scene, one that might have been captured on the canvas of a possessed painter. Henri Rousseau was famous for his jungle paintings, but they seem too tidy and muted next to the real thing. Hieronymus Bosch, the Dutch painter who covered canvases edge to edge with leering, misshapen creatures and mutant plants, might have captured it better. Or Bosch's surrealistic heir, Salvador Dalí, whose melting clocks, towers, and lampposts ape the rainforest's ambience of hanging and drooping, of stems curving down under the weight of glossy leaves and lianas undulating earthward from invisible celestial roots.

What confronts the walker in the rainforest is unparalleled biodiversity. No one knows how many plants and animals exist. But one thing is clear: here, biodiversity is run amok. Along the eastern slope of the Ecuadorean Andes, where the Amazon basin ends, there are thought to be as many as twenty-five thousand species of vascular plants, that is, practically speaking, the larger plants that are not lichen, moss, algae, or fungi. Down at the foot of those Andean slopes, in the lowland moist forest, where two to four meters of rain fall every year, the number of species reaches as many as fifty thousand. Here, over the aeons, the biological dice have been thrown uncountable times. Nature has then allowed the mutants, the experiments, to live on in profusion where, in harsher climates, they surely would have succumbed. The *Heliconia*, how bizarre a thing that is! Not satisfied simply to produce colorful flowers, the plant throws up a three-foot spike bearing a row of showy red, yellow, or orange bracts that look like lobster claws. Poking its petaled head out of each bract is a flower. The ungainly apparatus is designed to attract the plant's pollinator, the humming-bird, a lucky bird indeed to have such glorious color and shape created just for its pleasure. Or there are the ruthless strangler fig trees, who propagate from the seeds in animal droppings that collect in the crotches of trees. As they grow, they wrap their roots around the host tree in a woody lattice and send them down into the ground. Eventu-ally, the fig chokes off the supply of nutrients for its host, which starves, dies, and rots out from inside the fig. Sometimes several figs join to-gether to overcome a host tree in a sort of botanical mugging.

To grasp the extent of the world's biodiversity, biologists lay a sort of conceptual gridwork over the natural world by dividing it into "life zones." These are categories of habitat and climate that describe the way life parcels itself out over the Earth. Each zone has its own geo-graphical anchor — be it mountain slope, glacial valley, riverbank, or savannah — and its own characteristic forms of life. The tropical forest contains several life zones, such as the swampy, flooded *varzea* in Bra-zil, or the misty montane, or mountain forest, which absorbs moisture from clouds on slopes as high as ten thousand feet. Costa Rica, the size of West Virginia, has twelve life zones, one more than the entire eastern United States. Peru, on the western edge of the Amazon basin, has the most of any country, with seventy-eight at last count.

Along the slopes of the Andes, for example, the narrow band of montane and premontane moist forest, sometimes called cloud forest, is markedly different from what people normally think of as rainforest. If landscapes have mood, this one is of somnolence. The sky is usually overcast, and an almost unbroken dark green upholstery of low-lying herbaceous plants covers the precipitous rise and fall of cliffs, crags, and river gorges. The trees clump together in glades rather than in the massed formations of the lowland moist forest. Several hundred species of orchids grow hidden in the brush and the mist, for this is the land of the epiphyte, the piggyback plants of the forest. Perhaps the most intriguing are the spike-leafed bromeliads and aroids that live aboard trees. Huddled among the branches with seemingly no means of sustenance, these plants inherit rainfall, detritus, windblown soil, and insects and other animals that live and die amid their leaves. Some bear bright yellow edges like racing stripes on their leaves, others rich rose hues at their stems, and they dress up the forest like crepe paper for a woodsman's party. Arboreal epiphytes are among the least understood of tropical plants, since so many are beyond the reach of all but those who can climb or fly to them. They are also home to myriad creatures. A bromeliad's chief attraction is the well of rainwater that forms at the tight rosette where the leaves join at their bases. Birds sip from these wells, as do generations of tiny frogs with iridescent skin the color of limes or bananas. The frogs feed on the beetles and ants that forage and live within the bromeliad. The chain continues downward, with as many as three hundred different species of worms, protozoans, and microorganisms living in a single pool. The bromeliad is a miniature, aerial zoo.

Yet this thriving world is all but invisible to the 99 percent of humanity that long ago abandoned the forest. To most of us, the enormity of such a place, its indifference, its apparent immobility, either chills us or, more often, bores us. Aside from the indigenous peoples of the forest, those best equipped to really understand what they see in a walk through a South American rainforest are biologists, especially botanists. They have been coming to the Amazon like pilgrims to the Holy See since word of a new world overrun with exotic new forms of life returned with the ships of Columbus, Raleigh, Balboa, and Magellan. The naturalists marveled, described, collected, and returned to entertain the rest of the world with tales of adventure and exotica the newness of which this world will probably never experience again. Many died on their journeys, others lost their health, a few their minds, for it was arduous and dangerous work. Only someone bordering on the obsessive would have undertaken the jungle journeys of the early botanical explorers.

Perhaps the most famous was Richard Spruce, a nineteenth-century botanist with a yen for learning about the planet firsthand. The name Spruce is to tropical botanists what Sir Edmund Hillary is to mountain climbers. He was a hardy, stubborn Yorkshireman who spent seventeen years roaming the Amazon, twice traveling west from Belém up the Amazon River and its tributaries all the way to the Andes by boat, canoe, burro, and, mostly, by foot, for then as now the final demand the forest makes on the traveler is the muddy slope. Several times he came close to dying either by accident, disease, or treachery, all the while collecting thousands of plants never seen before by scientists. In a letter he sent in 1858 from the Amazon to his financial backers in England, Spruce gives a sense of the depth of his peculiar devotion as he describes a view from his dugout canoe:

> . . . I well recollect how the banks of the river had become clad with flowers, as it were by some sudden magic, and how I said to myself, as I scanned the lofty trees with wistful and disappointed eyes, "There goes a new *Dipteryx* — there goes a new *Qualea* — there goes a new 'the Lord knows what!' until I could no longer bear the sight, and covering up my face with my hands, I resigned myself to the sorrowful reflection that I must leave all these fine things "to waste their sweetness on the desert air."

As a plant-hunter, Spruce in turn drew inspiration from the experiences of those explorers who preceded him into the mysterious forests of South America. Their pedigree runs back through the visionary naturalist Baron Alexander von Humboldt, whose name is affixed to scores of tropical plants he first described in the Amazon and Andes, as well as to mountains, valleys, and ocean currents; the French scientist Charles Marie de La Condamine, who traveled widely among Ecuador's native peoples and introduced to Europe their exotic plants and customs; Don Antonio de Ulloa before him, the Spanish conquistadors' chronicler whose fanciful tales of man-eating serpents, ferocious insects, and hostile natives fed Europe's fantasies; and ultimately to the indigenous South Americans of uncounted centuries before any of them, for whom, like fishes, the forest was an infinite ocean.

Common threads tie together the histories of these explorers: bravery, imagination, persistence, acquisitiveness, sometimes arrogance. Above all, they were curious, fanatically so. First they were curious as naturalists. They poked into the corollas of orchids, measured the girth of monstrous trees, captured electric eels and beetles as big as snuffboxes. But they were also anthropologists. They collected tales from and about the native peoples of the rainforest, although in many cases they drew on hearsay from the Spanish colonizers and mestizos. But if they were amateurs in anthropological technique, they had the advantage of being among the first Europeans to encounter forest cultures in the tropics. Von Humboldt told of secret poisons cooked up by Indians from plants that, when applied to arrows and shot into a victim, killed in a most horrible and un-Christian manner. In 1736, La Condamine discovered natural rubber being tapped from trees by the descendants of shipwrecked slaves on the coast of Ecuador. One hundred and twenty years later, the Amazon rubber boom became South America's equivalent to North America's Gold Rush. Spruce reported potent vegetable potions that Indians swallowed to induce wild, grotesque hallucinations, and tracked down forests of mountain cinchona, the tree whose bark purportedly cured malaria.

This thread of curiosity about powerful plants is of a piece with the ancient tradition of medicinal botany. Two thousand years ago, medical practitioners were as much botanists as anything else, relying on their knowledge of healing plants to provide their materia medica. Until this century, in fact, plants and their extracts provided most medicines. Even as recently as the 1960s, 25 percent of the prescriptions filled in America contained one or more substances from higher plants as an active ingredient. Half of those come from the tropics. So the first rainforest plant-hunters were in their way medicine men. They whetted the appetites of Europe's physicians with stories and samples of fanciful febrifuges, magical poultices, saps that healed wounds, and decoctions that cured the ague. They started a quest for medicines from the rainforest whose hour, in our decade, has come round again.

Early European naturalists realized that the New World's biodiversity contained enormous potential for new products for the markets of Europe. Von Humboldt, after collecting several thousand new plants, returned to Europe in the first decade of the nineteenth century and hastened to correct the prevailing view that there might exist some fifty thousand or so plants in the world. "The thought rises involuntarily in the mind," he wrote in his book *Aspects of Nature*, "that we may not know yet the third, or probably even the fifth part of the plants existing on the earth!" His was a remarkably lucky guess: botanists now estimate the number of flowering plants worldwide to be about 250,000.

Spruce, with the benefit of seventeen years in the Amazon and Andes, added as much knowledge to rainforest lore as any single scientist before, and probably since. More than just a collector of herbarium pieces, he observed that tropical forests were not homogeneous thickets, but mosaics. The "virgin forests" were distinguished by "sombre foliage of the densely-packed, lofty trees, out of which stand, like the cupolas, spires, and turrets of a large city, the dome-shaped or pyramidal or flat-topped crowns of still loftier trees, overtopping even the tallest palms, both palms and trees being more or less interwoven with stout, gaily-flowering lianas." He described "white forests" with thinly set trees and bushes, odd-looking palms, and an abundance of ferns. There were also "recent forests" with low, irregular, tangled growth, paler foliage, and a weedy aspect.

What is extraordinary is that now, nearly 150 years since Spruce first set foot in the Amazon, scientists do not know that much more than Spruce did about tropical forests. Stewards of the Earth, we have built cities, tamed rivers, dissected the atom, even invented new forms of life, yet we do not know all the plants and animals that live here with us. Each time biologists go into the rainforests, they stand in awe, like Bulgarian shoppers magically transported from a bread line into an American supermarket. Each time the biologists emerge, they revise their species count upward again. Within the past decade, says Harvard biologist Edward O. Wilson in his book *Biophilia*, biologists have discarded their estimate of three million species on Earth and suggested ten. "Now," he says, "many believe that ten million is too low." The upward revision is due to the penetration of the last great unexplored environment of the planet, the canopy of the tropical rainforest, and the discovery of an unexpected number of new species living there. Truly, Wilson rhapsodizes, the rainforest is "the very heart of wonder."

Imagine that each species of plant and animal is a library stocked with a piece of our planet's life history. The tale of a bacterium lodged underneath your fingernail might represent a scholar's lifetime collection, with a thousand volumes or so, each volume being a gene. The humble white-blossomed periwinkle growing in your window planter would be the equivalent of a big-city library with tens of thousands of volumes. If you were to wander into one of the plant libraries, you would see signs guiding you from section to section: plant structure, growth rate, reproduction, geographic distribution, and so on. Climb the stairs to the second floor and into the stacks labeled "chemistry." Scanning the rows of leather spines on shelves swaybacked with the weight of information, you watch the titles pass: protein synthesis, carbohydrates, polysaccharides, cellulose. Now stop at the aisle labeled "secondary compounds." The titles may be vaguely familiar: alkaloids, terpenes, steroids, flavonoids, tannins. Pull out a book and let it fall open at random. On the page are written sentences in which a few key words are punctuated with lines of meaningless code. The words sketch the bare outline of an ancestral epic, while the unfinished sentences hint at some mysterious conclusion. But like glyphs on the tombs of an unknown civilization, the code reveals only fragments of the full message. You pull out another book, and it is the same, its meaning shimmering just beyond reach like a mirage.

Genes instruct an organism how to build cells, create or consume food, reproduce itself — everything needed to live. Since most of this activity takes place chemically, you could say that genes are the instructions that come with the chemistry set. The sheer number of genes in all living things is, for the foreseeable future, incalculable. Take the ants. There are about ten thousand ant species and no two are genetically the same. Or plants. Each of the 250,000 species of flowering plants is a genetic saga extending back millions of years. And each species contains scores, perhaps hundreds of chemicals that help it carry on the business of living. That includes defending itself against predators. In the rainforest, where there are so many ways to eat and be eaten, organisms have developed an elaborate arsenal of such chemicals that is more varied than anywhere else in the world. These chemicals are part of a class called secondary compounds, because they play no apparent role in the basic needs of growth and reproduction. They not only defend, however; they can heal. As scientists have peeled back the chemical layers of tropical life, they have discovered extraordinary substances — tree saps that kill viruses, seaweed that blocks cancer, spider poisons that combat neurological disease, even secretions from frogs that could treat depression and stroke.

Like the instructions included with Japanese appliances that are translated into English word by word, this genetic library of tropical life lacks syntax. Scientists have only just begun to decipher it. And from the far corners of the library, there comes the smell of smoke.

In 1979, about one percent of the world's rainforests were being burned yearly, mostly by slash-and-burn agriculture but also after logging and to create cattle pasture. That number has been disputed, as it is difficult to know exactly what is going on in all the far-flung forests of the world. Satellite imagery and aerial reconnaissance have improved the reliability of assessments, however. In 1989, scientists calculated that the rate of deforestation remained about the same as that of a decade earlier; some said it had risen to almost twice that rate. But at the very least, if all the rainforests put together will fit into the continental United States, then an area at least the size of Indiana is being deforested every year. Less than forty years from now, half of the remaining rainforests will be gone, and the rest will have been wiped almost clean by the end of the next century. And each year, a half of a percent of the species in these forests is becoming extinct.

What to do? Environmentalists berate the loggers and cattle ranchers and publicize the destruction. A few governments and wealthy conservationists actually buy up small reserves of rainforest by paying off the debts of Third World tropical countries. Scientists, most of whom have little money and whose clout generally evaporates beyond their university campus, fret and debate. The massive deforestation continues.

By the mid-1980s, the desperateness of the situation drove an unlikely group of people into an alliance unlike any seen before. It is a loose confederation — no name, no headquarters, no manifesto, not even a good slogan. Its participants, spread across the world, include cancer and AIDS researchers, Costa Rican bus drivers and housewives, executives of the world's biggest drug companies, college students, globe-trotting botanists in Land Rovers, and indigenous people living in remote rainforest villages. They often bicker with one another over how to go about their task, yet most of them share a common vision: that the way to save the rainforest is to prove that it is more valuable standing than cut down and replaced. They are gambling that the most valuable commodity in the rainforest is a cure for disease. Now, less than a decade after their search began, these medicine-hunters are bringing new green medicines back from the rainforest.

2

Green Medicines

who lived during the first century A.D. and whom history records as one of the first great medicinal botanists, describes uses for the mandrake, *Atropa mandragora*. The second prescription describes the use of sap from the Amazonian tree *Virola*.

Plus ça change, plus c'est la même chose. Today's plant-hunters are reviving a tradition almost as old as culture. Indeed, Dioscorides and Schultes went about their business in like fashion, needing little more than a rugged constitution and a good pair of eyes. Dioscorides traveled with Nero's army as a physician. Schultes explored the Amazon for the U.S. military and the Department of Agriculture during the 1940s, looking for sources of natural rubber. Both recorded the plant lore of the cultures they encountered and returned to their own countries with plants and prescriptions to improve their own peoples' health and welfare.

While plant-hunters extended the reach of medicine, few won much of the credit handed out by historians of medicine. The discovery of antibiotics, for example, was attributed to Louis Pasteur and Alexander Fleming, not to the healers in ancient Greece and Rome who discovered how certain molds stopped infections. Perhaps that is to be expected of history, whose profile is mapped like an almanac's guide to a mountain range, noting its highest peaks, not its contours. Moreover, historians of science have gravitated toward the world's great laboratories, they being more accessible than the godforsaken swamps, steppes, and tundras where medicinal botany is practiced. For it is essentially a foraging activity, followed by trial-and-error experimentation. Our culture has become a stargazing one; we fix our eyes on faraway black holes, elementary particles of matter, or the molecular structure of life itself. The chemistry of plants is in the middle distance, and studying it has rarely earned anyone wealth or fame.

But remarkable in the history of medicinal plant-hunting is tha despite thousands of years of experimentation, humans have bar touched what nature has to offer. Even the known is forgotten and rediscovered. Take the crocus, for example, one of the plants lis Dioscorides's famous herbal. Dioscorides recommended that a of the flower then called *Ephemera*, later given the Latin name C *parnassicum*, be soaked with wine as a poultice for treating tu plant, from the lily family, in fact contains colchicine, an alk which a powerful treatment for granulocytic leukemia is Even the world's most common medicine can be traced t from the white willow that Dioscorides recommended fo eighteen hundred years for chemists to find what gave analgesic effects. It was a compound called salicin. Salicin was modified to become salicylic acid, which was effective against skin diseases but which could not be taken internally. Eventually, in 1899, German chemists turned salicylic acid into acetylsalicylic acid. They called it aspirin.

Dioscorides would have to concede that he stood on the intellectual shoulders of many plant-hunters before him. Among them were Mithridates VI Eupator (circa 131–63 B.C.), ruler of Pontus, and his physician, Cratenus. Mithridates earned the title "the Great" for challenging Rome and taking over much of what is now Asia Minor, but he also had a reputation for learnedness, having described most of the plants of his kingdom, especially poisons and their antidotes. Any monarch who knew poisons improved his odds of survival. In fact, Mithridates is said to have built up an immunity against poisons by regularly ingesting small amounts of them, and in the Middle Ages the word "mithridate" meant a potent antidote.

Another fourteen hundred years back in time, an Egyptian laid down what was known then about pharmaceuticals in a document now called the Ebers Papyrus, which dates to the mid-sixteenth century, B.C. The Papyrus was bought by Egyptologist Georg Moritz Ebers in 1872 from an Arab who said the six-meter-long scroll was found between the feet of a mummy discovered at Thebes. The document included a prescription for heart disease made up of dates, bulbs of squills (Mediterranean sea onions), amamu plant, sweet beer, and tehebu tree. This was to be boiled, then strained and taken for four days. Turning the clock back another millennium, the greatest Chinese herbalist is said to have been the emperor Shen Nung, who reigned at about 2700 B.C. He left behind a book of medicine now called *Pen Tsao Kang Mu*, which lists 365 plant medicines. Among them was Chinese rhubarb, consisting of a few species of the genus *Rheum*, whose roots were used as a purge. Its fame was so widespread and durable that in sixteenth-century France such roots were worth ten times the price of cinnamon, and the plant is still cultivated and used widely in China. Plants were even considered valuable booty in wartime. According to an inscription found in what was then called Mesopotamia, the Sumerian king Sargan in about 2500 B.C. crossed over the Taurus Mountains into the heart of Asia Minor and brought back as a prize of conquest, among other valuables, trees, vines, figs, and roses for acclimatization to his own land.

In a world that was largely built, fed, and medicated from the raw tissue of nature, curing plants were among the most highly prized.

There was one plant so precious to ancient Greeks and Romans that its value was said to exceed its weight in silver. It grew only in the North African city-state of Cyrene but was traded throughout the Mediterranean, and its image was carried on Cyrenian coins. Farmers tried and failed to cultivate it in Greece and Syria, and it was eventually harvested out of existence. Historians believe that the plant, called *silphion* by the Greeks and *silphium* by the Romans, may have been the ancient world's most effective oral contraceptive, either by preventing pregnancy or by inducing early-term abortion. Botanical descriptions suggest that it was a species of *Ferula*, or giant fennel. Extracts of related species such as *Ferula assa-foetida*, which grows in North Africa, and *F. jaeschkaena* have been shown in experiments with rats to prevent implantation of fertilized ova from 40 to almost 100 percent of the time.

Ironically, some of history's most valued medicinal plants belonged to the pharmacopoeias of women, who were for the most part excluded from the official practice of medicine. Women certainly had their own herbal treatments, especially for those needs exclusively female. Among the plants taken to prevent pregnancy or induce abortions were juniper, rue, pennyroyal, squirting cucumber, artemisia, and Queen Anne's lace. Some of these are toxic, pennyroyal lethally so, and may have induced abortions simply because of that. Whether others were more efficient is difficult to tell since both abortions and accounts of how to perform them have been suppressed for so long.

The earliest evidence of a female pharmaceutical practice harks back to the sixth century A.D. The physician's name was Metrodora, and she left for history's edification a record known as the Metrodora text: an alphabetical listing of cures, aphrodisiacs, and beauty tips. Translated by classics scholar Holt Parker at the University of Cincinnati, the text includes the following prescription for a contraceptive: "One dram pomegranate flower, four drams pomegranate peel, two drams oak gall, one dram wormwood. Make everything smooth, take up in cedar oil and after giving her a douche after her period, apply for two days and after another day let her have intercourse, but not before. This is infallible; based on much experience." Metrodora's materia medica includes treatments for uterine cancer, infections and diseases of the breast, infertility, difficult childbirth, keeping breast size small, and restoring the appearance of virginity, the latter a procedure that nowadays would no doubt require hefty malpractice insurance.

Regardless of sex, healers have always had a special place in society. In primitive societies, there often were hierarchies of healers, not unlike the specialists that have subdivided modern medicine. At the apex of the order stood the shaman. The word *shaman* derives from the Tungus culture of Siberia, and, technically, it is in Siberia and central Asia that shamanism has been known the longest to ethnographers. The shaman, says the French scholar and historian of religion Mircea Eliade, "is the man who knows and remembers, that is, who understands the mysteries of life and death." In a worldview that separates the universe into the sacred and the profane, the shaman is the link with the sacred, and his primary role is, in essence, as a technician of ecstacy. While societies have their priests, their magicians, and their healers, the shaman stands above them in that only he (traditionally shamans are male) can transport his soul from his body and ascend to the sky or to the underworld, where he can communicate with the spirits whose invisible hands shape the turning world. Shamans are thus separated from their societies in the intensity of their own religious experience; indeed, they are not so much officers of a religion as they are a mystical elite.

Shamanism spread throughout the world, and although variations have arisen spontaneously, its basic nature remained the same from Asian steppe to Amazonian rainforest. Anthropologist Michael J. Harner, who started studying shamanistic customs in South America in the 1950s, describes the shaman of South America's forest-dwelling people as a man "who is in direct contact with the spirit world through a trance state and has one or more spirits at his command to carry out his bidding for good or evil. Typically shamans bewitch persons with the aid of spirits or cure persons made ill by other spirits. . . ." Among other things, shamans find lost or stolen objects, identify people who have committed crimes, or foretell the future. South American shamanism contains some of the most archaic characteristics of the phenomenon: initiation of the shaman through inheritance or through a personal quest, belief that illness is caused by intrusion of a magical object in the patient requiring a suctioning of these invisible objects out of a patient's body, and sometimes the loss of the soul from illness. Even the symbols of shamanism echo each other around the world. The South American shaman drinks a brew from the liana, or vine, *Banisteriopsis*. Its hallucinogenic powers are his vehicle to heaven, and the vine's form is sometimes described as a ladder up which the shaman ascends to find knowledge. On the other side of the world, the Altaic shaman of central Asia ritually climbs a birch tree in which steps have been cut, each one representing a stage of heaven through which he must pass.

In order to treat the sick, shamans often employ plants in either or both of two ways. First, they may administer plant medicines directly to their patients, although this task is often shared with others who are not shamans but are trained in a culture's herbalism. In some cultures, a patient will go to a herbalist first, and if that course of action fails, to a shaman for stronger medicine. The second and principal skill of a shaman, however, is to intervene in the spirit world. This requires magical and often hallucinogenic plants, such as mushrooms, cactus, or any of the myriad vines and barks with alkaloids found in South America. The ingestion of hallucinogens may be accompanied by the beating of drums, fasting, drinking of alcohol, smoking of tobacco, or chanting. While under the influence of these plants, the shaman experiences visions and may do battle with spirits or even voyage to the world of the dead to retrieve a sick person's soul. In some cultures, such as the Jívaro of Ecuador, the daily world one sees is believed to be a lie, while the true world is the supernatural realm experienced while under the influence of magical plants.

As pastoral society began to replace nomadic life, the importance of shamans dwindled. The ascendancy of new religious themes, such as ancestor worship and multiple divinities, and the eventual rise of the organized church ultimately pushed shamanism and the use of intoxicating plants into obscurity and disrepute. During the Middle Ages, it was witches and sorcerers, not respected healers, who prepared strange brews and ointments from the likes of belladonna, henbane, and the mandrake root, and usually for ill purpose. In Europe, the mandrake was believed to have the power to kill just by being pulled from the ground. In New England, witches were suspected of using a fungus, ergot, to induce mass hallucinations. Even though powerful plants continued to be the source of medicines, their connectedness to things spiritual dissolved. Perhaps the desire to enter so directly into contact with the sacred was overwhelmed by the fear of renouncing the simple human condition. In any event, the eighteenth century's age of reason, or the Enlightenment, as Immanuel Kant dubbed it, further buried the spiritual role of medicinal and magical plants. It rolled over mythology and folklore on the wheels of universal doctrines like Newton's *Principia Mathematica*. The universe now had knowable rules and empirical scientific methods employing observations and experimentation with which to discover those rules. The workings of the body were seen as mechanisms and there was no room for the likes of shamanistic healing.

Official medicine nonetheless helped itself to the collective experience of folk medicine and appropriated it frequently. An example was the "discovery" of digitalis, a potent heart medicine still used today. It comes from a little garden plant commonly called foxglove. After serving as an underground remedy for centuries, it got a proper coming out from a country doctor in Shropshire in the late 1780s.

William Withering, a protégé of Erasmus Darwin, grandfather of Charles, began practicing medicine in the midland town of Stafford in 1766. Withering was an amateur botanist who was fortunate in having come to adulthood after 1753, when the Swedish naturalist Carl von Linné, or Carolus Linnaeus, published the seminal work of botanical science, the *Species Plantarum*. If it is true that to know something you must first name it, then Linnaeus made the plant kingdom knowable. He organized plants into a hierarchical system based on paired Latin names, known as binomials, and laid the groundwork for the science of taxonomy, the system for describing the kinds and diversity of organisms and the relationships between them. Inspired by Linnaeus, Withering studied plants as well as medicine: physicians were not blind to the fact that useful medicines might sometimes be found among the clutter of newt's tongue and yew bark.

Among the ailments Withering commonly treated was dropsy, an accumulation of body fluid in cells or body cavities (now called edema, usually caused by congestive heart failure, the inability of the heart to pump blood at sufficient pressure). In Withering's time, neither cause nor cure was known. In 1775, Withering treated a woman with dropsy but advised her family that she probably would not survive. When she recovered weeks later, Withering asked the patient's family how this had transpired and was told that she had taken a secret potion prepared by an old woman in Shropshire who practiced herbal medicine. Withering investigated and found the potion to contain about twenty herbs, one of which, his botanical eye told him, was probably the cure: a lovely biennial with purple, trumpet-shaped flowers hanging from a spike. It was foxglove, common all over England and Europe. Linnaeus had called it *Digitalis purpurea*, though it was commonly called "dead man's bells" in Scotland, and in Wales, "goblin's gloves." It often caused vomiting and purging, and was a diuretic. Overdoses were common and sometimes fatal. Withering found that the leaves were the most potent and should be picked when the plant was in full flower in its second and final year of life. In his mansion in Birmingham, he would dry his leaves over a fire and grind them into a fine powder. The powder could be taken safely in doses of a grain or two (an aspirin contains five grains) and would eliminate the swellings that accompanied dropsy. At the time, Withering did not realize that foxglove actually did nothing for the underlying cause of dropsy, but for patients who suffered its depredations, that hardly mattered. Withering published his findings in 1785 and became an international sensation. He never knew exactly how foxglove worked, only that it seemed to have some power over the motion of the heart.

It remained to others over the next two centuries to find that the compound in foxglove, called digitalis, was a cardiac glycoside. It increased the force of systolic contractions and lowered venous pressure in hypertensive heart ailments. The dried leaves are still used today in capsules or pills for heart patients, as well as other more powerful compounds from the digitalis leaf such as digitoxin. For many years, most digitalis came from a farm in the Pennsylvania countryside operated by the company S. B. Penick, one of the leading sources of plant-based drugs in the United States.

Cardiac glycosides are only one of many phytochemicals — chemicals from plants — that have medicinal value. The largest group are the alkaloids. These are a large class of phytochemicals that always contain a nitrogen atom and are so named because they are alkali-like, or basic. Over four thousand are known, and about 20 percent of all vascular plants contain at least one alkaloid. A single plant species may contain fifty different alkaloids. They range from the relatively benign, like caffeine, to the more stimulating, like cocaine from the coca plant, to the addictive morphine of the opium poppy and nicotine from tobacco. It is believed that most alkaloids are secondary compounds — that is, they appear not to be required for a plant's essential functions — and they are heavily represented in the tropics — one study found that 45 percent of tropical plants have them — where year-round attacks from the host of insects, fungi, and bacteria is the norm.

The most famous alkaloids are those that act along the neurological divide that splits pleasure and pain. Like fire, they are gifts of nature that carry a high price. Opium was first described by a Greek, Theophrastus, a disciple of Aristotle who wrote a history of plants. Some four hundred years later, Dioscorides explained how opium was derived from the heads of the poppy plant. A few days after the petals fall, a green pod about two inches high and equally thick develops that, when gently slit, causes the pod to exude a milky juice that is crude opium. Dioscorides prescribed it for pain and insomnia but warned that too much will make the imbiber lethargic or kill him. Galen, the great Greek-born physician of the second century (known for his axiom "Nature does nothing in vain"), treated several emperors with opium.

In 1753, Linnaeus gave the species from Asia Minor, the only one that produces the drug, its current scientific name, *Papaver somniferum* — the sleep maker. By then it had already cut a swath through Europe. The Swiss chemist Paracelsus in the sixteenth century helped popularize it when he created a tincture of opium with alcohol, which he called laudanum. In Britain, it was the secret of Dover's powder, a medicine that British buccaneer Thomas Dover, captain of the H.M.S. *Duke* (and famed rescuer of "Robinson Crusoe") foisted on the public. To a poet like Samuel Taylor Coleridge, opium could be the inspiration for fantastic visions, but at great personal expense. The ghostly passenger that sailed the derelict death-ship across a windless sea in his "Rime of the Ancient Mariner" might well have been Coleridge's lament on his own addiction: "Her lips were red, her looks were free / Her locks were yellow as gold: / Her skin was white as leprosy, / The Nightmare Life-in-Death was she, / Who thicks man's blood with cold."

Opium, however, led to anesthetics. Moreover, it was the raw material for a young chemist to whom the credit for isolating and characterizing alkaloids must go. Twenty-year-old pharmacist's assistant Frederich Wilhelm Adam Sertürner, from the village of Paderborn in Germany, isolated the compound in opium that gave it its power. He called this alkali-like substance *morphium*, now known as morphine. With what Sertürner revealed in 1803 about the chemical nature of this alkaloid, drug hunters could better guide their search for valuable plants by testing them for alkaloids. In short order, the pure alkaloids in numerous useful plants were found and replaced the crude extracts from which they came: strychnine in 1817, caffeine in 1820, nicotine in 1828, atropine in 1833, and cocaine in 1855. Sertürner had sowed the seed from which modern pharmacology grew.

As scientists were unraveling the secret chemical life of plants, explorers in the tropics continued to bring back new and ever more exotic flora for them to puzzle over. From the New World, one of the most extraordinary was the rubber tree, *Hevea*. In 1736, the French explorer Charles Marie de La Condamine arrived in Esmeraldas, in what is now Ecuador, on a mission to measure the curvature of the Earth. While his companions proceeded to Quito by a traditional route from the port of Guayaquil, La Condamine, encouraged by friend and fellow adventurer Don Pedro Vicente Maldonado, governor of Esmeraldas Province, decided to investigate the coastal villages first. It was the Frenchman's first experience with equatorial rainforests, and he wrote with astonishment of the variety of life he encountered. He collected plants for his colleague Joseph de Jussieu, the botanist on his expedition, as he canoed up rivers to visit the Tsachali, who still paint their bodies head to toe with red dye as La Condamine described them. Among the forest products he encountered was an amazing substance called *caoutchouc*, a cloth that stretched and was waterproof. Esmeraldans showed him how they tapped the rubber tree and drew out a viscous, white milk that they called *jebe*, which was poured between shaped plantain leaves and then left to solidify into almost any shape. La Condamine had a rubber pouch made for his scientific instruments, which bore up well when he and Maldonado made an arduous trip up the Río Esmeraldas to Quito. Although rubber and the latex-bearing trees had been reported by earlier Spanish explorers, it was La Condamine who took rubber samples back to Europe and who performed the first scientific experiments on it.

It was killer plants that most intrigued the first explorers in the New World, however. As long as there has been poison, men have endeavored to find ways to deposit it in prey or enemy (although apothecaries knew that poisons in small doses could cure as well as kill). Take the word *toxic*, meaning poisonous. It comes from the Greek word *toxon*, which means "bow" or "bow and arrow." The Greek *toxicon* was a poison in which arrows were dipped. The Greeks did not invent the idea of poisoned projectiles, however. They probably learned from the Scythians, an earlier nomadic people who established themselves around the Black Sea about three thousand years ago. They were said to have mixed snake venom with human blood and smeared the concoction on their arrow points. Earlier still are written Sanskrit references from the Vedic period in India, three and a half thousand years ago, that banned poisoned weapons. Archaeologists have pushed the practice still further back in time, to the last Ice Age, when bone blades bore carved notches or grooves that are believed to have carried poison into wounds.

In Europe, aconite, also known as wolfsbane or monkshood, a plant with blue, purple, yellow, or white flowers shaped like hoods, contains an alkaloid called aconitine that slows the action of the heart and may have served as an arrow poison. The personal physician of Roman emperor Claudius I is credited with using this fast-acting poison to kill his royal patient. Another ancient killer was the plant hellebore, the common name for *Veratrum*, which grows in swampy areas and has distinctively ribbed leaves and small, star-shaped flowers. Parts of the plant are now used as an insecticide. That artful collector of myths and practices, William Shakespeare, described a veritable bouillabaisse of poisons in the cauldron prepared by the three witches in *Macbeth*. Their recipe included eye of newt, toe of frog, adder's fork, blind-worm's sting, a toad kept under a rock for thirty-one days and nights, filet of snake, and root of hemlock. One ingredient, "slips of yew," returns us to the Greek toxon, for not only were the yew tree's red fruits poisonous, its wood was the favorite of English bow-makers.

But the floral armamentarium of Europe and Asia paled next to what the tropics' biodiversity had to offer. Explorer David Livingstone reported in the nineteenth century that East Africans tipped their hunting weapons with juice from *Strophanthus*, from the family of plants that gives us periwinkle and oleander. Yet another heart medicine with a digitalis-like action came from the African arrow poison ouabain, known to its users as *wabayo* or *ouabaio*. It works even faster and in smaller quantities than digitalis. And from West Africa, in the southeastern corner of Nigeria, missionaries came across an unusual plant near the seaport of Calabar. Indigenous people who lived in its upland regions called the plant *esere*. It was a woody vine growing about twenty meters long with small, pink flowers, and was used as an ordeal poison. A prisoner accused of a crime was made to drink a brew made from the kidney-shaped Calabar bean. If he died, then he was, of course, guilty. If he vomited, or somehow survived, he was innocent. Scientists named the plant *Physostigma venenosum*, and isolated the alkaloid physostigmine from it. It can be effective against the eye disease glaucoma or myasthenia gravis, a progressive, wasting neuromuscular disease, and led to a synthetic drug, neostigmine, with a host of medical uses.

As for indigenous peoples of the Americas, they dispatched game and each other with diabolically inventive concoctions. Philip Smith, in his book on curare, describes a practice of the Dakota Indians that began by pinning down a rattlesnake with a forked stick and allowing it to sink its fangs into the liver of a deer. The liver was then wrapped in hide and buried for a week until it rotted. Dug up and dried, it was mixed with blood and dried once more. A paste from this *foie gras vipérin* served for both warfare and for hunting. South American Indians were no less imaginative, having at their disposal a much wider variety of sources, including not just plants but venomous animals too. The Cholo Indians of Colombia, for example, dipped their blowgun darts in the excretions from the skin of a yellow and black striped frog, one they called *kokoa*.

Travelers with Columbus's second expedition to the Americas in 1493 may have been the first Europeans to experience South American poison-tipped projectiles. An account of the voyage published in 1553 in London, based on the writing of a German monk and geographer, Sebastian Münster, described a battle in the Caribbean islands in which one of Columbus's sailors perished from a poisoned arrow. A similar report appeared in Pietro Maitre d'Anghera's *De Orbo Novo*, published in Spain in 1516, describing the death of a soldier by arrow, from which a liquid substance oozed when extracted from the corpse. Farther south, one of Ferdinand Magellan's men was killed in Patagonia, now Argentina, by a poisoned arrow.

What these poisons were actually made from was not easily discerned. During Sir Walter Raleigh's voyage ascending the Orinoco in 1595 in what is now Venezuela, the expedition came upon a tribe of people called the Aroras. The trip's historian, Richard Hakluyt, described pitched battles during which those wounded endured "the most insufferable torments in the wound, and abideth a most ugly and lamentable death, sometimes dying stark mad, sometimes their bowels breaking out of the bellies, which are presently discoloured as blacke as pitch, and so unsavoury as no man can endure to cure, or to attend them." No Spaniard knew of a cure, and few Indians either, said Hakluyt, who wrote that there nonetheless were "soothsayers and priests who do conceale it, and only teach it but from the father to the son." Like so many others from the age, this account could not be confirmed, as Hakluyt no doubt knew. But the story, and some preparations from poisonous herbs that Raleigh's group brought back to England, launched a legend that lasted 350 years. When its secret was finally revealed, it became one of the most famous rainforest drugs ever found.

The legend's name came from a young lieutenant of Raleigh's, Lawrence Keymis, who published a book about what at the time was called Guiana. He described poisonous herbs the party had encountered, including one called *ourari*. Ourari's reputation grew, and along with it the number of its pursuers. La Condamine collected specimens of what he called curare and described its use by a people on the Amazon River called the Yameos, who could bag game with blowguns from as far as forty paces. "They cover the points of these little arrows, as well as those used with the bow, with a poison so active that, when it is fresh, it will kill in less than a minute any animal whose blood it has entered," La Condamine wrote. He noted that there was no danger in eating the flesh of animals so killed. "The poison only kills if it enters the blood; but is no less mortal to man than to animals. The antidote is salt, but of safe dependence, sugar."

The Frenchman assayed a few of his own experiments with this curare. With Brazil's colonial governor and a physician among the observers, La Condamine wounded a chicken with a dart he had been given by an Amazonian thirteen months before. The bird died in less than ten minutes. For a test of the supposed antidote, he wounded another chicken, this time with fresh curare, then forced sugar down its throat. It died anyway. When La Condamine returned to Europe, he repeated his demonstrations before eminent doctors and scientists. He never proved that sugar worked as an antidote, but he dined out on the story often enough, and the supplies of curare he brought back served as the first material European physicians could experiment with. La Condamine was of little help discerning the source of curare, however; he reported only that one Amazonian group from whom he got the poison, the Ticunas, used about thirty different herbs and roots to make it. The most important ones, he said, appeared to be vines.

In that assessment, La Condamine was correct. It was enough of a clue for Friedrich Wilhelm Karl Heinrich Alexander, Baron von Humboldt, the tireless engine of early-nineteenth-century natural history, to track down the likely vines. Von Humboldt arrived in South America with his partner, botanist Aimé Bonpland in 1799. He spent over three years wandering the continent, from Mount Chimborazo in the Ecuadorean Andes, where the altitude made his eyes and gums bleed, to the meandering switchbacks of the Orinoco River. It was near the Orinoco that he claimed to have located the source of curare. At the settlement of Esmeralda in Venezuela, he found native people who had collected lianas to make the poison. He observed a *brujo*, or healer, as he prepared the secret substance with what von Humboldt noted was "that self-sufficient air and tone of pedantry of which the pharmacopolists of Europe were formerly accused." Indeed, the brujos sneered at the white man's hunting weapons. Von Humboldt quoted one as saying that "the whites have the secret . . . of manufacturing the black powder that has the defect of making a loud noise when used in killing animals." Curare, the brujo pointed out, is superior because "it kills silently, without anyone knowing from whence the stroke comes."

The German explorer noted that the vine was pounded into fibers to make a yellow, runny mush, which was poured into a funnel of rolled palm and plantain leaves. Water was added, then allowed to evaporate until the material was as thick as molasses. "There is no danger in tasting it," von Humboldt wrote, "the curare being dangerous only when it comes in immediate contact with the blood stream." When mixed with the juice of another plant, the material turned black and sticky enough to adhere to darts and arrows. Von Humboldt took some back to Europe and the laboratories of armchair chemists as La

Condamine had done. Physiologists, who had already poisoned all manner of animals with it, found that it would first stupefy and then asphyxiate its victims. As for how it worked, they had no idea.

Von Humboldt failed to make a botanical identification of the crucial vines, so the hunt continued. Next to add to its lore was the explorer Charles Waterton. Waterton was a rough-and-ready Yorkshireman like Spruce but disdained science and the trappings of intellectualism, traveling barefoot through the forests of northeastern South America and bringing back numerous specimens of plants and animals that he had shot. The latter he stuffed and preserved, often reassembling their parts in unusual configurations and naming them after British gentlemen he disliked. In British Guiana, Waterton observed indigenous people (the Macousis) making curare from lianas. The Macousis added stinging ants to their brew, the fangs of the fer-de-lance viper, pepper, and cuttings from a vine and a bitter root. For the most part, the process was much the same as what von Humboldt had seen. Waterton took some of this curare back to England and to Benjamin Collins Brodie, a Wiltshire physician who already had tried curare on guinea pigs and cats. Waterton and Brodie administered this new curare on a donkey, a report of which made the rounds of the medical cognoscenti of the time and delivered the two of them a small measure of fame. The poison, which they called by the Guianese name for the essential vine, *wourali*, was administered in the animal's shoulder. The donkey collapsed and stopped breathing in a matter of minutes. Brodie made an incision in its windpipe and kept its lungs going for two hours with a bellows, at which point the donkey sat up. When Waterton lay down the bellows, the donkey collapsed again. Eventually, the poison wore off and the donkey survived, to be renamed Wouralia and put out to pasture as a reward for her contribution to science.

One other explorer in the early nineteenth century added a crucial chapter to the curare saga. Sir Robert Hermann Schomburgk, a Prussian who adopted England as his home and became one of its leading naturalists, covered some of the same ground in British Guiana as did Waterton, though with a finer knowledge of what plants to look for. During the early 1830s, he trekked into the forest with an Indian guide who promised to show him the vine used to make the poison. Indeed he did, but it was not in flower, making its botanical identification tentative. It had a crooked stem, about as thick as a man's forearm, with rough, ashen bark and thin branches that climbed into the trees. Its leaves were dark green and it produced a berry about the size of an apple, of a bluish-green color and filled with a jelly-like pulp. Schomburgk decided it must belong to the genus *Strychnos* (which is now known to contain over three hundred species), and named it *Strychnos toxifera*. Denied permission to watch a shaman prepare curare from it, he boiled some of the bark down himself and succeeded in killing a chicken with it in half an hour. It was the first time a European had personally pinpointed a botanical source of curare.

By Schomburgk's time, the remarkable medical potential of tropical plants had taken hold of Western science's imagination. Indeed, explorers were then on the trail of a plant that, if not as mysterious as curare, was certainly more valuable, perhaps the most valuable medicine ever to come from nature.

The longest and most exhaustive plant-hunt in the world began in what is now Ecuador. Driving the hunt was the world's most sedulous killer and crippler, malaria, a disease that over the centuries had taken more victims than the plague, pneumonia, or influenza. The tree that could cure it, or at least palliate its symptoms, was *Cinchona*. Its name comes from the oft-told but unverified story of Europeans' first encounter with it, in the person of an ailing countess and her doctor. The woman was the Countess of Chinchon, Doña Francisca Henriquez de Rivera, wife of the Viceroy Don Geronimo Fernandez de Cabrera, Bobadilla y Mendoza, Conde de Chinchon, who governed Peru from 1629 to 1639. Like many who made South America their home, the countess contracted fever, a catch-all term that usually meant malaria. During the countess's time, no one could have known that it was caused by a protozoan in the stomach of the female *Anopheles* mosquito. There was no known cure, although physicians were fond of bleeding patients to loose their patients' ill humors. To his everlasting credit, the countess's physician, Juan del Vega, was open-minded enough to try a treatment known in the province of Quito (later to become part of Ecuador) as the "quina bark." He and the ailing countess dispatched themselves to the city of Loja, where, as the story has been recounted over the centuries, the lady's fever abated after drinking a brew made with the bark. (The doubt that has been cast on this story stems from research suggesting that the countess never lived in South America.)

The bark reputedly was an ancient Andean cure for intermittent fevers prevalent there, yet no historian had observed local people using it. One account held that the Quichua Indians had learned of its effectiveness from jaguars, who cured themselves of fevers by gnawing on the bark of the quina tree. Not that indigenous medical traditions would have made much difference to quinine's lineage; as was and still is common practice, the bark was only deemed to have been "discovered" when Europeans first used it. In any event, it became known as "Countess's bark" in Europe. Among its promoters was a Cardinal de Lugo, Procurator-General of the order of the Jesuits, who spoke of the remedy during a journey through France and recommended it to his superiors. Thenceforth, the Jesuits began a lively trade in quina bark from South America, which they obtained from their missionaries. "Countess's bark" soon became "Jesuit's bark" or "Jesuit's powder." The new name was an unfortunate choice, for Protestants despised most everything espoused by the Jesuits, and Protestant Europe and England shunned the bark as a Catholic fetish.

No fetish, cinchona was in fact the first specific remedy for a specific disease, and probably worth more to the world than all the gold and silver brought back by the Spanish from the New World. Ironically, it was a quack who finally popularized it. Robert Talbor was an apothecary's assistant, like Sertürner, the German discoverer of morphine, but no scholar or chemist, just a clever opportunist. He earned himself a reputation as a healer of the ague in the late 1660s in London. He called himself a "pyretiatro," or feverologist, and cured his patients, mostly the high-paying aristocracy, with a secret remedy. Nothing would induce him to reveal the ingredients, but, like Br'er Rabbit pleading not to be thrown into the briar patch, he insisted that it contained none of that foul and dangerous Jesuit's powder. This was good enough for King Charles II, who came down with malaria and called on the famous miracle healer. Talbor's medicine relieved the King's symptoms, much to the dismay of the upright Royal College of Physicians, and Talbor soon became Sir Charles. With England conquered, he moved on to France at the request of King Louis XIV, who with his son was suffering from the fever. Talbor promptly cured the both of them, and the Sun King made Talbor a very rich man. But he extracted a promise in return: Talbor would tell him the ingredients, which would be held in confidence until Talbor's death. Talbor agreed and returned to England, his reputation enlarged as the man who saved two kings, but died shortly thereafter, at age forty. Louis immediately revealed the secret: rose water, lime juice, wine . . . and Jesuit's powder.

Cinchona's Catholic stigma soon fell before the intense demand for the Peruvian bark. Over the next 150 years, a huge trade in bark developed. Meanwhile, chemists sought to find the substance in the bark that performed this medical miracle. In 1820, two Frenchmen, Pierre-Joseph Pelletier and Joseph-Bienaimé Caventou, isolated the compound, another alkaloid. They called it quinine, after the bark quina.

The cinchona story took a turn back to Ecuador in the mid-nineteenth century. By then, harvesting was literally outstripping supply and cinchona bark began to grow scarce. At the same time, Europe's empire-builders were creating an ever-greater demand as they sent their soldiers and administrators out to subdue and manage tropical colonies. What they needed were seeds to grow in those colonies, seeds from the very best plants. Such seeds, it was said, came only from the slopes of the northern Andes. Many explorers already had tried unsuccessfully to secure cinchona seeds. La Condamine and his botanist de Jussieu acquired a large cache of seeds that de Jussieu intended to take back to Europe, but these were stolen in 1761, and the two explorers were only able to describe the tree to the French Académie. The Spanish had similarly bad luck. In 1777, explorers Hipólito Ruíz, José Pavón, and José Dombey gathered samples and an exhaustive record of Andean cinchona, only to have it lost at sea. Shipwreck was listed as the cause of the loss, according to Margaret Krieg's account in her book *Green Medicine*, but the collection turned up almost a century later in the British Museum, suggesting that the seeds had been hijacked by British pirates. And von Humboldt and Bonpland, never ones to pass up a legend, found cinchona trees during their trips across the continent. Von Humboldt's descriptions of the leaves and distribution of the tree were highly valued. His warning that if South America did not conserve the quina tree, "this highly esteemed product of the New World will be swept from the country," was not.

Chance in the cinchona hunt finally favored the most prepared mind — the itinerant Briton, Spruce. In 1859, he was in semi-retirement in a mountain village in Peru, nursing a body ravaged by eight years of wilderness living in the service of tropical botany. A letter arrived asking him to proceed to Ecuador to collect the seeds of cinchona, the Red Bark tree, or *cascarilla roja*, as the local people called it. Duty to country, like quiet suffering and afternoon tea, was the very pith of Britons like Spruce: of course he agreed.

The job almost killed him. It did kill Spruce's most beloved companion during the first leg of the journey. His dog, Sultan, went mad after the entire party was capsized in a rapids on the Río Huallaga, and Spruce had to shoot him. The botanist grieved the loss no less, however, than the destruction of the plant specimens he had collected along the way. The expedition had turned northwest onto the broad expanse of the Río Pastaza, and for two hundred miles Spruce and his hired

Quichua fought a six-knot current in their twelve-meter-long dugout canoe. The lowest ebb came when he had to placate his companions, who were not only physically spent but querulous over Spruce's inhuman attachment to the heavy bales of rotting plant specimens and bags of paper for pressing them that the Briton insisted on bringing. They frequently threatened to quit the expedition and leave him stranded until, several days from the next village and reduced to boiling a few fruits with the rest of their sugar for a meal, Spruce relented and surrendered the supply of paper that he used to press his plants. He noted with chagrin how gleefully the Quichua danced around the bonfire they made of it.

After three hundred kilometers, the explorers saw the great volcanos of Sangay and Cotopaxi and the summit of Chimborazo high above the treetops. The group walked from the Río Pastaza to the settlement of Canelos, where Spruce met his first Jívaro headhunters. They turned out to be quite friendly and open, true to Spruce's rule of thumb that the "shirtless Indians," those least influenced by Europeans, were the most honorable. They showed him what they called *varvascu*, the roots of a plant used to stun fish. He studied and named the vine *Banisteriopsis*, the vine of the souls used to make the holy hallucinogen *ayahuasca* and the subject of Schultes's studies a century later.

The Jívaro directed the party to a path along the Pastaza, where they set out for the last leg of the trip to Baños. This was the most difficult part of the journey. In his journal, Spruce wrote: "June 26 — Rain again from midnight, but about nine in the morning it abated so much as to allow us to get under way. Road dreadful, what with mud, fallen trees, and dangerous passes, of which two in particular, along declivities where in places there was nothing to get hold of, are not to be thought of without a shudder." Food was scarce, and at several junctures Spruce overheard his Quichua companions debate whether to turn back and leave Spruce to find his own way. To botany's everlasting benefit, they did not, and the exhausted expedition finally dragged itself into Baños in July.

From Baños Spruce made his expeditions through the cold Andean *paramos*, or high plateaus, to explore for cinchona. In forests that clung to the Andes between three thousand and ten thousand feet, where rain and mist shrouded the slopes almost constantly, Spruce found seeds and young plants of a superior race of quina tree, a species called *Cinchona succirubra*. The trees, with their startling ruby-red bark, had been preserved by local Quichua and colonists, who sold the bark. They believed that it was used in Europe as a coffee- or chocolate-colored dye. "I explained to the people," Spruce wrote, "how it yielded the precious quinine which was of such vast use in medicine; but I afterwards heard them saying one to another, 'It is all very well for him to stuff us with such a tale; of course, *he* won't tell us how the dye is made, or we should use it ourselves . . . and not let foreigners take away so much of it.' "

Spruce was not the only agent in the international conspiracy to corner the quinine market. Five years before Spruce's hunt for cinchona seeds, Dutch entrepreneurs had sent a naturalist, Justus C. Hasskarl, to South America for the same treasure. Hasskarl, posing as a tourist, collected seeds of *C. calisayas* in Bolivia and sent them to planters in the Dutch colonies in Java to start plantations. The trees they produced, however, were almost devoid of quinine. British planters in India had much the same experience with Spruce's seeds. The *succirubra* that he risked his life to collect and send to India turned out to be rich in alkaloids but rather poor in quinine, only about 3 percent, too little to be worthwhile.

It was in fact almost by accident that plant-hunters finally succeeded in securing a renewable supply of cinchona. The credit goes to an Englishman who lived on the shores of Lake Titicaca in Peru, Charles Ledger, and his Indian *cascarillero*, or bark collector, Manuel Incra Mamaní. Ledger was a trader in cinchona bark, and knew as well as Mamaní which trees were the most potent. He asked Mamaní to gather seeds from one particularly fecund source, a forest in Bolivia near the headwaters of the Río Beni. Manuel refused and left, but returned four years later with six kilos of the tiny seeds — at about one hundred thousand seeds to the ounce, enough to plant a whole country. He was subsequently arrested for exporting this national resource and thrown in jail, where he eventually died. Ledger, however, had by then sent the seeds to his brother George in London, who offered them to the British government. His timing was terrible. The government had just failed again, embarrassingly, to get seeds from South America to grow into cinchona-bearing trees, and declined the offer. George Ledger went to Holland and offered the six kilos of seed to the Dutch, who bought half a kilo. Ledger finally sold the rest to a British planter from India.

The British planter sold the seeds in India to colleagues who tried to grow them. They never germinated. The Dutch, however, had better luck in Java. In 1872, cuttings from the young trees' bark proved to contain 10 to 12 percent quinine, three times the usual amount. The Dutch set about locking up one of the biggest pharmaceutical trades in history. First, horticulturalists isolated the Ledger trees to make sure no other cinchona trees cross-pollinated with the superior strain, which they called *Cinchona ledgeriana*. They grafted Ledger seedlings onto some of the roots of Spruce's more vigorous variety. Seeds were harvested and distributed to planters, who were encouraged to grow cinchona instead of tea and coffee. The plantations soon became the world's principal source of quinine and the Dutch had themselves a monopoly that lasted until World War II. Then, the invention of DDT to kill mosquitoes lowered the incidence of malaria and the need for quinine. Also, two synthetic drugs were created that treated the symptoms of malaria (neither quinine nor any of its replacements can cure the disease) as effectively as quinine.

Still, the demand for cinchona continued to fuel international intrigue. In 1942, Java and its plantations fell to Japan, which cut off the Allies from much of their quinine supply. So the U.S. government sent botanists to Colombia to set up a bark-harvesting system. More than a dozen species were known to grow in the Andes, each with different quinine content. It turned out, however, that the need for seed would be filled through stealth. In the early 1920s, Americans in the Philippines had paid a smuggler to bring them seeds of cinchona from Java and a plantation had been started in the province of Mindanao. When the Japanese were closing in on the Philippines in 1942, a U.S. intelligence officer with the Luzon Force, Lieutenant Colonel Arthur Fischer, hatched a plan to take out as much bark and seeds from this plantation as possible. The U.S. military dispatched a B-17 Flying Fortress to rescue key Philippine personnel, one of whom was Fischer carrying a bagful of seeds. These made their way back to the U.S. Department of Agriculture and thence to plantations in Central and South America.

Quinine was finally synthesized by two American scientists, William E. Doering of Columbia University and Robert B. Woodward of Harvard, in 1944. It was too expensive a process to be commercialized, but it led the way for more synthetic drugs that, while lacking the ability to cure malaria, now control various stages of the disease.

While most of the European medical establishment had dismissed the "primitive" lore of New World peoples, explorers like La Condamine, von Humboldt, Waterton, Schomburgk, and Spruce were more open-minded. They not only revealed a new botanical realm but a world of healers and shamans who knew the tropical pharmacopoeia. They joined botany with anthropology, and in so doing inspired future generations of medicine-hunters to study tropical forests and their inhabitants. True, the flora of the temperate world had delivered the likes of morphine, codeine, colchicin (an anti-inflammatory from the plant *Colchicum autumnale*), aspirin, digitalis, and a handful of other useful medicines. It was the equatorial tropics, however, with their breathtaking biodiversity and remoteness, and the arrow poisons and herbal medicines of their indigenous peoples, that promised to be the richest trove of pharmaceutical wealth. Adventurers, like fish drawn to a coral reef, began to school there, and a rainforest medicine-hunt was born.

3

The Arrow Poison
and the Yam

Ethnologists who came to the Americas encountered a native people with an acute understanding of nature. Explorers who knew something about botany discovered a huge variety of economic plants used for food, textiles, building, weapons, and medicines. In 1895 one such botanist from the University of Pennsylvania gave the study of native peoples and their plants a name: ethnobotany.

By then, much had been published about the useful plants of North America's peoples. Indeed, in that sincerest form of flattery, purveyors of medicine wagons and sideshow barkers found they could turn a tidy profit by imitating Native American herbalists. If most of what they hawked was bunkum, some was based on chemically solid ground. Bloodroot (*Sanguinaria canadensis*), for example, was used by Native Americans as an antiseptic; recently, it has become an ingredient in toothpaste. The Penobscot Indians in Maine got rid of warts by rubbing them with the root of the mayapple (*Podophyllum peltatum*). In 1984, a compound from the plant, etoposide, was approved for use against testicular cancer.

Far less was known about South American ethnobotany, though

the continent's allure had grown as reports filtered out of its rainforests. As North America's attentions turned toward its southern neighbors, expeditions were mounted to hunt for new plants there. Most were for horticulture or new crops, but soon fortunes would be made from tropical plant medicines. Two of the most famous were curare, whose mystery would finally be solved by Americans, and steroid hormones. Their stories are emblematic of plant-hunting for medicines: maverick adventurers worked outside of mainstream science and relied instead on shamans and Indian healers, only to be cast aside once they turned their discoveries over to the drug business. Moreover, the indigenous peoples whose ancestors perfected these marvels of plant chemistry got beads, mirrors, and machetes in return.

The mystery of the Amazonian Indian arrow poison, curare, continued to tantalize the world into the twentieth century. In an astonishing show of solidarity, the indigenous peoples who made it, regardless of their region, language, or culture, refused to reveal its manufacture. It might have been the only thing that the warring Amazonian peoples could agree on.

By the 1930s, botanists thought they had narrowed the active ingredients down to a handful of plants. Chemists and physicians had small amounts of the end product, enough to whet their appetites. Still, no one knew for sure what went into this gooey black paste, and which of its ingredients packed the chemical jolt that paralyzed so perfectly.

Then, in 1938, an American emerged from the rainforests of eastern Ecuador with what he said was the answer. His name was Richard Gill. He had risked his life to get it, for in addition to the usual hazards of travel in tropical forests, Ecuador's Oriente was still headhunter country. Gill said his cache of curare would provide the raw material for a miracle drug that would change the practice of medicine. Gill had another, secret agenda as well. If curare's molecular puzzle could be solved, he believed, among the first lives that it might save would be his own.

Gill was born in 1901, the son of a physician in Washington, D.C. He grew in his father's image, a handsome, brown-haired boy who was bright, hardworking, and interested in medicine. He went off to prepare for medical school at Cornell University, and he seemed destined to follow his father's career. He lasted two years before he quit school and ran.

Gill went to New Orleans, where he boarded a steamer headed for

South America. He ended up along the docks by the River Plate in Buenos Aires. This was Argentina's golden era: the quays bustled with the loading of beef and grain headed north to New York, London, and the Mediterranean, and the unloading of machinery, bolts of fine linen, and European furniture for the country's land-rich ranchers. Even in an emporium like Buenos Aires, though, Gill must have drawn stares, standing six feet six and thin as a cattail, his curly hair like a handful of autumn leaves, squinting against the Argentine sun and reeling from the head-clearing stench of the tanneries. Gill did not tarry there long; he soon got a job as a deckhand on a whaler bound for the Antarctic. He spent a year there, his frame filling out from the kind of labor his father had never intended for his scholarly son. The experience was to change him forever.

Gill returned to North America and took another stab at medicine, but it held little interest now. He was infected with a traveler's chorea that could only be mollified by setting foot in faraway places. After earning a degree in literature in 1924, he got a job teaching English at Lafayette College in Easton, Pennsylvania, but quit after three years and took a job as a salesman for a rubber company doing business in South America. He was married now. Ruth Gill was slim, dark-haired, and as charming and pretty as Gill was impetuous and dashing — he had met her on a blind date. They spent two years discovering Peru, Bolivia, and Ecuador.

The couple soon found financial backers for a ranch that they wanted to start in South America. After eight months of looking, the Gills found their spot: in the valley of the Río Pastaza, on the eastern slope of the Ecuadorean Andes, a day's ride on horseback from the town of Baños — one of the towns from which Richard Spruce made his expeditions for cinchona.

In two years, the Gills built themselves what they jokingly called their "tropical barony" out of trees that grew on their land. The house had twelve-foot-high ceilings, seventeen rooms, a veranda, a library, an imported stove, a radio, fine-grained *canelo*-wood furniture, and showers from a hot-and-cold running water system. Dinners were by candlelight with silver candlesticks. Though rustically royal, the house was perched at the littoral, a place where Gill could almost put one foot in the mountains and the other in the forest, the one world combed to a facsimile of European neatness and the other a tangle of animism inhabited by the Quichua and Jívaro peoples. The Pastaza was the most reliable route east into the wilderness and to its indigenous cultures, and it was to be a way station for the pith-helmeted from the north and the feathered and painted from the forests. Gill called his hacienda Río Negro, the first South American dude ranch.

Gill's ranch hands were mixed-race peones and full-blooded Quichua, and Gill set himself to learning the Quichua language and culture. "When you are living, as the Niña [Ruth Gill] and I were, in a permanent ranch," Gill wrote, "the Indians become something more than anthropological curiosities." Friendship with the local people would in fact lead Gill into ethnobotany and, eventually, to the secret of curare.

Gill's interest in medicinal plants came about, literally, by accident. While hiking, Ruth fell down a steep slope. She had about sixty splinters and a badly wrenched knee, what Gill diagnosed as a slipped ligament. Gill decided his wife would have to be taken out on a litter for professional treatment of the knee. A mestizo woodcutter, known to the Gills only as "Old Lopez," suggested there might be another way. He said he had learned many healing traditions from the brujos, and even, he confided, from the Jívaro, the headshrinkers.

Figuring that it could do no harm, the Gills consented to let Lopez try a little brujo healing. Lopez and his assistant, Teresa, an equally old and jungle-wise mestiza, mixed some powdered leaves with tallow from the fat of a guinea pig and applied them directly to the splinters, which they then bandaged. Then Teresa greased the knee with more of the tallow while Lopez built a small fire in the middle of the bedroom floor. Lopez massaged the knee lightly for a few minutes, then threw a handful of herbs on the embers of the fire along with some green leaves, which filled the small bedroom with a pungent, aromatic vapor. Lopez combined the burned leaves with tallow and applied them, along with some paprika, to Ruth Gill's knee, and finally wrapped it in rags. Much of the procedure was accompanied by prayers in various Quichua dialects and Spanish. The brujos also held two live guinea pigs while they administered their cure. "I already knew," Gill wrote in his journal, "how the little animals are used in such cases. They are rubbed until suffocated against the injured part to 'absorb the hurt.' Then, when the thing is done in real Indian style, as a brujo sacrifice, one has its throat cut over the fire used to heat the medicaments; the other is split open, eviscerated, and applied 'as is' to form a ready-made poultice." When Gill asked Lopez why he had diverged from this tradition, Lopez explained that "the Niña would be very *delicada* in such a matter." Gill, suppressing a smile, agreed that indeed she might.

Pig evisceration or no, Ruth Gill was walking normally within a week. Gill dismissed the brujos' incantations as nothing more than hocus-pocus, but from then on he carefully noted the plants used in the local materia medica. Such was the beginning of his career as an eth-nobotanist.

What Gill wanted most were the secret ingredients of curare. By the 1930s, a procession of researchers had raised some plausible explanations for curare's action. It had been postulated that the junctions between nerve and muscle possess something called an end plate, essentially a row of nerve cells facing a row of muscle cells with a tiny gap in between. When the nerve cells receive a message in the form of an electronic impulse from the central nervous system, they release chemicals — neurotransmitters — that crisscross the gap like swimmers in a relay race. These stimulate the muscle cells to contract or relax. With this new neurochemical model, scientists went back to look at curare and proposed that it worked by blocking the receptors on the muscle cells that neurotransmitters, in this case acetylcholine, connect with. So the voluntary muscles shut down. The result: death by relaxation.

Although the action of curare was now fairly well understood, its source was still murky. Explorers were now bringing back curare that they said did not come from *Strychnos*, the vine identified a century before by Schomburgk, but from another vine that was used in the western Amazon basin. A German plant collector, Guillermo Klug, said the plant looked like another genus of vine, *Chondrodendron*. Only two species of this large, woody liana were known to exist. The search intensified in 1935 when a British chemist, Harold King, finally isolated the active ingredient in curare. He had only twenty-five grams of raw material to work with, taken from a museum specimen of unknown origin. From this, King isolated one gram of a crystalline alkaloid that he called *d*-tubocurarine chloride, the "tubo" from the fact that it was the type of curare kept in a bamboo tube (gourds and tin pots were also used).

With an active compound in hand, scientists needed the active botanical ingredient to make consistently pure material so that physicians could try it on the millions of people suffering from a host of horrible and debilitating conditions. Most any convulsive malady was a candidate: epilepsy, rabies, chorea (a nervous disorder causing uncontrollable spasms and tics), forms of spastic paralysis, the rigidity of joints and limbs caused by Parkinson's disease, and multiple sclerosis, to name just a few.

But Indians made arrow poisons with as many as eight different types of plant, plus various animal parts. Confounding the problem was the fact that so many of the samples were collected by amateurs. Typical was a supply of "cuare" brought back by Giles G. Healey, described in a news report as "the youthful Yale explorer" who obtained six pounds of the stuff from South American natives "by barter, through the sign language." Healey did not determine what plants or other substances went into it, but did relate to rapt listeners at the Yale Club in New York City how, when his food ran out, "I ate ants several times and found them fairly appetizing . . . including the giant ant, one-and-a-half inches long, which is roasted like coffee and tastes like kerosene, and the Yellow Tamari, the Due-Due, and the Bachaco-Bravo, which is as hot as tabasco sauce." Drug companies, understandably, were skeptical of such "suppliers," and without drug companies, curare would never be more than a plaything of academics.

It was Gill who, quite literally, fell to the task. By 1932, he had established himself comfortably at the Río Negro ranch and had made friends with several members of local Indian groups, in particular the Canelos Quichua. One man in particular, Severo Vargas, a trader and head man of a nearby group, had visited Gill often at the ranch. They had exchanged gifts and confidences, and at Gill's invitation many of Vargas's people had camped by the river near the ranch, where, in exchange for trade goods, they had shared with the inquisitive Gill their traditional way of life. Gill impressed the Canelos brujos with his own magic, such as the trick of storing sunlight in a tube — his flashlight — and releasing it at night. In return, Gill was invited to go hunting with the men and watch them shoot poison-tipped darts from blowguns into the tree canopy, silently bringing down birds and monkeys with an accuracy the American found uncanny. He spent hours practicing himself: using the jawbone of a piranha to groove the points of the ten-inch-long darts; winding their butt ends with the vegetable silk, *kapok*, to form an airtight seal when the dart was inserted into the nine-foot-long blowgun of metal-hard *chonta* palm; and firing it at a target nailed to a post like a dartboard. "I was most impressed with the humaneness of this method of hunting," wrote Gill. "There is no pain other than the slight prick of the needle-like dart, and, above all, there is no escaping of wounded animals to crawl off into the bush and gasp out their lives in agony." Gill also learned a few of the methods for preparing curare, but he did not witness the entire process. The ingredients, he noted, were "jealously guarded by the medicine men, for it has largely been the basis of their influence among their tribesmen."

The Canelos who camped at Río Negro eventually returned to the forest. Gill planned further investigations, but first he was to return to the United States for a vacation. A few days before the Gills were to depart, Gill went riding on his horse Chugo near the ranch. Something spooked the horse and Gill was thrown, landing heels first on a flat rock. Though dazed, he seemed intact, and returned to the ranch, dizzy and feeling sick, but on his own two feet. That night, however, he experienced an unnerving tightening sensation around his waist. Over the next few days, he suffered other strange symptoms: his hands shook, he dropped a cup of coffee, and he had trouble lighting his cigarettes. He and Ruth were able to travel, however, and they returned to the States as scheduled. But the symptoms worsened. Then one morning Gill woke up to find the entire right side of his body was paralyzed. A week later his left side went limp too. "I was just a bodiless head on a pillow," he wrote. "For months on end I never knew where my body was, or even whether my legs were lying straight or bent, or my arms were crossed or at my sides."

Ruth took Gill to his father's house by Rock Creek Park in Washington, D.C. A neurologist diagnosed his affliction as multiple sclerosis, a wasting of the myelin tissue around the nerves that causes tremors, paralysis, and eventually death. There was and still is no treatment.

Gill refused to believe the diagnosis, insisting instead that it must have been the fall from his horse. Whatever the cause, however, his dream of Eden in Ecuador was smashed. As the months passed, he slipped into a morbid sentimentality. He remembered the toucans that had called to each other outside his windows at Río Negro. "Dios te dé, Dios te dé," their call went . . . "God gives you, God gives you." His father's house was within earshot of the Washington zoo, and every day, just before their feeding time, the big cats and the wolves howled in anticipation and the birds in the aviary set up a screeching counterpoint. It was a painful reminder of the wildlife with whom Gill shared Río Negro. Here, the animals were more like him, their future occluded, their days and nights an ordained ritual of feeding, pacing, defecating, and sleeping. Luckier than he, they at least did not know that this was all there was to be.

One fall afternoon Gill lay watching the leaves drift past his window as his doctor scraped his skin with pins, looking for sensation. When the doctor had finished, he sat down to discuss the patient's future. He said that if Gill were lucky, he *might* walk again. Then the doctor said something peculiar. He said he had heard of a substance that the Indians in the Amazon made, a deadly arrow poison that had a powerful relaxing effect on the muscles. It was something the neurological community was fascinated with but could not get reliable samples for experimentation. It was a pity, he said, for although it could not cure Gill's disease, it might relieve the symptoms. If only we knew more about it, the doctor kept saying.

Curare! Gill yelped. He knew as much about how it was made as anyone in the country. He swore that if he could learn to raise himself up off the bed, he could train himself to walk, and if he could walk, he would find a way back to Ecuador and bring back curare.

Gill devised exercises. He would pick up marbles from one cereal bowl and transfer them to another, or tie reef knots in rope. He paced around his room on crutches specially made for his long legs, learned to walk with a cane, and then to walk on his own again. When he was not pushing his body, he was pushing his mind. He relearned to type and pecked out magazine articles about Ecuador and the Indians, and of course about curare and its promise as a medicine. And there were botany, physiology, and medicine to study. After five years, his efforts paid their first dividend. Early in 1938, a letter arrived from a wealthy Massachusetts businessman named Sayre Merrill. Merrill had read one of Gill's articles and was interested in backing an expedition to obtain botanically verified specimens of curare and the plants it was made from. Gill redoubled his efforts. He visited museums and drug companies and consulted scientists and medical experts to learn how to identify, collect, and dry plants in the field. He asked them how much to bring back, found botanists who agreed to identify them, and got lists of companies that might be convinced to take on the pharmacological research. He went over his old, yellowing maps of Ecuador, their corners punched with thumbtack holes, and his own sketch maps of the Río Pastaza and environs. Then weeks were spent laying in supplies: machetes, fishhooks, necklaces of colored beads, and other trade goods; pharmacist's scales and plant presses for samples; tents, compasses, rubber boots; and photographic equipment to record the journey, for Gill remained very much the journalist with an eye for making history.

By May 1938 the Gills sailed for Ecuador. Gill kept a close record of his efforts. He made a film, took numerous still photographs, and kept a log of the journey. Many of those papers now lie in a filing cabinet in the Arthur E. Guedel Memorial Anesthesia Center in San Francisco. They describe a heady voyage into a part of the Ecuadorean forest that Gill would never identify, either because, as he argued, he wanted to protect the Indians from a stampede of opportunists, or because he planned to monopolize the supply of curare. In any event, the trip was to be the climax of Gill's career. The explorer could not have predicted that in fact he would succeed in finding a new drug, only to see people and forces far stronger than he extract curare from his limp hands.

"Once more it was the ranch, the jungle, the soft rain . . . and the horse Chugo. I rode him in from the end of the automobile road, and very suddenly I was at ease with the world again." So Gill remembered his return to Río Negro. The forest had closed in around the trails and retaken the fields of coffee and corn. The hacienda was in a sorry state. A week of the Gills' enthusiasm, however, put it back much as it had been. Now the plant-hunter settled into his mission. They would need thirty mules and six horses, seventy-five porters, several machete men, and four trail managers to look after the porters. They would head east, into a region called Pacayacu, provisioned to live for several months in the forest. Once they reached the end of the Pastaza trail, four days by pack animal, they would travel by foot. In a few days, according to Gill's maps, they would reach a river, down which they and their considerable cargo would ride in a dozen dugouts handled by *bogas*, or canoemen, hired from local villages.

For Gill, still hobbled by his neurological illness, the terrain was a test of strength. He walked with two staffs, each the length of one of the Canelos' lances. He held the effortless agility and strength of the porters as a standard for which to strive, though even the older women and children who accompanied their men could have passed him in a moment. He may have written with disdain about amateur Abercrombie & Fitch explorers mincing through the bush, but he cut just such a figure in his many-pocketed khakis, a red bandanna around his neck and a pith helmet bobbing on his head. Unable to balance well enough to manage the steep, root-ribbed embankments, he tied himself to a rope and had two strong men stand at the top of each slope to lower him down. He was grateful when they reached the first river and poured their considerable luggage into an armada of dugouts, although hauling the canoes across gravel bars and portaging around the worst rapids was hardly easy passage.

Gill never revealed which streams and rivers the expedition followed, or even the indigenous group he sought. He described the "zone" he was interested in only as a place ignored both by early explorers and the Ecuadorean government. The only scientifically trained voyager he knew of who had spent time there, Gill said, had been a botanist of great fame who had passed through in 1860 on his way out of the Amazon valley. That would probably have been Spruce, during his trip up from Iquitos to Baños along the Río Bobonaza on his way to collect cinchona seeds. Gill's journal notes that he collected his own plant specimens near the Conambo and Bobonaza Rivers, which puts his expedition about 150 kilometers east of Baños, in lowland moist forest. Gill's contacts were primarily with the Canelos who had visited his hacienda in years past, and on occasion the Jívaro. A taller, more isolated population of truculent, independent people, the Jívaro were well known as never having been subjugated by either the Spanish or the Europeanized Ecuadoreans. They were also known as master makers of curare. It was along the margin that separated these two groups that Gill finally settled, in what he described as a "lovely, forest-lost, straggling village" along a river. He called the people there Parayacus, probably a people that have since been absorbed into the lowland Quichua or Jívaro.

Trade goods by the boxload were offered to the *curaca*, or village leader, for his community, and Gill's party was duly welcomed. Gill had a large camp of six Amazonian-style *malocas* built, the open-sided, thatched-roof, high-peaked houses with split-bamboo and cane floors common to the region, into which he unloaded his gear. The Gills' quarters were practically a village unto itself, with a platform for drying plants on sunny days and a laboratory where some simple field tests and curare experiments on animals would take place. Once established in a level of comfort that would be the envy of modern-day ethnobotanists, Gill began winning the local peoples' confidence. He traded tales with the village elders, revealed bewitching new objects from his cache of oilskin-covered ammunition boxes (the most rugged conveyance Gill could find), and asked about medicines. He was as persuasive with the Amazonians as he was with the North Americans he had cajoled into backing his adventure. Word spread that this bearded white brujo would barter goods for knowledge of herbal medicine. Soon Gill's camp was filled with more cures and contrivances than the explorer had imagined possible. In all, Gill collected about seventy-five different botanicals. There were gargles and inhalants for sore throats, emetics and stomachics for gastric pains, snakebite and scorpion-bite remedies, antifungals, and medicines for toothache. There was *guayusa*, a tea-like preparation made by steeping leaves in boiling water and prescribed for rheumatism; *avelina rosada*, crushed pink roots that were mixed with water and used by women to wash their lustrous black hair; *avelina blanca*, a white root that reputedly removed hair permanently; and *copa maria*, a leaf that when powdered was used to clean wounds.

Most important, of course, were batches of curare. Gill eventually convinced several brujos to show him how they prepared the poison. This was done with great ceremony, for the making of curare was the work of a specialist and not to be done without the proper deference to tradition. Gill's field notes describe one such episode with a brujo named Emilion Mayanchi.

Five days to gather materials. Uses three large, pointed-bottom *ollas* [yellow clay jugs] for first general cooking. Concentrates mess down after first day so that on second day all enters one of the smaller of the three ollas . . . must be cooked away from his household, as the poison would damage the house, and also the household in general would have a weakening effect upon the drug.

Goes into the "sacrifice" for the days of actual cooking: No food, aji, chicha, etcetera, and salt is especially forbidden. Even I as mere witness, must wait twelve hours after eating own meal with salt before I can return to the fires . . . [the brujo is] not permitted to sleep with wife. The visit to the scene of a pregnant woman will spoil the poison; others who might accidentally pass by don't matter.

Over the first day, almost twenty kilos of stems from three types of vine, *tonispa pala ango, lamas ango,* and *tonispa* were bruised with stones, passed three times around the brujo's head as a nod to the spirits, and boiled in water. Brujo Mayanchi added bark from another woody plant, then spent the day boiling the whole thing down to half its volume. The next morning, the fire was relit and two more types of bark and a root, which Gill recognized as a poison used to stun fish in the rivers for easier catching, were added. More boiling followed, until the contents of the ollas became like a thin honey. This was strained through a cloth into another pot for more boiling, until it was a black syrup, at which point foam "like a black-brown egg white which has been beaten" formed at the surface. Readiness was determined by consistency; the brujo drew the stuff into points with the tip of a dart, as one might test cake frosting. At this point, just before the stuff gelled, Mayanchi deemed it fit for a test. Toucans and water toads were favorite victims. Gill wrote: "*Birds:* Shot with blow-gun arrow; flies at once to nearby branch. If overcome while alighting, poison is good. *Frogs:* Equivalent of intra-muscular injection in hind leg with arrow forced in by hand while frog is held. Frog then released and prodded into jumping. Frog must die — or at least be totally paralyzed — within six to eight jumps." Otherwise, the poison was deemed too weak.

By comparing the ingredients used by several brujos, Gill narrowed down the sources of curare's potency. Mayanchi and two other brujos he watched had only one plant in common in their recipes: *tonispa pala ango*. It was a woody vine, a climber that could grow as thick as a man's thigh and wind for dozens of meters through the trees. Gill collected many specimens of it. It was not *Strychnos*, that much he knew. In fact, it would later be identified at the New York Botanical Garden as *Chondodendron* (sometimes spelled *Chondrodendron* and first associated with curare by the explorer Guillermo Klug). It was a genus of the moonseed family, Menispermaceae, a tropical species described by eighteenth-century botanist Antoine L. Jussieu. Indeed, one brujo, Felipe Aguinda, told Gill that he could make curare using only tonispa palo ango. Gill got hold of one such batch of curare and tested it on a guinea pig. Given a dose of .15 cc injected into the hind leg, a guinea pig weighing half a kilo was paralyzed in just over one minute, and dead in two. This, indeed, was the real thing.

The Gills spent three months at their forest encampment. Richard attended healing ceremonies by the shaman of the village, who drank the hallucinogenic ayahuasca, gave some to his patient, and pretended to suck pebbles and frogs — the incarnations of evil spirits — from the patient's mouth. Ruth Gill learned some of the "women's plants," remedies that were especially shrouded in ritual and among the most secret. One was allegedly an oral contraceptive, used by the unmarried women who had sex with various men in the village. The Gills also joined villagers on fishing trips. The Indians fished with the barbasco root, *Lonchocarpus utilis*, also the source of the insecticide rotenone. In 1938, one and a half million pounds of the plant were imported into the United States. It was highly toxic — one part in thirteen million would kill a goldfish — but it was relatively harmless to mammals. The fishing party would fill a canoe with the root and paddle it to where the stream was wide and the water slow-moving, where they would pound the root with clubs while rocking the canoe to fill it with water. This created a white, soupy froth that was tipped into the stream. Within minutes, stunned fish would float to the surface, and the laughing Parayacus would snare them with lances as casually as litter-collectors spearing trash in the park. As for the curare, Gill amassed about twenty-five pounds of the gummy paste.

On their last night in the village, the Gills were honored with a farewell ceremony of celebration and chanting, at which, Gill noted, most everyone danced, drummed, and got falling-down drunk. His informants, the brujos who had shared their knowledge, sent him home with mementos of their culture: a headdress of orange and blue bird feathers, a necklace of iridescent green beetle wings, and a quiver of blowgun darts.

Gill made the trip home in good health, his botanical specimens intact, and his ambitions soaring. Once in New York, he sent his botanical samples off for identification to the best in the business, the eminent tropical botanists Boris A. Krukoff and Albert C. Smith at the New York Botanical Garden, in the Bronx. He set up a corporation in a suite of rooms at Gramercy Park Square, a pocket of brownstone elegance in Manhattan built around a landscaped park. He churned out brochures advertising "Hacienda Río Negro," a place where vacationers could learn how to use the Jívaro blowgun, hunt and fish, trek into the forest, or while away the hours talking to jungle rats over a gin and tonic. He promoted a "Río Negro Ranch School" to teach young Americans about Indian cultures and their tropical flora and fauna. This was to be his jungle entrepreneurship, with himself as procurer of everything from package vacations to 250 pounds of curare a year.

Krukoff and Smith at the New York Botanical Garden soon identified the plants in Gill's curare as *Chondodendron iquitanum* and *C. tomentosum*. Krukoff, who had observed Brazilian brujos preparing curare from *Strychnos*, remarked that the Ecuadorean brew was rather different, in that brujos used the entire stem, rather than just bark as was done in Brazil, and that the Ecuadoreans boiled it rather than soaking the material in cold water. Gill was the first to have collected *Chondodendron* in that part of the Amazon, and scientific attention shifted to this new source of curare. Gill, of course, was overjoyed. With a sure botanical identification in hand, he knew he could go back to Ecuador and secure the best plants for curare. In the meantime, Gill owned the largest supply of curare outside of the Amazon rainforests, as well as the most detailed description of its manufacture. He gave samples from his cache to Merck & Company for analysis. He also gave some to doctors and chemists who promised to pick apart its complicated chemistry. In the meantime, he set out on the lecture circuit to extol curare's virtues, and wrote articles about it and his adventures acquiring it.

The first doctor to request samples from Gill was Abram E. Bennett of the University of Nebraska. Bennett was a psychiatrist who thought curare, if it could be formulated into a standard compound, could be used to treat people who suffered the horrible tremors and muscular rigidity of several diseases generally characterized by spastic paralysis. Bennett was a conservative man who was sometimes embarrassed by

Gill's flights of enthusiasm. Nonetheless, he became the explorer's staunchest ally. He asked a colleague at Nebraska, Archibald R. McIntyre, who also had an interest in curare, to perform the chemical analysis of Gill's curare. In the meantime, he developed a procedure using rabbits that would allow physicians at least to standardize the raw material's potency so they could keep from killing patients with it.

As in the nineteenth century, attempts by physicians to cure with curare had failed. In 1930, an English doctor, Ranyard West, used it to relieve the convulsions from tetanus in dogs. By 1932, he had similarly treated about thirty cases of spastic paralysis in humans with curare. Sometimes the arrow poison relaxed limbs that had been crabbed and frozen for years. It only worked temporarily, however. Moreover, curare had dangerous side effects, such as sudden constrictions of the windpipe called bronchial spasms that could suffocate a patient. West warned that some types of curare caused convulsions instead of relaxation of the muscles, and that in general its effects were dangerously unpredictable. Across the Atlantic, a young orthopedic surgeon in New York, Michael Burman, had received a small sample of curare from the Merck Institute of Therapeutic Research. Burman tried it on human patients in 1934. These were the backroom cases, people whose bodies were ruined, either rigid like statues or, in the case of children with cerebral palsy and similar neurological diseases, in a state of ataxia, an uncontrollable, constant motion. It was with great frustration that Burman watched curare relieve these symptoms for a matter of hours, only to see them recur when the drug wore off.

Curare's fickle behavior led Merck to hire Krukoff at the New York Botanical Garden in the mid-1930s to collect ingredients in Brazil, in the hope that its chemists could isolate the paralyzing ingredient. The company also had curare samples from the German cavalry officer Klug, who got them from Peruvian brujos who claimed it was made from the genus *Chondodendron*.

This was the situation when Gill arrived in 1939 with his suitcase full of curare. He had expected Merck to usher him in on a red carpet, especially since he had more curare and better botanical evidence than what Klug had. Merck, however, was lukewarm, having failed to standardize the material it already had. So Gill looked elsewhere, and in July 1939 he signed a multiyear contract with the drug company E. R. Squibb & Sons to supply them with enough curare for two hundred thousand doses. Squibb balked at sending Gill back to Ecuador, however. Company executives had yet to see medical results exciting enough to justify further investment in curare. They kept Gill in suspended animation, neither accepting nor rejecting his travel plans.

That was not nearly good enough for Gill. He had kept some of his original cache and he also had sources in Ecuador who continued to supply him. In the early 1940s he started to farm out curare to others to engender more demand for it and to place himself at the source. His solicitations were always sunny and infused with a can-do spirit, his letters peppered with as many exclamation points as periods and with jolly, cajoling Anglicisms. "It would be perfectly grand of you," he would write for support; or, "You're an awfully good egg to help"; or, referring to the doubters, "I'm no end disappointed in their view," and so on. He could flatter shamelessly. "Someday, you know," he wrote Bennett on January 12, 1942, "if I can keep on writing, I shall be hounding you for the data on your biography. I'm not alone in thinking that you are one of the great contributors to modern medicine." Bennett affectionately referred to Gill as his "expansive manic."

Curare was Gill's one and only trade-good. He had been luckless in winning buyers for his other forest pharmaceuticals. At first, a few companies wanted supplies of Ecuadorean *Lonchocarpus* because it yielded twice the average rodenticide, rotenone, that they had been getting from tropical plants, but their interest did not last. *Avelina rosada*, the root used as a shampoo by the Quichua, impressed one Joseph Parentini, a pharmacist with Pioneer Cosmetic Company in New York City, whose sworn affidavit stated that he had cured dandruff with it. Bald men also wrote Gill thanking him for samples and saying it helped them grow hair, and Gill noted enthusiastically that it removed nicotine stains as well. No one, however, would sign Gill on as a regular supplier.

Meanwhile, Bennett had tried curare on several human subjects. His first was a nine-year-old boy with spastic paralysis. The boy could not walk because his legs were permanently drawn up almost to his chest, his arms were rigid, and his fingers clawed and useless. Surgery had failed him, as had attempts to straighten his limbs by casting them in plaster. Within minutes of being injected with curare, the boy's limbs became flaccid and flexible. Sadly, as the curare wore off, they contracted again. Bennett watched patient after patient respond the same way. As Burman had discovered, the benefits were cruelly fleeting, and it seemed that curare had been oversold.

Bennett had another idea, however. It occurred to him that curare might work in a new treatment for another baffling disease, *dementia praecox*, or schizophrenia. At the time, a new treatment was in vogue, electroshock therapy. It provided some long-term relief, but the convulsions from the shocks often broke patients' bones. Bennett and other psychiatrists found that patients dosed with curare did not suffer these violent convulsions. He pioneered its use on scores and then hundreds of electroshock patients during the early 1940s, and although it was not immediately accepted, the fact that curare could be administered without killing or maiming people kept Squibb and other drug companies interested. For this, Bennett earned his place as the first person to take curare out of the laboratory and into the clinic.

It was on January 23, 1942, however, that curare was fully redeemed. On that day, a Canadian doctor and anesthesiologist, Harold Griffith, discovered that curare achieved an even, complete muscular relaxation when used in conjunction with a general anesthetic. This was far more important than it might seem. Abdominal surgery had always been a problem because the abdominal muscles are difficult to relax; nitrous oxide and other anesthetics only put a patient to sleep and deaden the sensory nerves to pain but do not affect the motor nerves significantly, at least in doses that are safe. Griffith had been fascinated with curare's potential to assist anesthesia but had been warned that it was too dangerous. In fact, during the operation in which Griffith first tried curare, on a young plumber with appendicitis, he informed neither the surgeon nor the patient that he was using it. Fortunately for all concerned, it worked. As more anesthesiologists tried it, they discovered that patients on curare required less ether or other powerful anesthetics for chest and abdominal surgery, all of which have unpleasant and sometimes dangerous aftereffects.

Drug companies like Merck and Squibb now were seriously interested. After all, the first effective anesthetic, cocaine, had come from a South American plant. Squibb developed a more precise biological test to standardize it and began distributing ampules of a formulation they called Intocostrin for anesthetic experiments. As demand for curare surged, Squibb needed new supplies. To Gill's dismay, Squibb passed him over. The company said his curare was too low in potency and too contaminated with other substances to work with. Squibb now got its curare and *Chondodendron* supplies from August Rabaut, an explorer who collected it in the Amazon basin, and from Astoria Pan-Americana, Inc., a company that had its own botanist in Peru.

It was a crushing rebuff for Gill and arrived at a time when he was recovering from an attack on his integrity. By the early 1940s, the price of curare had leapt to almost four dollars a gram, and plant-hunters were packing their bags and heading south in search of *Chondodendron*. Many were hopelessly naive — Amazon grocers and jungle rats, Gill called them. He struggled, in vain, to find backers to put up three hundred thousand dollars for his own expedition to Ecuador. He began to suspect that Squibb and others were trying to convince the public that Gill had had nothing to do with the cache of curare that had fueled the revival of interest in the arrow poison. Hope came, however, in the form of a proposal by the federal government to support a collecting expedition to the western Amazon. Gill applied for the grant, considering himself the ideal candidate to lead such an expedition.

That was not, however, the view of Robert Griggs. Griggs was a senior scientist at the quasi-governmental National Research Council in Washington, D.C. He claimed that the Ecuadorean government had asked the NRC to put together a team to explore for *Chondodendron*, and that he and his own team were best suited. Griggs threw Gill a bone, offering him a position as a field assistant on his team. Gill scoffed at the idea. There followed a bitter exchange of accusations between the two. Griggs said Gill was withholding curare from patients, and belittled him because he was not a trained scientist. "Perhaps he [Gill] cannot afford to give up the idea of profit and adopt a detached scientific interest exclusively for the benefit of the patients who need the drug," Griggs wrote in a letter to the State Department, which had the task of choosing the leader of the fifty-thousand-dollar expedition.

Gill would not let such accusations stand unchallenged. He prevailed on the network of researchers whom he had supplied with curare to come to his aid. Through some political connections of Bennett's, he won a hearing in Washington, D.C. In April 1941, Gill made his case before a committee of State Department experts. It was a judicial setting, with a panel of scientists and foreign policy experts convened to weigh Gill's impassioned self-defense. Gill hobbled in on his cane — his illness was one of the few things that had kept pace with the man since his return from Ecuador — carrying with him letters and documents to bolster his case, maps of Ecuador, and accounts of his travails in the jungle. Politically conservative and an ardent believer in American government and the scientific establishment, he approached the witness table somewhat dazzled. Once into his presentation, however, his enthusiasm — to many, his obsession — with curare quelled his nervousness. He said Griggs was part of a cabal of people that had been trying to find out the source of his curare since he had returned from South America, and had even offered his assistant a job in return for what she knew about the poison. They called themselves the "Andean Anthropological Expedition," yet none of them had been there and none knew anything about *Chondodendron*, curare, brujos, or the Amazon.

It was Gill's most dramatic moment in the public eye. Here was someone who had started as an engaging misfit seeking provender and providence in the jungle. Now he sat in a State Department hearing room in Washington, D.C., defending his right to give the public this marvelous substance he had discovered. In a letter he wrote to Bennett before the hearing, he swore he would "vanquish the opposition." Indeed, the "expansive manic" may well have convinced the State Department's doubters. The performance, however, was typical of Gill's entire plant-hunting career: high drama made moot by prosaic events offstage. At the time of the hearing, Griggs had already backed off and sent a letter to the State Department withdrawing the NRC's proposal. Gill had already won.

The victory was as hollow as one of Gill's Jívaro gourds. The State Department did not give Gill the assignment, and he never got backing to return to Ecuador. He remained a gifted and imaginative amateur who thought he could keep curare within his grasp when, in fact, his very success in publicizing the arrow poison ensured that he would lose it. Once the pharmaceutical companies realized curare had value in the marketplace, Gill became a footnote. He was no match for commercial interests with huge resources doing what they do best — capitalizing on new drug discoveries. In the end, Squibb would tip its hat to Gill, but essentially as just a soldier of fortune.

Gill moved to California and spent the rest of his life trying to turn curare into a cure. There was always a supply from his friends in Ecuador to sell to European companies for a little money and for his own experiments. These he performed in his garage. His dream was to formulate an aqueous solution of *d*-tubocurarine that could be administered over long periods of time to patients, like himself, with debilitating disorders of the nervous system. For Gill, the memory of lying like a rag doll in his family home in Washington was still sharp. He wanted a cure from curare, not just an anesthetic. As for his own illness, the diagnosis was never sure; it was either atypical multiple sclerosis or amyotrophic lateral sclerosis. Gill treated himself with a variety of diets and massive doses of penicillin, and reportedly with curare as well. The disease finally killed him in 1958. By then, curare had become an important part of anesthesia, and a molecule on which other valuable anesthetics, such as the faster-acting succinylcholine, were based.

Gill believed he never got the recognition he deserved for his contribution to medical history. He left behind a red-blooded legend, however. Among those who still float down tropical rivers and live in remote villages in pursuit of new plants, his name is still remembered. While a self-promoter and dramatizer, he was also a rare man for his time, who believed in and respected the indigenous peoples who lived primitively in the rainforest yet knew things of great scientific value. Besides his books, articles, and a few letters and field notebooks, mementos of Gill's adventure lie in a single cardboard box sitting on a shelf of a library in San Francisco: a headdress of orange and blue bird feathers; a necklace of iridescent green beetle wings; a quiver of blowgun darts; and a gourd, at the bottom of which can still be seen the traces of the gummy, resinous, coal-black arrow poison of the Oriente.

Gill may have died without fulfilling his dream, but he reminded practitioners of Western medicine that people they deemed primitive had more to offer the world than wooden carvings and feathered headdresses. In fact, when Gill was first popularizing curare, the public was being introduced to a striking new discovery of an ancient and sophisticated pharmacopoeia. In 1940, a magnificent manuscript was uncovered after 350 years of obscurity. The book revealed a pharmacological sophistication among the indigenous peoples of the New World that had been lovingly recorded, illustrated, and preserved, only to be forgotten for centuries.

The book was called the Badianus Manuscript. The author was an Aztec physician, Martin de la Cruz, who had been an assistant at a Spanish school for Aztecs, the College of Santa Cruz at Tlaltelolco, in mid-sixteenth-century Mexico. De la Cruz had been asked by a Spaniard, Don Francisco de Mendoza, an avid botanist who was credited with introducing cloves, pepper, ginger, and other spices to the New World, to write down all that was known about Aztec medicine. The herbal was completed in 1552 and translated from the Aztec Nahuatl into Latin by another Indian, Juan Badiano, hence its name. With scores of color illustrations, it detailed what had never been written down in one place before, the huge materia medica of the Aztecs.

The manuscript was soon shipped to Spain. One hundred years later, it was acquired by the Vatican library, where it lay unnoticed until an American professor from Baltimore found it in the 1930s. Johns Hopkins University published the first English translation in 1939. The manuscript listed 251 plants and described a system for testing them on humans, for creating medicinal gardens, and for preparing a wide assortment of medicaments for specific ailments, including several expressly made "for the fatigue of those administering the government and holding public office." Many of the plants depicted are still used by *curanderos* in Mexico today.

As the world was learning about the Badianus Manuscript, an American drug-hunter was planning a secret plant-hunting expedition to Mexico. He sought a plant — one identified, in fact, in the Badianus Manuscript — that he believed could transform what was then a medical novelty into one of the biggest drugs in the world. He would be right about the plant — it would remake not only medicine but sex as well. Yet, typically, he would be forgotten while his discovery changed the world.

Russell E. Marker had been a very good chemist at Pennsylvania State University. Besides his academic tasks, he worked part-time for the pharmaceutical firm Parke, Davis & Company, specializing in steroids. *Steroid* means "like a sterol" (from the Greek *sterros*, or firm), which is a solid alcohol that occurs widely in plants and animals. Steroids as a group have a core skeleton of carbon and hydrogen atoms arranged in four fused rings. Hundreds of natural and thousands of synthetic steroids are based on this structure. Cholesterol is a steroid. So are products of the adrenal gland that are essential to life: the male and female sex hormones and the corticosteroids. Marker dedicated his life to learning their chemistry. By 1943, he had written over 160 scientific papers and had taken out more than seventy-five patents (assigned to his financial backer, Parke, Davis), mostly about steroids.

At the time, medical scientists were also infatuated with steroids. They believed the sex hormones like estrogen, progesterone, and testosterone, and the corticosteroids (the latter so-called because they are made in the outer layer, or cortex, of the adrenal gland) might be useful as medicine. It had been observed, for example, that women with crippling rheumatoid arthritis got better when they were pregnant, a time when their level of progesterone was high. But steroid hormones were prohibitively expensive to get. Small quantities of the sex hormones were being produced by a cartel of European drug companies that controlled the patents on the process and set prices that made gold look cheap. Progesterone, for example, cost two hundred dollars a gram. Everyone wanted to find a way around the monopoly. Rumors helped fan the hunt. One, never substantiated, held that Nazis were injecting Luftwaffe pilots with steroids so they could fly at higher altitudes without suffering oxygen deprivation. In 1942, a team of scientists in Switzerland isolated a corticosteroid they called cortisone, followed shortly thereafter by two American teams, who called the substance Compound E. These efforts would later win the discoverers the Nobel Prize in 1950. In 1942, however, there was not enough cortisone to fill a Coke bottle. What existed had been extracted from tons of animal adrenal glands at a cost that would have balked a Rockefeller.

Marker, however, believed he could make steroid hormones and cortisone by the ton. In 1942, he abruptly quit his position at Penn State and Parke, Davis. He told his family he had to travel for an indefinite period, alone. Then he dropped out of sight. He resurfaced in a suburb of Mexico City. There he rented an old pottery shed, set up a crude chemistry lab, bought himself some good boots and a machete, and went plant-hunting. He was after a plant called *Dioscorea*. It was the true yam, not the sweet potato that is often called a yam. Hundreds of species exist, more than fifty in Mexico alone. Some are edible while many others are quite poisonous. *Dioscorea* belonged to the order Liliales, whose plants were rich with sterols, and was related to the yucca and agave, which had been used by Native Americans to clean fabric. The "cleansing" chemical in these plants is saponin. Marker predicted that saponin and a variant, sapogenin, which he had isolated from sarsaparilla root in Mexico, could also be used as a starting point to make sex hormones. And he suspected that certain Mexican yams were bursting with them.

Marker knew a great deal about Mexican yams. In previous years, he had spent vacations roaming the Mexican countryside, querying indigenous people and campesinos who used the yam about its location and abundance. They told him what to look for: a small, shrub-like plant with spindly branches that grows from a half-buried rhizome (an underground stem) that looks like a large, scaly lump of coal. It was usually found in tropical savannahs and especially in abandoned fields or second-growth vegetation in areas with over a meter of rainfall yearly but with a distinct dry season. Mexicans called it *cabeza de negro*, or black's head. The rhizome usually grew to about two kilos but could attain the weight of a full-grown man. It wasn't much to look at, but Marker thought the plant was among nature's most beautiful, for it contained a highly concentrated saponin called diosgenin.

That the yam had medicinal use was no secret: the Badianus Manuscript described it, and country people in Mexico used some species as an antirheumatic, expectorant, or diuretic. In the nineteenth century, a substance made from dried yam root, called "dioscorein," was sold in the United States by the drug company W. S. Merrell, as a remedy for colic, as an expectorant, and to induce perspiration or vomiting. The question was, could anyone turn crude diosgenin into sex hormones and cortisone? In fact, Marker had figured that out in 1940. That year, he published a paper that described a five-step method to convert diosgenin (first isolated by Japanese scientists from a Japanese species of yam in 1937) into progesterone. He expected drug companies in the United States would bankroll him in a scheme to manufacture cheap progesterone in Mexico. They would not. Perhaps they viewed a flood of cheap progesterone as a threat to their profits, or simply were leery of the vicissitudes of getting regular supplies of plants from tropical countries. In any case, Marker, a man described by those he worked with in Mexico as temperamental and secretive, decided to do it himself. He set up a collecting network among campesinos to supply his Mexico City lab, where he not only worked but slept. He suspected he was being spied upon, not an unreasonable notion given the level of competition in the drug industry, so he carried his paperwork with him whenever he left his laboratory.

In 1943, an unkempt, bald, and clearly agitated American walked into the Mexico City office of Laboratorios Hormona carrying two packages wrapped in brown paper under his arms. He was shown into the office of the company's chief scientist, Frederick Lehmann, a young German who, with another expatriat, Hungarian Emeric Somlo, had created the company to manufacture medicines and hormones eleven years before. How much do you charge, the visitor asked, for a gram of progesterone? Lehmann said about eighty dollars. The visitor unwrapped one of his packages and set it on Lehmann's desk. It was a glass jar, and within it, he said, were a thousand grams of progesterone. He unwrapped the other package. Another kilo. Total value: $160,000.

The visitor was of course Marker. Not only did he sell Hormona his progesterone, he was enticed to join the company, with 40 percent ownership. The new company became Syntex, a combination of "synthesis" and "Mexico." Syntex began manufacturing and selling progesterone at a few dollars a gram, and broke the monopoly held by the European cartel. Syntex set up a huge collecting system to harvest wild *Dioscorea* by the trainload. It imported European scientists and also paid Mexico's National University to start a training program for young chemists to fill the company's growing ranks. It set out to use diosgenin as a starting point for the scores of other hormones and corticosteroids in the steroid family. Marker, however, did not see most of this. He was a difficult man to work with, and within two years Somlo and Lehmann had had enough and suggested he either buy them out or vice versa. Marker chose the latter. He took his share and started one company after another to make hormones, and he also consulted for drug companies. He even found more potent sources of diosgenin in another species of *Dioscorea* known locally as *barbasco*. None of his companies made a dent in Syntex's control of the industry. Marker remained in Mexico but avoided publicity, and little is known of him after his falling out with Syntex.

Syntex, meanwhile, vaulted from a $100,000-a-year pip-squeak in 1945 to an $8 million-a-year enterprise in 1950. With what Marker had taught the company's chemists — he had not patented his technique in Mexico — they created a flow of new steroids. The biggest fortune would come to whoever learned how to make the super-steroid cortisone. Merck & Company had developed a dauntingly complex synthesis starting from animal bile in 1944 that rendered ounces at great cost. Demand became almost hysterical after 1949, however, when Philip Hench, a scientist at the Mayo Clinic and one of the 1950 Nobel Prize winners, showed movies of helpless arthritics too crippled to stand who, a day after getting cortisone, got up and danced. Cortisone and its family of steroids were being recommended for over thirty illnesses and conditions, from snakebite and burns to asthma and cancer. Drug companies upended the chemical literature looking for other compounds like diosgenin. Two companies, Upjohn and S. B. Penick, sent a large expedition to Africa in a fruitless attempt to get a potential candidate compound, sarmentogenin, from *Strophanthus*, the poison arrow plant that David Livingstone had written about almost one hundred years before.

Syntex, however, would scoop the world again. The little Mexican company that North American competitors had first regarded with disdain, then with annoyance, and finally with grudging respect, hired on another genius. Carl Djerassi was a steroid chemist like Marker who was looking for someplace adventurous to pursue his career when he took a job with Syntex. In 1951, under his guidance, Syntex made its first synthetic cortisone from diosgenin. Djerassi eventually led the company to an even greater discovery: the oral contraceptive. Along with cortisone, Syntex had synthesized a hormone it called norethindrone that inhibited ovulation. It was now possible to stop pregnancy before the egg even had a chance to be fertilized. Just over ten years later, Syntex would be supplying the hormones for half the world's market in oral contraceptives.

Syntex had become the world leader in steroid chemistry. It had drawn great European and North American scientists to Mexico, where many of them became citizens, and it helped train a generation of

Mexican chemists. The Mexican government had put stiff export duties on the raw yam and diosgenin to ensure that the sophisticated, and most profitable, processing techniques developed in Mexico. Syntex had also created a local industry of yam collectors, processors, and eventually cultivators, and had started subsidiaries in New York and Puerto Rico. The company had shown that a developing country, albeit with some help from European scientists, could run with — indeed, outrun — the big dogs of the world's pharmaceutical industry. And they did it with the lowly yam.

The company's Mexican coloration would soon begin to fade, however. In the late 1950s, the drug company Eli Lilly committed itself to fund half of Syntex's research for five years, giving Syntex patent ownership and choice of research topics but getting co-marketing rights for discoveries (similar to a deal Lilly would cut with a small California company, ethnobotanically oriented Shaman Pharmaceuticals, in 1992). In 1959, Syntex was bought by Allen & Company, a New York investment banking firm, and went public, becoming one of Wall Street's greatest success stories. The research operation, however, was moved to Palo Alto, California, where Djerassi had become a faculty member at Stanford University. Syntex was now a multinational, a creature of no single country. Then in the late 1960s, a new Mexican government decided to nationalize yam production. Mexico was at the time still the foundation of the huge steroid market, selling tens of millions of plants to several international drug companies. The reason the government gave for its nationalization decision, Djerassi recalls, was to get more money for the working peasant. "This was chemical OPEC thinking," Djerassi wrote in *Science* magazine in 1992, "with one fatal flaw. While it may take decades to come up with economically attractive alternatives to petroleum as an energy source, it took the international pharmaceutical companies only a few years to come up with other alternatives . . . that transformed the Mexican diosgenin-based steroid industry into a minor player on the world stage — a transformation from which Mexico has never recovered."

Gill, the gifted amateur, and Marker, the maverick scientist, were thoroughly Western, scientific soldiers of fortune. Their attitude toward nature and the people who lived close to it was pragmatic, more like that of art dealers than painters. Yet both men proved that there was more to the lore of indigenous peoples than voodoo and incantations. Gill especially applied himself to learning the Indian way of medicine, and he gave his teachers credit. Moreover, the two men showed that medicinal botany and ethnobotany were not necessarily *passive* disciplines of collecting and classifying, but instead were dynamic, *active* interactions with the natural world.

As their fates attest, the relationship between naturalist explorers like Gill and Marker and the pharmaceutical industry was as mercurial as that between a court jester and his king. Wandering botanists with mud on their shoes waved a dirt-caked root and recited a tale of a marvelous native cure effected overnight by a loinclothed witch doctor. Much of the time, these people were well-meaning and wrong, yet a few were right often enough to engage the drug industry, at least in fits and starts. For example, while Gill was preparing for his first trip to Ecuador, two New Delhi chemists isolated several interesting and apparently unknown crystalline substances from the root of a plant known scientifically as *Rauwolfia serpentina*. Common to tropical climates, the plant in India resembles an azalea, with dark, glistening leaves and clusters of white to yellowish-pink flowers. For three thousand years, it had been called *sarpagandha*, or snakeroot, and was used as a folk remedy in India to treat nervous disorders, insanity, and snakebite. The mongoose, according to legend, would eat the leaves before attacking a cobra.

The crystalline compounds were alkaloids. By the 1940s, Indian physicians were reporting from experiments with plant extracts that it was an excellent sedative and treatment for hypertension, or high blood pressure. Reports of these findings made their way to the West, and in 1952, E. R. Squibb & Sons sponsored experiments with snakeroot and soon marketed a standardized version of the extract called Raudixin. Eventually, its active ingredient, reserpine, was isolated and became the backbone of numerous drugs for hypertension and psychiatric illnesses. By 1960, prescriptions for reserpine-based drugs were valued at $30 million a year, and reserpine-based drugs are still widely prescribed today.

Such serendipity in drug discovery happened again in the late 1950s with the rosy periwinkle, *Catharanthus roseus*. Canadians at a research laboratory in Toronto had heard that periwinkle was employed as a diabetes treatment in Jamaica. About the same time, chemist Gordon Svoboda from Eli Lilly & Company in Indianapolis found that species of the same genus were used for diabetes in the Philippines. The plant actually did nothing for diabetes, but luckily Lilly scientists discovered that it killed certain kinds of cancer cells. Alkaloids from the plant, also known as *Vinca*, became fabulously successful cancer drugs called vincristine and vinblastine. They turned childhood leukemia and

Hodgkin's disease from almost sure killers to among the most treatable and least lethal of all cancers — and made Lilly lots of money.

Stories like these made plant-hunting for medicines seem like found money. In neither case were there clear "owners" of these substances with whom Western scientists and drug-makers shared profits (although Lilly paid for bulk supplies of periwinkle from Madagascar for some time before bringing the plant to the United States for cultivation). In reality, however, for every reserpine and vincristine, tens of thousands of plant extracts were tested and rejected. The plant-hunting trade was littered with disappointments and, occasionally, ineptitude. A story is told by Norman R. Farnsworth, a professor of pharmacognosy (the study of natural drugs and their chemical constituents) at the school of pharmacy at the University of Illinois in Chicago, and one of the world's experts on medicinal plants. A physician convinced a drug company to send him, for a large sum of money, into a tropical forest to observe medicine men using plants as drugs. He would diagnose the patients, assess the effects of the herbal remedies, and collect those that worked. The physician went off, and at first all went as planned. He collected several large samples of plant material, including with each one a voucher specimen, the sine qua non of botany, consisting of the leaves and wherever possible the flowers or fruits of the plant, pressed between sheets of paper and dried to prevent decay. He identified each voucher by writing a number on one of its leaves in ink. The bulk material and vouchers were sent to the drug company. When they arrived, the voucher specimens had dried and crumbled, and the identifying numbers were, of course, illegible. The entire expedition was a waste.

Some expeditions, such as one to the Amazon by adventuress Nicole Maxwell, were amateurish, and produced frothy travel books but no serious drug leads. Others were backed with large investments and experienced chemists like Robert F. Raffauf, a seasoned plant-hunter and now professor at Boston's Northeastern University's school of pharmacology. As in his Amazon days, Raffauf is a compact, neat man with a rich sense of irony and a formidable knowledge of plant chemistry who enjoys skewering nostrums of rainforest riches falling from the vine. "I was with Smith, Kline & French, from about 1950 to 1965," he remembers. "I spent a lot of time wandering through jungles, in South America and Africa. There was a guy like me at Ciba, another one at Squibb. Everybody was doing it in those days because of reserpine, from *Rauwolfia*, and that was a great thing. Well, we'd go down in the Amazon and we'd meet the representative from Abbott or

Ciba at the same bush, right? We were all plodding the same ground. Then we'd go to the air-conditioned hotel and sit and have drinks and have conversations like, 'Well, what did you find today, Al?'

" 'I didn't find anything, did you?'

" 'No, I didn't find anything either. But what the hell, it's lot's of fun, isn't it?'

" 'Yeah, it's lots of fun. Let's have another drink.' "

Although Raffauf laughs at the story, he looks back fondly at his ten years spent hunting for plant drugs in the world's rainforests. Unfortunately, only about ten compounds from the effort were deemed potentially useful, and none became a drug. "The toxicologists would say, 'You can't put this stuff in man!' " Raffauf remembers. "So you'd come back and say, 'But sir, this plant and its leaves and roots have been in man for four thousand years, whaddya mean you can't put it in man?' Then they'd just say, 'Okay, if you want to live in the Amazon and have a life expectancy of thirty-eight, go ahead.' "

Raffauf believes rainforests are worth saving for their inherent value. "And if people find a few drugs along the way, that will be icing," he says, but they should realize that medicinal plants are damned hard to find. "I looked at thousands of plants," he says, many of them hacked from the rainforest in the company of his friend and colleague Richard Schultes. "Someone might go back and find some new drugs this time, but the statistics are against finding a lot. They are looking at the same plants we did in 1956." That is partly because drug companies never revealed much of what they found out, so no one really knows what plants have been tested for what properties. "It reminds me of something I read in the *Botanical Gazette* from 1889," says Raffauf. " 'Thus we, for lack of knowing what has been done, grind over and over the same grist.' "

Even when they found a drug candidate, pharmaceutical companies had to contend with plant shipments that varied biologically and chemically, leading to unpredictable laboratory results. Supplies of bulk material were subject to sudden price increases, natural disasters like plant diseases or floods, irregular transportation, and the uncertainties of *baksheesh* politics practiced by epauletted dictators, family-run governments, and grasping foreign bureaucrats. So companies increasingly turned to the newfound wonders of synthetic chemistry. Their feeling was that synthetic chemists could turn out candidate compounds for drugs much like so much beer. Chemists, it was decided, could do almost anything that nature could, right in the lab between nine and five with two coffee breaks and lunch.

By 1974, the last cycle of plant-hunting for medicines was ending. Of the $1 billion the pharmaceutical industry spent that year on research and development, only $200,000 went into phytochemical research. Rainforests were something for *National Geographic*, and the ancient science of medicinal botany tottered near obsolescence. There seemed to be no place in science anymore for green medicines.

4

Ethnobotany

Three times a week, the seventy-six-year-old explorer climbs the wrought-iron staircase at Harvard University's Botanical Museum to his high-ceilinged, fourth-floor office overlooking Oxford Street. Straight-backed and broad-shouldered, his necktie tied in perfect Windsor symmetry, he greets all with a vaguely anglicized "good morning." To the staff, he is "Professor Schultes," curator, storyteller, authority on hallucinogenic drugs, and emeritus professor. In his sunny office, Schultes removes a crisp white lab coat from its hook and slips it on over his tweed suit. At his desk beside the picture window, he settles into another day's work turning a half-century's experience in ethnobotany into books, articles, and speeches that together make up a kind of requiem for a disappearing breed of scientist-explorers. Schultes is a vestige, a throwback to the age of naturalist-explorers, a man who uses words like "motor car" and who does not type. Yet he also is a bridge, a man who kept the venerable practice of medicinal plant-hunting alive until a time when it could flourish again. There is no one like him left on the planet. They know that at Harvard; in his laboratory across the hall from his office, the instructions from his last lecture, five years ago, are still chalked on the blackboard.

Ethnobotany is mostly messy, muddy, unpredictable, and disease-ridden work, especially when pursued in the tropics, where Schultes did most of his work. True, there is a certain romance to living in a shack in a remote jungle village. A seven-day romance, perhaps. Soon the heat, the will-sucking humidity, the monotonous food, and the war with the insects subdue all but the most ardent. Success brings little fame, and the pay is lousy.

Why would anyone want to do this?

Schultes, perhaps the only living ethnobotanist to whom notoriety has come, says simply that it is the most fascinating thing there is to do. His many books and papers rarely indulge in the greater meaning of it all, although he elaborates in a roundabout way in the foreword to his book *Where the Gods Reign: Plants and People of the Colombian Amazon.* He writes: "The explorer, especially the scientific explorer, has, more often than not, stood at the vanguard of penetration into unknown regions and has usually been the means of acquainting the world with these remote parts of the planet." Such was the way Schultes lived much of his life, although he credits another man as father to the thought: Richard Spruce. Spruce, says Schultes, "was fired by a God-given urge to live with nature and to try to understand the mysteries of earth's green cover . . . of no man can Juvenal's words be more truly spoken: 'Everyone wants to know, no one to pay the price.' "

Paying the price is part of the ritual for each new generation of ethnobotanists, like drinking a tribal ordeal medicine or digging botfly larvae out of one's ankles. Schultes paid his during thirteen years in South America's rainforests, a good part of it spent living among the indigenous peoples of the northwestern Amazon. At the time, almost no one knew what he was doing there. Other than as a potential source of rubber, the rainforest was then of little commercial interest to North Americans, and was left to storytellers, biologists, and a few anthropologists who liked to live in thatched huts. Quietly, Schultes changed that. He brought back plants of great mystery and possibly of great value, plants used for millennia by forest peoples as food, fiber, building materials, and medicines. Many of the plants were purely therapeutic, like tree saps and barks to treat fungal infections or to rid the intestines of worms. Others were far more mysterious, like ayahuasca and *yopo,* the powerful shamanistic hallucinogens used to contact the spirit world. It was in that world, Schultes explained, where the answers to these peoples' most fundamental questions lay. "Primitive cultures," Schultes says, "usually have no concept of physically or organically induced sickness or death: both result from interference from the spirit world. Therefore, hallucinogens, which permit the native healer and sometimes even the patient to communicate with the spirit world, often become greater medicines — the medicines *par excellence* — of the native pharmacopoeia."

Schultes returned to Harvard from the Amazon and recreated economic and medicinal botany through his writings, his encouragement of drug companies to experiment with tropical plants, and most of all his enormously popular lectures at Harvard. He and his students and others who followed him have now succeeded in drawing the world's attention to the rainforest and especially to its people. They have created a renaissance, one whose precepts include the belief that instead of dismissing the botanical knowledge of native peoples as a novelty, it should be respected. Certainly, Schultes the scientist matched the alkaloids and cardiac glycosides and lysergic acids to their respective exotic plants. But he also learned that the holy snuff of the Amazonian Tukano people, taken from the bark of the tree *Virola*, came from the penis of the Sun, and that it enabled its user to contact Viho-mahse, the "snuff-person" who dwells in the Milky Way and controls life on Earth. Both chemistry and mysticism were fair subjects and ones that could be uttered in the same sentence. For there was more than science in the medicinal and hallucinogenic plants of the rainforest; there was art, art in the way the writer Aldous Huxley, himself an experimenter with hallucinogens, described it — a means by which people transport themselves to another place, another world.

The lives of many medicinal plant-hunters have had an epic quality. These explorers were self-styled green knights on a quest for some Holy Grail to be snatched from the wilderness and brought back to civilization to cure the sick. Of course, a certain amount of personal fame and wealth in return was not to be sneered at; these were real people, after all, not fairy-tale characters. Yet William Withering, Richard Gill, or Russell Marker would not have been satisfied with wealth earned by cobbling together man-made things like factories, art, or the law. They chose to enlarge themselves by drawing from something greater than themselves. Not being clergymen, they chose nature.

Richard Schultes was a different breed of plant-hunter. The following is an entry from one of his field journals:

Vomiting continuously, very weak, probably mostly from malnutrition — we have had no warm food, only a tin of sardines for supper last night. A strange accident happened this morning. About five a.m. there was a jolt and a loud crashing and splitting of wood. The barge had run into a leaning tree along the river's edge and the already badly damaged cabin was smashed. With my flashlight, I saw that the tree was in young fruit, with a recently fertilized ovary, that is, so I broke off a few branches to put in the press later. When dawn came, I examined the plant — it was *Micrandra minor*, which I am especially anxious to collect! Naturally, all on board were highly amused at my joy in collecting branches from a tree that had caused them so much fright.

This was the kind of observation that marks the lyrical plant-hunter Schultes had been in the western Amazon for six years when he experienced this little epiphany, yet the flush of satisfaction from a new find was as fresh as if he had just stepped off a plane from Cambridge. The lyrical plant-hunter meets nature with an innocent enthusiasm and that simplest of hopes, the joy of the experience. Nature's taxonomic hierarchy is his medium, through which he moves from one discovery to the next almost unconsciously, like a hummingbird skimming from flower to flower. He is not unmindful that what he uncovers might become a valuable commodity. Yet he enters the forest like a painter facing a blank canvas, with the credo of the father of botany, Linnaeus, to guide him: Live innocently; God is here.

When Schultes went to South America in search of plants in 1941, eyewitness tales of jungle expeditions were regular newsstand fare, their accounts bursting with narrow escapes and punctuated liberally with hyperbole and exclamations of wonder. *National Geographic* magazine extolled plant-hunters with stories like "Into Primeval Papua by Seaplane: Seeking Disease-resisting Sugar Cane, Scientists Find Neolithic Man in Unmapped Nooks of Sorcery and Cannibalism." Even bureaucrats were romanticized. The exploits of U.S. Department of Agriculture botanists who were seeking new crops for American farmers were serialized in a newspaper cartoon strip called "Uncle Sam at Your Service," depicting pith-helmeted explorers bartering with spear-carrying natives in loincloths.

Schultes had little in common with the swashbuckling characters portrayed in most of these stories. His paternal grandparents had emigrated from Prussia, and his engineer father, Otto Richard Schultes, earned the family's living in the Roxbury section of Boston installing steam vats in breweries. His mother had descended from English sheep farmers and was no stranger to hard times. Her mother and two older sisters had had to go to work when her father, a mechanic, fell off a bridge and drowned, and she attended secretarial college and worked in an office before marrying. The Schultes were hardly cosmopolitan, their foreign traveling experience consisting of Otto's one-year stint in South Africa helping to build a brewery there.

It was not long after Richard Schultes was born in 1915 that Otto Schultes was thrown out of work by "that S.O.B. President Wilson" and his Prohibition, the younger Schultes recalls, and had to switch to the plumbing and heating trade. Otto Schultes worked at that until he was seventy-six, and only quit when his wife and son convinced him to slow down. At ninety-three he still went to fetch the daily newspaper, and it was on that mission during one particularly heavy Boston snowstorm that he got stuck in a snowdrift and had to be rescued. "He came back wet up to his hips," Schultes remembers. "He died shortly after that of pneumonia."

Schultes attended public schools in East Boston. He was not an outstanding student, he says, and his parents felt it necessary to fortify their son's education by reading to him at home. One of the books his parents took out of the library was a formidable two-volume history called *Notes of a Botanist in the Amazon and Andes*, the account of Spruce's Amazonian travels. Schultes says that at the time the book did not shape his plans for the future, but after winning a scholarship to Harvard, he soon chose to study biology. Moreover, he helped pay his expenses by working in the Botanical Museum on Oxford Street on the Harvard campus — the very museum he one day would supervise. He filed documents and generally helped out the man who soon would launch his career, Professor Oakes Ames. Ames ran the Botanical Museum and taught the botanical course at Harvard, Biology 104. He was an economic botanist as well as a committed taxonomist and orchid expert. Again, Schultes recalls being less than a standout in class, but the young man's interest in the southwestern cactus peyote and its role in rituals of Native Americans impressed his professor. When Schultes proposed writing a thesis on the subject, Ames bankrolled a trip for his student to the Southwest out of his own pocket, as Schultes later learned.

The journey was an eye-opener. It was Schultes's first exposure to the world outside the Northeast, and landed the twenty-one-year-old on a reservation in Oklahoma where, among other things, he had his first encounter with an hallucinogenic substance. His account of eating peyote mescal buttons is dryly scientific for a young Bostonian having the first hallucinations of his lifetime. He describes the sensations as "macroscopia, depersonalization, doubling of the ego, alteration of loss of time perception, and other rather unearthly effects. . . ." Fanciful he was not. He did not, nor would he ever, take psychedelic substances for kicks. In later years, he would condemn even the term *psychedelic* as etymologically unsound and part of the jargon of recreational drug-takers. He prefers the term *psychotomimetic*, meaning "mimicking a psychosis," or *hallucinogenic*, meaning the chemical stimulation of changes in perception, thought, and mood, often but not necessarily accompanied by visions. Schultes actually was interested in the medical uses of these plants as well as their fantastic effects. Peyote, for example, was prescribed by Native Americans for a wide variety of conditions, including tuberculosis, diabetes, influenza, and even venereal diseases. To treat illness with these plants made perfect sense, Schultes concluded. "The only explanation for their unearthly effects contrasted with the great majority of plant species," Schultes says, "is that these few psychoactive plants are the homes of spiritual forces."

The Southwest drew Schultes back several times, and he wrote his Ph.D. thesis on the economic use of plants in Oaxaca, in southern Mexico. Especially interesting was the bridge formed between medicinal and hallucinogenic plants and the cosmologies of indigenous peoples, and it was this subject that would become his life's work. He uncovered and still translates obscure historical accounts of useful plants and hallucinogens, especially in the New World. Libraries and museums held troves of evidence that hallucinogenic plants were common among the Inca, Aztec, and other New World civilizations. When the Spanish came to the New World, however, they repressed these practices. They called peyote "satanic trickery" that caused "diabolic fantasies," an attitude that, Schultes notes unhappily, still exists toward native use of ritual hallucinogens. "Spanish ecclesiastics were intolerant of any cult but their own," says Schultes, who in his own travels, like Spruce, expressed his dismay at how the church converted indigenous people from proud, independent people into cultural misfits in ragged shirts and tennis shoes.

From the outset, Schultes participated in shamanistic rituals. He went on peyote hunts and watched the elaborate ceremonies and dances that accompany peyote's use by the Huichol, Tarahumara, and Cora Indians of Mexico. Later, in South America, he took part in the three-day *Kai-ya-ree* dance of the Colombian Yukuna that reenacts the evolution of the tribe from the primordial anaconda egg. One of the many photographs that record his South American journey shows Schultes prepared for the ceremony, dressed in grass skirt, tunic, and a huge, painted mask, only his six-foot-tall frame giving away his identity among his Yukuna hosts. He found in culture after culture the same pattern. "There are two types of 'medicines': those with purely physical effects (i.e. to relieve toothache or digestive upsets); and the medicines *par excellence*, that put the medicine man into communication, through a variety of hallucinations, with the malevolent spirits that cause illness and death." Sometimes, as anthropologist Michael Harner found among the Jívaro, these communications can be used to kill enemies or protect the tribe from danger. Most were life-affirming, however: Schultes remembers the description, enigmatic perhaps to Western ears, of a peyote ceremony by a Huichol shaman: "It is one; it is a unity; it is ourselves."

In his travels, Schultes observed the use of *teonanacatl*, the hallucinogenic mushroom of the genus *Psilocybe* whose Aztec name means "divine flesh." There was also *ololiuqui*, from two herbaceous plants of the Southwest and Central America, *Ipomoea violacea* and *Turbina corymbosa*, both commonly known as morning glory. Its seeds were ground up and drunk with liquid to produce vivid hallucinations in the service of shamanistic medicine. There was the San Pedro cactus, *Trichocereus pachanoi*, sacred to the Incas and the Nazca of the Andes and source of the widely used hallucinogen mescaline (which stimulated Aldous Huxley's visions described in his books *The Doors of Perception* and *Heaven and Hell*). And there was of course the narcotic but also psychoactive *Cannabis*, source of marijuana, on which Schultes has occasionally been called upon to testify as a courtroom expert.

For the most part, the active compounds in these plants were alkaloids. There were intriguing similarities between these and neurochemicals that transmit signals from one nerve cell to another. Psilocybine in sacred mushrooms was similar to the neurotransmitter serotonin. The alkaloid mescaline, from peyote and San Pedro cactus, resembled the neurotransmitter norepinephrine. In morning glory, the hallucinogenic compounds were forms of lysergic acid, which had earned a fearful reputation long before their recreational use began in the 1960s. Large amounts of the compound were contained in ergot, a fungal infection of cereal grains that had been named St. Anthony's fire for causing mass hysterias, hallucinations, gangrenous disfigurations, and deaths in European villages where it was inadvertently eaten.

Straight taxonomic botanists often tittered at all that shamanistic stuff and were downright suspicious of a man of science who consumed drugs. At Harvard on a clear, icy February morning in 1992, Schultes can look back and chuckle at those critics, most of whom are long gone. "They thought I was a bit eccentric," he recalls as he stands amid a swirl of children in the echoing atrium of the Botanical Museum, where its famous collection of glass flowers is on display. The exhibit has been overtaken by a busload of kids with field-trip fever, who ignore the old man's requests for a little less shouting. Schultes seeks refuge in an exhibit room in the neighboring Museum of Comparative Zoology. Someone has laid out cookies on a table, directly underneath a model of an octopus with twelve-foot-long tentacles that hangs threateningly from the ceiling. "Zoologists get all the money, you know," Schultes remarks as he scoops up a couple of cookies in his large hands. They are steady hands, although he fidgets with them as he talks, as if he were still itching those insect bites he learned to live with in the rainforest. He is partly deaf in one ear and turns his head slightly to listen, but there is little bend in his frame, and he exudes a sense of physical strength. The wire-rimmed glasses he wore while among the Amazonians are still there, but the crew cut is gone. "I suppose I should have found a cure for baldness while I was there," he says as he strokes his shining head.

Schultes found the hallucinogens to be chemically fascinating. Moreover, they served a vital purpose to forest-dwellers. The geographer Yi-Fu Tuan in his studies of "topophilia," meaning the love of topography or scenery, notes that forest people live not so much on the Earth as within an all-encompassing element. Perspectives are curtailed, everything is short-range, and life is a continuum with barely noticeable seasonal changes. Plants are their medium, their firmament. But learning which plants are powerful and why is no summer field trip. "To do ethnobotany," Schultes says, "you have to 'waste' a lot of time, at least *they* [traditional botanists] considered it a waste of time, just talking and being nice and jolly, telling jokes to Indians and acting like a fool."

Fortunately, Schultes was to have lots of time to do that. When he arrived in Colombia in 1941, fresh from Harvard and Mexico, he was supposed to investigate the plants that produced the arrow poison, curare, on a grant from the National Research Council. He was in the field only a few months before Pearl Harbor was bombed. By foot and canoe, he made his way to the American embassy in Bogotá to volunteer for service. "I was asked to join, agreed to do so, and was promptly sent back into the jungle," Schultes recalls, to find rubber trees for the U.S. Department of Agriculture and the war effort. Far from being upset at the interruption of his research, Schultes was elated. "Besides the chance to explore the secrets of the rubber tree," he says, "it would permit the study of hundreds of rare, unusual plants, some of which had never been known to science."

The assignment was an ironic coincidence, as if the lifelines on the palms of Schultes and Spruce had taken the same jagged turn. (Schultes, in fact, is fond of pointing out that their initials are the same.) Spruce had been called by the British government to the Andean Amazon to gather cinchona seeds to create a British supply of quinine. Now Schultes was called by his country to find natural rubber in case the supply from Asia should be cut off. The botanist would spend ten years doing this, in the process collecting thirty-five hundred specimens from the rubber-tree genus, *Hevea*, and literally tons of seed. He would become botany's modern rubber baron, and to this day he is still consulted by rubber-tree growers all over the world.

The assignment allowed Schultes to explore Amazonian economic botany on the government's nickel, one of the best values for money in the annals of research. Living was cheap. When he was traveling, Schultes slept wherever he could stretch out. He ate whatever the local people ate: deer, monkey, the rodent capybara, lots of fish, and the staple, a sort of tapioca paste. "That's why my wife has one order," he says. "No tapioca pudding." He traveled in an eighteen-foot, fifty-three-pound aluminum canoe powered by outboard motor, slept in a hammock, and carried most of what he needed on his own broad back. Teenagers from villages along his path were his guides and assistants, whose talents as climbers, river navigators, and cultural guides Schultes still marvels at. Schultes learned several local languages, won the friendship and respect of Colombia's scientific community, and amassed his stockpile of plants. Much of the lore that goes with them is still in his field journals and notebooks, in his neat, cursive handwriting. "They are all stained from being dragged through the mud," Schultes explains. "My son says I should put them on computer, but computers and I are not friendly." Indeed, Schultes still writes letters by hand.

When he returned in 1954 to Harvard, Schultes began immortalizing what was in those notebooks. Much of it appears in a series he entitled *De Plantis Toxicarus E Mundo Novo/Tropicale Commentationes*. He insists on the proper Latin nomenclature for botanical work. When Timothy Leary, a faculty member at Harvard during the 1960s, sought to enlist Schultes in an effort to allow undergraduate students to try hallucinogenic substances, Schultes declined, noting with pique that Leary incorrectly spelled the Latin names of plants. Schultes also spent the 1950s courting a young woman named Dorothy Crawford McNeil, a professional singer of Scottish descent who also had an advanced degree in economics. They were married in 1959 and have three children.

Of the several books that Schultes has filled with his Amazonian discoveries, the most comprehensive is *The Healing Forest*, written with Robert Raffauf. The authors list over fifteen hundred plants used as medicines and hallucinogens by Amazonians. Many were first described by Spruce, and Schultes is diligent in noting the Yorkshireman's precedence. Indeed, he describes Spruce's three-year marathon from the Brazilian port of Manaus up the Río Negro and its tributaries and back as the "pinnacle of botanical expeditions in South America." Both Spruce and Schultes were plant men first, eventually embracing the human connection when it thrust itself upon them. They differed though in regard to the hallucinogens. Of the vine of the soul, known as *caapi* to the Indians living along the Río Uaupés, Spruce took one cup during an Indian celebration and described it in his diary as a "nauseous beverage." The local head man, he wrote, being "desirous, apparently, that I should taste all his delicacies at once . . . came up with a woman bearing a large calabash of *caxirí* (mandiocca-beer), of which I must needs take a copious draught, and as I knew the mode of its preparation [fermented chewed manioc], it was gulped down with secret loathing." Next, a two-foot-long cigar was thrust into his hand, from which the nonsmoker took several polite puffs. "Above all this," Spruce continued, "I must drink a large cup of palm-wine, and it will readily be understood that the effect of such a complex dose was a strong inclination to vomit, which was only overcome by lying down in a hammock and drinking a cup of coffee. . . ."

While no gourmand of Amazonian delicacies, Spruce recorded the first detailed description of *caapi*'s manufacture and source. As for true medicinals, Spruce was an interested skeptic who nonetheless tried to track down rumors of rainforest remedies. He was once tipped off to the arrival of a renowned brujo in a village on the Río Negro where he was staying. As soon as the medicine man, or *paye*, learned that a white medicine man was there, Spruce wrote, "he and his attendants immediately threw back into the canoe his goods, which they had begun to disembark, and resumed their dangerous voyage down the river in the night-time. . . . I could only regret that his dread of a supposed rival had prevented the interview which to me would have been full of interest; the more so as I was prepared to barter with him for the whole of his *materia medica*, if my stock-in-trade would have sufficed."

Spruce suspected that most native curing was simply invocation of the supernatural under the influence of narcotics. Schultes, ninety years later, would show that there was actually a chemical logic to these herbal medicines, which he could demonstrate in the laboratory. As for their supernatural inhabitants, Schultes says, "I suppose if the school of divinity here at Harvard ever asks me to lecture, I'll be able to draw those gods, which is better than they can do. It's the same idea as communion, in imbibing something great — the spirit that is in the plant."

Near the end of his Amazon years, Schultes investigated a plant that was as true a combination of the medicinal and supernatural as he had ever found. Moreover, it is a plant that soon may become part of Western medicine. Schultes was traveling near the Río Apáporis in Colombia. Amazonians from several cultures had been brought there to tap rubber, and Schultes found that many of them spent off-hours inhaling a kind of hallucinogenic snuff. It had several names: *yákee* among the Puinave, *yáto* among the Kuripako, or *paricá* among the Tukanos. Schultes tracked down the source — the resin of at least two trees of the family Myristicaceae, *Virola calophylla* and *V. calophylloidea.* Tracing its history was more difficult. South Americans had used various psychotropic snuffs for centuries, but accounts of their use by Europeans were confusing. Alexander von Humboldt reported seeing something called *yopo* made from beans of a tree and lime from snails (he believed it was the snail lime that produced the narcotic effects). Spruce later described a snuff called yopo, or, in Venezuela, *niopo* (which has since been found to contain bufotenin, the same alkaloid as is found in the skin glands of poisonous toads). Other explorers reported snuffs made of everything from tobacco leaves to tree sap. None, Schultes complained, bothered to affix Latin names to the plants associated with these drugs (Spruce excepted).

In Colombia, Schultes befriended the makers of the yákee, who led him to the tree from which it came. It was a tree Schultes was quite familiar with: *Virola*, from the same family as nutmeg and mace (both of which can have narcotic effects). A Brazilian botanist, Adolpho Ducke, had first linked it to Amazonian hallucinogenic drugs early in the twentieth century. But Schultes was the first scientist to observe not only its manufacture but its remarkable healing powers as well.

The bark was peeled in early morning, the Puinave told him, because the sun's rays weaken its narcotic effects. It was then placed in water for about half an hour, after which the soft inner layer, with beads of red latex congealed on its surface, was rasped off and the fragments thrown into an earthen pot. Water was added, and the mass kneaded and squeezed until the water turned brownish. This was strained several times and the liquid simmered over a low fire. From time to time a dirty foam was scraped off the surface. After about three or four hours, a dark brown syrup took semi-solid form in the bottom of the cooking vessel. This was ground into a fine powder, mixed with ashes from a wild cacao tree, and put into a bag or a large snail shell (empty, one would hope). A bone tube stopped with feathers and pitch at one end served as the conduit from shell to nose.

"It may be of interest," Schultes writes with scholarly detachment, "to append a few observations which I was able to make personally after taking yakee-snuff." As with ayahuasca and other hallucinogens that Schultes tried, he took much less, in this case about one-quarter, of what his informants inhaled. The object was not to get high but to get a glimmer of what the plant was capable of doing to a human. "Within fifteen minutes a drawing sensation over the eyes was felt, followed very shortly by a strong tingling in the fingers and toes. The drawing sensation in the forehead rapidly gave way to a strong and constant headache. Within one half hour, there was a numbness of the feet and hands and an almost complete disappearance of sensitivity of the finger-tips; walking was possible with difficulty, as in a case of beriberi [a vitamin B deficiency that Schultes suffered from]. Nausea was felt until about eight o'clock, accompanied by a general feeling of lassitude." Schultes eventually fell into a fitful sleep until the next morning. He woke with a headache and "a profuse and uncomfortable sweating, especially of the armpits, and what might have been a slight fever lasted from about six o'clock all through the night." Schultes also observed the effects of a full dose on medicine men: they mumbled deliriously in their sleep, shouted incoherently, experienced visions of spirits and wild animals that were interpreted by an assistant, and sometimes experienced uncontrollable twitching of the fingers and facial muscles and popping of the eyes.

Virola turned out to be much more than a bad trip, however. Schultes found groups like the Kubeos and the Tukanos treating fungal spots on their skin by clipping off a piece of *Virola* bark and "painting" the spot with the bark's sticky latex. After fifteen or twenty days of this, the infection disappeared completely. Schultes also observed Brazilian indigenous people far to the east who treated babies' colic with a decoction of the bark. All in all, *Virola* was a remarkable tree, and one that Schultes encouraged his students to take an interest in when they made their own trips to South America. One who did was ethnobotanist Mark Plotkin, now with the Washington-based group Conservation International. Plotkin found indigenous people in Suriname who also use a species of *Virola* for fungal infections, and he has traced this use back to 1775, when a French botanist recorded that natives in French Guiana used it to treat thrush, a fungal infection of the tongue and roof of the mouth (and which now frequently infects people with AIDS). Another former Schultes student, Wade Davis, reported that the Waorani Indians of Ecuador used it against fungus too.

The alkaloid tryptamine in *Virola's* resin and bark has been identified as the cause of the hallucinogenic effects. Variations on such tryptamines cause the hallucinogenic effects of Mexican mushrooms, yopo, and ayahuasca. As for *Virola's* antifungal effects, the source is likely to remain a secret for some time. Schultes sent some bark to various labs in the United States, including Smith, Kline. No one found anything of use in it; Schultes suspects that this was because the samples were not fresh when tested. However, Schultes and Plotkin were invited by the ethnobotanical drug company Shaman Pharmaceuticals, shortly after the company started business in 1989, to give them ideas for new drug compounds. The two ethnobotanists recommended investigating *Virola*. Shaman sent its own ethnobotanist to the Amazon to investigate, and by 1991 Shaman had isolated a compound from the tree bark that one year later was being investigated as a treatment for fungal infections. If it passes muster, Americans may soon be able to treat athlete's foot with an hallucinogenic plant — truly a prospect for happy feet. More important, it could help in the treatment of the fungal infections that plague people with AIDS.

During the 1960s, the world's fascination with recreational drugs put Schultes in the spotlight. Students and a few faculty assumed he might play Virgil to their Dante and lead them on a guided tour of the hallucinogenic underworld. The professor's detailed descriptions of ceremonies with ayahuasca made lurid reading even in his careful scientific prose, and his laboratory at Harvard was a museum not only for economic botany but home to perhaps the world's largest collection of the tools and icons of the narcotic and hallucinogenic. In glass cases, neatly arranged and labeled as all things Schultesian, were hookahs, a marijuana leaf embedded in a solid block of plastic, snuff tubes made of bird bones, dried psilocybe mushrooms, beads for peyote ceremonies, opium pipes, desiccated poppies, shards of bark, dried leaves from *Belladonna* plants of the nightshade family, ropy strings of the ayahuasca vine, gourd rattles, and diagrams showing the chemical structures of numerous drugs that no doubt were committed to memory by those undergraduates whose short-term memories were still intact.

But Schultes was more Heifetz than Hendrix. Not that he was oblivious to the spiritual. He dug deeply into the rituals and cosmologies of ancient and indigenous cultures, from the Hindu Rig-Veda (which, Schultes notes, has 120 hymns devoted to *soma*, believed now to be the mushroom *Amanita muscaria*, or fly agaric), to the Zuni Indian legend of the origin of the holy and hallucinogenic plant *Aneglakya*, from *Datura inoxia*. Schultes chewed coca leaves almost daily for years while in the Amazon — as the local people have for millennia, as a stimulant and to suppress hunger — and chides moralists for trying to suppress that use of it. But he left most experimentation with drugs in the laboratory to his colleague Albert Hofmann, who discovered LSD in 1938 while working at Sandoz Laboratories in Switzerland. Hofmann became an advocate of the use of hallucinogens as stimulants for psychiatric patients, especially those with deeply repressed traumatic experiences, a medical use that never gained wide acceptance. Rather than advocate the use of plant hallucinogens in his own culture, Schultes would haul a two-meter-long blowgun to his classes and demonstrate his prowess (never as good as the worst Indian, he would avow) at shooting darts at a target on the wall of the lecture hall. The fuss over hallucinogens, in fact, was often quite an annoyance to him. "You couldn't keep a text on the subject in the library," he recalls, "because people kept stealing them."

Schultes's office at the museum is now the center of his ethnobotanical world. The notebooks filed away in rows of green cabinets that surround his desk have been steadily finding their way into his books and the lectures he is constantly asked to give all over the world. Though chronically busy, he rarely seems hurried; he is, he acknowledges, without quibble, a man with a certain nineteenth-century air. The man is old enough, and charming enough, that women forgive the jokes that by current campus standards are sexist, and except for the tools of chemistry, his science has changed less than most since the last century. Yet in one thing modern Schultes has learned to believe: conservation. According to his students, he was not friendly with the environmental movement when it coalesced in the early 1970s. By the 1980s, his views had changed. His book *The Healing Forest* decries the disappearance of the world's rainforests and their cultures. "When I first went there," Schultes says of the Amazon, "the Indians were wearing loincloths. Now they wear khaki pants, carry transistor radios, and work for the oil companies." He claims he never encountered hostility from indigenous people in the Amazon, and he always traveled unarmed. "Primitive people are very close to nature, and plants are dear to them. When they see you collecting plants they love, they can't resist talking about them. They are interested in anyone who is interested in *their* work." He lauds Colombia for its efforts to conserve its rainforests and native cultures, but he is unlikely to return; his wife, he says, worries that he is likely to get shot by some drug runner. He is an honored man there — the Colombian government has named a huge park after him, and he is the only foreign scientist to receive Colombia's highest decoration, the Order of the Cross of Boyaca. He is likewise honored in North America, not only for his unique work in the Amazon but for reviving a dying discipline. Perhaps the most lasting thing Schultes accomplished was to train, entertain, and inspire a new generation of ethnobotanists. It was a career more propitious than the outwardly retiring and conservative professor could have imagined, for these students have emerged from the chrysalis of his laboratory at a time when the rainforest and its inhabitants most need them.

It is not the rainforest that has been calling Schultes, however, but England. In 1992, he went there to receive perhaps his greatest honor, the Linnean Gold Medal of the Linnean Society, the premier award in botany. He had been making pilgrimages to England for decades, however, drawn by the ghost of Spruce. A man with many stories and a lust for telling them, Schultes is perhaps most pleased by his account of his discovery of Spruce's cottage, as if he had stumbled on an unknown Inca tomb in suburban Bogotá.

Schultes was in London in 1950 on business and, having some extra time, decided to track down Spruce's last home. Spruce, with little money and in ill-health, had spent his last seventeen years in a one-room cottage in the Yorkshire village of Coneysthorpe, where he died in 1893. He lived on a small government pension, having lost his own money in a South American bank that failed. Schultes found the village and the approximate location of Spruce's house — one of about twelve cottages around a green. He rang the doorbell of one that advertised itself as the post office. "They called it the 'pust uffice,' " Schultes says with a credible Yorkshire accent. "I'd learned to pronounce the Yorkshire dialect from a couple of Yorkshiremen in a boarding house in Bogotá. Anyway, I said to the 'pust uffice' lady who answered the door, 'Would you know where Mr. Spruce once lived?'

" 'No,' she said, 'Who is he?'

" 'He was a famous botanist. I thought you might know, being postmistress.'

" 'No.'

" 'Is there anybody here who might know?'

" 'No.'

" 'He died so long ago, I supposed nobody would know him.'

" 'No.' "

As Schultes was about to give up, the postmistress mustered up a few syllables and suggested that he ask at the Castle Howard, where "his Lordship" might have records, since he owned the cottages. Schultes went up to the great door of the castle and rang the bell. The butler who answered the door listened to Schultes's plea, invited him in, and fetched his employer, Lord George Howard.

"Well, in came this man," Schultes recalls, "at least three hundred and fifty pounds, and dressed in the most ridiculous clothes. In fact, he was known for ridiculous clothes. He had on an Hawaiian shirt with a palm tree on it and purple trousers." Lord George welcomed Schultes and said yes, he knew the house where Spruce had lived, and he would be happy to drive Schultes back and show him. "So this three-hundred-and-fifty-pound man and I — and I'm not small — get into this Volkswagen. So what does he do? Starts right over the lawn! They have signs saying Stay off the Lawn, and the people who had paid two pounds to go in and have a picnic, not knowing who he was, are shouting at him. And he gets a kick out of this."

When they arrived at the cottages, Lord George stopped and pointed out the correct one but said he would wait in the car. "My tenant is a bitch," he told the American. "She'll throw a broom at me." Schultes got out and walked up to the cottage. No sooner had he taken out his camera than a very old woman opened the door and shouted, "What're you doin'?" Schultes apologized and explained who he was and why he was there. She opened her door wider. "Mr. Spruce, I knew 'im," she told Schultes. "Come in. Kittle's on, we'll have some tea."

Over tea, Schultes discovered that the woman's mother had been Spruce's housekeeper and cook. She said Spruce wrote a lot during that time, and was visited by old colleagues and friends. He was tall and dark, and thin as a wren's bone. "He'd ask me to fetch his slippers. He was very sick. I had to fetch his fiddle and play it every night." Then she said something that made Schultes's heart skip a beat. "You know," she said, "in my attic . . . he used to write a letter to everybody, and there are a lot of his letters up there in two boxes." Schultes's first thought was that if this lady left the cottage, someone might move in and burn them. He begged her to save them, thanked her for her hospitality, and raced back to the Royal Botanic Gardens at Kew, near London, the center of botanical study in Great Britain. Officials at Kew acquired the letters shortly thereafter.

Schultes is often called the father of ethnobotany, a title that embarrasses him, says his former student Michael J. Balick. "He is simply a gentleman," says Balick, "doing what he enjoyed. He never thought of himself as a hero." Says Robert Raffauf, Schultes's longtime collaborator: "He is essentially a Victorian. Dick Schultes doesn't live in this century, and he has affectations that make him unusual even on the Harvard campus. His papers are written in British English and he's as much British as I am Chinese. But he had the experience. He introduced the Indians to me, as real people, and they were just as charming as anybody else. We'd stay in settlements, we'd get stuck, and they'd let us hang our hammocks in their *malocas*, although it was better when you brought along a carton of cigarettes or a bottle of rum."

Schultes is actually more intent on being the caretaker of Spruce's legend than becoming one himself. He returned to Yorkshire to straighten Spruce's tombstone and once again to help place a memorial plaque on the man's tiny cottage. And if one reads Spruce's obituary in the February 1, 1894, issue of the journal *Nature*, one might conclude that the man still lives, having simply reemerged from the Amazon in 1954 with a different name — with the same initials. "Richard Spruce was . . . dignified in manner, but with a fund of quiet humour which rendered him a most delightful companion. He possessed in a marked degree the faculty of order, which manifested itself in the unvarying neatness of his dress, his beautifully regular handwriting, and the orderly arrangement of all his surroundings. . . . It was this habit of order, together with his passion for thoroughness in all he undertook, that made him so admirable a collector. He was full of anecdote, and even when suffering from his complicated and painful illnesses, an hour would rarely pass without some humorous remark or pleasant recollection of old times. He was a man who, however depressing were his conditions or surroundings, made the best of his life."

It is at the New York Botanical Garden, three stops on the Metro North line out of Manhattan's Grand Central Station, that the Schultes tradition is likely to be remolded for the twenty-first century. Verdant and cloistered, the Garden is a fortressed oasis of biodiversity camouflaged by the sooty tenements and abandoned warehouses of the Bronx. Behind its tall fences and palisades of trees resides Michael Balick, former Schultes student and director of the Garden's Institute of Economic Botany.

Economic botany is the study of economically useful plants, and while the term fairly describes what Balick does for a living, the forty-one-year-old scientist also claims the title "curator of philecology." *Philecology* does not appear in dictionaries; it is a hybrid word grafted from the Greek *philos*, meaning love, and *ecology*, the study of the biological forces that interact to create what we generally call our natural environment. The word resonates with a certain spirituality that Balick finds more descriptive of his life's work.

Balick is an influential man in a field that most people know almost nothing about. At the Garden, he has helped organize the world's largest collection of ethnobotanists under one roof. Gentle in his movements, Balick is a soft-spoken man of concentric shapes: an oval face within an oval reddish-brown beard atop a comfortable, oval body. His smile is a little uncertain, the kind that causes small children to walk up and hold his hand. A study in concentration one moment, his mind may suddenly wander off on a tangent if pricked by a random or amusing observation. This is the kind of fellow you might imagine standing before a row of rhododendrons, clippers in hand, reassuring them that what he has to do is going to hurt him more than it will hurt them.

But that would be quite off the mark, and Balick would be the first to say so. "Actually, I happen to be as interested in people as in the plants themselves," he says. Specifically, people for whom plants are still a major part of their lives. Also, people who want to support what he is doing. Professional botany, especially ethnobotany, is no bed of roses. Up until the last few years, government and industrial funding for this line of work numbered in the thousands of dollars, not the millions. Small rewards pursued by well-educated, ambitious men and women breeds fierce competition. For all his gentleness, Balick is a competitor, one who keeps his best moves to himself.

Running the country's premier corps of ethnobotanists means spending one week sitting cross-legged in a thatched hut with hill tribes in Thailand, the next with gray-suited foundation executives in a Manhattan skyscraper. Balick prefers doing the former but knows it cannot happen without the latter. His Institute, which he cofounded in 1981 with the eminent British botanist Ghillean T. Prance, has drawn much of its financial support from foundations, the U.S. government's Agency for International Development, the National Institutes of Health, and commercial and industrial donors. By no means is that enough to sustain economic botany, so Balick is on the move a lot. Like F. Scott Fitzgerald's Hollywood character Pat Hobby, he is a man in a constant state of negotiation.

Balick credits Schultes with keeping ethnobotany alive. "Schultes laughs when they call him the patron saint of ethnobotany," he says. "But each of us in this field has strong links with him." It is among indigenous, forest-dwelling cultures, he says, that science now has its best chance of finding new medicines from plants. "Some people think I'm nuts," he says, smiling at the thought. Indeed, people have stood up in scientific meetings and asked Dr. Balick why he, a respectable botanist, would bring shame to Western science by running off into the woods to ask some barefoot witch doctor if he has a cure for AIDS. Balick thinks these people underestimate traditional healers. To prove his case, he has established one of the only full-time field ethnobotanical stations in the world, in a remote part of Belize. There, he and his colleagues collect medicinal plants and study traditional Mayan medicine, as practiced by the few remaining healers who have kept the practice alive. So far Balick has gathered over twenty-five hundred plant samples from Belize. "A thousand years of practice by the Mayans has got to yield some clues," he says. "Besides, this is our last chance. We've got maybe ten or fifteen years left. It's not just the forests that are going. The traditional medicines of the world are disappearing as these cultures die out."

The Botanical Garden is a good place to talk about plants, especially out on the patio at the entrance to the domed, four-columned Beaux Arts administration building. Rows of tulip trees march up to the lip of an outdoor café surrounded most of the year by pots of wildflowers and graced by a twenty-foot-high statue of a cherub on a horse planted in a large fountain. Balick likes to take his lunches here, where he can look out over the expanse of green. "Look, there are a quarter of a million higher plants on the planet," he says, gesturing out toward the thousands that grow right here. Estimates of the number of plants thoroughly examined for medicinal value range from less than one to about 10 percent. Balick thinks the number is more like half a percent. "And if half a percent of the plant kingdom has given us twenty-five percent of all our drugs, you don't have to be too deep to understand that you could go out there and collect the other ninety-nine point five percent and just through the odds find something that's of use."

As the U.S. government and drug companies reconsider nature as a source of new medicine, they come to Balick. He tells them that it is a different world now from the one Schultes canoed through. "The framework under which the discipline was carried out fifty or one hundred years ago is being changed completely," Balick insists in his quiet but pressing way. "It is now being linked to conservation, to nutrition, to health, to development, to drug development, to intellectual property rights for indigenous peoples, and to human rights issues. It is a new synthesis that won't really be mapped out for five or ten years."

Many of those who are mapping the new ethnobotany can be found buzzing around Balick's Institute like bees around their hive. There are senior collaborators at the Garden like the serious, phlegmatic Brian Boom, a veteran of numerous journeys through some of the Amazon's least-traveled territories, and the gregarious, urbane Manhattanite Douglas Daly, an historian of ethnobotany and a connoisseur of rare coffee as well as exotic plants. There are Balick's durable young recruits, like Hans Beck, a lean, blue-eyed explorer who shuttles between Rastafarian villages in Dominica and the remote rainforest hideaway of Ecuador's Awá people, where he is the first Western scientist to have been admitted to Awá healing ceremonies; or like outdoorsman Bradley Bennett, a guitar-picker and self-proclaimed redneck from Florida who learned how to survive off the land in the swamps of the Everglades.

And while these few explore the tropics for the nectar of their trade, the line of people waiting to see what they come back with is now lengthening. The line forms, for the most part, on the couch outside Mike Balick's office: scientists looking for voucher specimens and samples, drug company executives, government officials, and, most recently, journalists who sense a hot story. Balick has a hard time saying no, is constantly overbooked, and grouses about the paperwork that keeps him office-bound. He frequently turns to his secretary, Elizabeth Pecchia, to ask, "Am I in trouble? Have I missed a meeting or anything?" Newspaper articles call him "The Medicine Man of the Bronx" and "Earth Father," giving him the kind of attention he says he hates. Yet publicity means money and support. And as he tells everyone who comes through his office, time is running out.

"I was in a taxicab a few months ago in Belize," he recalls, "and the driver said, 'My grandmother was a wonderful healer and knew a lot about the plant world. She passed on some information to my mother, who was knowledgeable, but I know very little. I've heard about a few plants, but I'm more interested in cars.' " So, insists Balick, someone must to take care of those plants. He spent several years doing so in Brazil, where he specialized in palms like the babassu, whose hard-shelled nuts are used to make bread, a milk-like beverage, cooking oil, and, in a pinch, motor fuel. In fact, he has been messing around with plants since he was a toddler. "I was always a gardener. My earliest memories are of growing plants. This is what I have always done, this is what I am here for." He has written several scholarly books on tropical botany and plans to write a popular version of his ethnobotanical experiences and philosophy as well. It will *not*, he says, be called *Medicine Man*.

"When I first started working with ethnobotanists and tribal healers," Balick says with a trace of defiance, "I was told that this was looked at as a little bit flaky." Sometimes it did look that way. He once watched a Colombian snake-doctor who treated a man bitten in the leg by a fer-de-lance. A physician had tried antivenin and antibiotics, but the venom had spread throughout the victim's body: his blood pressure was very low, his kidney was failing, and his liver was enlarged. The man was dying, and he knew it. Agreeing that it would do no harm, the doctor let the Guahibo snake-doctor perform his rituals: blowing tobacco over the patient, chanting, and sprinkling him with tobacco water. Almost immediately, the patient was calmed and his condition improved (although two weeks later gangrene cost him his leg). Balick holds it up not as evidence of magical spirits but of a strong psychological response in a case of trauma. It shows, he says, that people "have a demonstrated psychological need to identify with their own culture during medical treatment."

The tools of the ethnobotanist's trade — a plane ticket, a plant press, a camera, a machete, and good boots — remain much the same as they have for centuries. The rest of the world, however, has changed drastically. Economic development of the tropics, North-South politics, the struggle for rights by indigenous peoples, and even the way medicines are manufactured are dragging medicinal botany out of the horse-and-buggy era that persisted even to Schultes's time. "The conventional method has been to go into an area, collect plants, and say good-bye," says Balick. That is now viewed as exploitation, a throwback to the imperialist days of Cecil Rhodes and Rudyard Kipling. "Our intention is always to give back more than we take from the healer, the tribe, the community, and the society." Balick was taught that medicine men have persisted for good reason: they get results. Among the axioms Schultes has left behind is this: "The naturalist, interested in plants and animals — both close to the Indian's preoccupations — usually is immediately accepted with excessive collaborative attention. These leaders are gentlemen, and all that is required to bring out their gentlemanliness is reciprocal gentlemanliness. Until the frequently unsavoury veneer of western culture surreptitiously introduces the greed, deception, and exploitation that so often accompanies the good of ways foreign to these men of the forests, they preserve characteristics that must only be looked upon with envy by modern civilized societies."

Central America's only ethnobotanical research farm lies several dusty kilometers from pavement down a rutted road in the Cayo district of Belize. Here, on the slope of a gentle hill overlooking a curve of the Macal River, a small and unorthodox family of visionaries collect unusual plants, record their ancient medicinal lineage, and prepare extracts of them to treat patients and to send to scientists in North America.

Ten years ago the farm was secondary forest abutting a resort hotel called Chaa Creek, built and run by two homesteaders, Mick and Lucy Fleming. The thirty-seven acres that would become the farm had changed hands in a card game in Belize and the new owner had no use for the land. He asked the Flemings if they wanted it. They did not, but they knew someone who might. They called Rosita Arvigo.

Arvigo was a lanky, dark-eyed woman of the counterculture who was looking for a way out of the United States. Born in 1941 in Chicago, she spent much of her twenties in a commune in the San Francisco area called Black Bear Ranch. When her boyfriend, the commune's chief gardener, was faced with going to Vietnam or to jail, she moved with him to a remote region of Mexico. After seven years, having studied local techniques of herbalism, natural hygiene, and healing through diet, she moved to Florida to work in a natural health spa. Her employer there soon sent her to Belize to run his fruit-growing operation, but she returned to the United States when he died and enrolled in the Chicago National College of Naprapathy, which teaches a form of therapy that claims to improve the body's resistance to disease through manipulation of connective tissues and diet. There she met and married Gregory Shropshire, a former paramedic who had decided to add naprapathy to his practice of homeopathy.

Conventional medicine had no time for Arvigo and Shropshire, nor they for it. They sought a place where they could homestead and practice herbalism and other alternative forms of healing without risking a jail sentence. When the Flemings called and offered to sell them a tract of jungle in a country where 80 percent of the population still sub-scribed to herbal medicine, they took the leap. In 1983, Arvigo, Shrop-shire, and Arvigo's five-year-old daughter, Crystal, came to Belize with about one thousand dollars in hand and a dream in mind. They cleared the land, built several whitewashed adobe huts with conical thatched roofs, put in rainwater tanks and butane for their stove, and farmed organically to produce food and a few medicinal herbs. They supported themselves by practicing alternative medicine in San Ignacio, a town about twenty kilometers from the farm. They gave their farm the name Ix Chel, for the Mayan goddess of healing.

In 1984, a man with a terribly scarred leg that would not heal hobbled into Ix Chel. Doctors had told him that the lower leg would have to be amputated. Arvigo could do little for him, so the man went to a famous local healer, Don Eligio Panti. Panti was a *curandero* in the Mayan tradition, a man in his nineties who still practiced herbal heal-ing along with all its spiritual trappings — prayers, chants, amulets, and icons, some strictly Mayan, others borrowed from Christianity. Panti treated the man with jackass bitters, castor oil, and other herbs. After several weeks, the man returned to visit Arvigo, his leg healed.

Arvigo was intrigued. At the time, her healing practice was in trouble. The herbs she and Shropshire had brought from the United States grew moldy in weeks, and they could not get suppliers to replace them. "I had to find someone to teach me about the medicinal plants in Belize so I could incorporate them into my daily practice," she recalls. She traveled to Don Eligio Panti's village of San Antonio, about fifteen kilometers away, and asked him if he would teach her. He said no, he would not teach a foreigner, who would simply take his knowl-edge and leave. The knowledge, he said, was not transplantable. Arvigo set about changing his mind.

"I slept on the floor, cleaned his house, chopped medicine, mas-saged him, made tea, whatever I could to help," she says. He was still reluctant. One day, after months of this, she volunteered to help him harvest corn from his milpa, or corn, field. She had participated in many harvests in Mexico, and she brought in as much corn as he did. He was impressed, and as they sat together under a tree eating an orange, he took a long look at her.

"Just what is it that you want to know?" he said.

"Don Eligio, if you teach me and let me be your apprentice, I will work hard and study."

He stood up, looked down at her, and shook his finger at her.

"Do you promise to be patient and kind and take care of my people? And do you promise that if I take the time to teach you, that you won't leave Belize?"

Arvigo promised. They began that day. "I got into it only for the medicinal plants, although I was quite charmed by him," Arvigo says. "I wanted to be his friend. His wife had died three years before, and even though he was surrounded by a big family he was lonely." Arvigo, who has a phobia against driving cars, walked more than two hours each way, three days a week, to Don Eligio's house. She learned the herbs and how to collect and prepare them. She also learned the prayers that would invoke the spirits of Mayan folk medicine. Don Eligio taught her to treat him with prayer as well, for he was suffering *pesar*, the Spanish word for grief, which is viewed as a spiritual illness in Belize. "He pulled at my heartstrings," she says.

Don Eligio had learned his practice while working in a chicle camp. The sapodilla tree was a source of chicle, used to make chewing gum, until the 1930s in Belize. Tapping the trees was rough work in remote places, and camps needed doctors. Doctors, however, did not need chicle camps. So bush doctors, traditional healers of Central America, took care of the workers. Don Eligio studied with one of the last, a man named Jeronimo Requena, who made his student give the same promise that Don Eligio demanded of Arvigo. Now at 101 years of age (by his count; Arvigo calculates that he is probably ninety-six), Don Eligio still practices healing in a two-room cement block house no bigger than a small garage. It sits beside a dirt road surrounded by rotting fruit from an orange tree and a roaming family of pigs that have spilled over from a neighbor's pen. Chips of bark are spread out on burlap bags to dry in the sun. In the house, Don Eligio owns two stools, two chairs, and one table. Hung across the entryway to his bedroom is his most cherished possession: an embroidered orange sheet on which, shortly before she died, his wife stitched the words "God Is Love." Electricity has lately come to the village, bringing with it twenty-four hours a day of loud music from a radio across the street.

"Fighting off age and death" is how Don Eligio responds sardonically to a query about his health. Yet he spends hours each day working cross-legged on the floor of his workshop, a dark hut of scavenged boards and rolled tin sheeting a few paces from his house. Bags of herbs hang from the ceiling, spiders crawl in the corners, and the darkness is thick with the odor of skunk root, balsam, and Billy Webb bark. With numbing rhythm and the metallic ring of his machete, he chops the vines and herbs collected under his direction by Arvigo and a new apprentice.

"The doctors from Belize City learned from books," he says. "*I* learned from the plants, the herbs, the spirits. I am one hundred and one years old. I still start work every day at five-thirty in the morning." He smiles at Arvigo, perhaps the only outsider he really trusts. "When she came to study with me she was strong, she could swing a machete, carry bags from the hills," he says. And, he adds, stroking a patchy new beard he has decided to start, "she was good-looking." Don Eligio does most of his talking to the rest of the world through Arvigo. It has become a big job, for the outside world has begun to take notice of this old man. The reason lies partly in a frame hanging on the wall of his house. On its parchment in eloquent script is written an appreciation for Don Eligio's contribution to biological science. Along the top of the certificate are the words "The New York Botanical Garden."

The plants that Don Eligio Panti has used for decades are now being chemically picked apart at the National Cancer Institute (NCI) in Frederick, Maryland, courtesy of the New York Botanical Garden. The arrangement began in 1987, when Arvigo heard that the Garden had received seven hundred thousand dollars from the NCI to explore traditional medicine in the neotropics for leads for new drugs. She wrote Mike Balick and within a month he was standing on their doorstep. Thus began a collaboration that has become one of the largest permanent, international ethnobotany projects in the world. Balick recruited Arvigo and Shropshire to begin a lengthy inventory of the plants used by Don Eligio and other traditional healers. With hired Belizean assistants, they locate patches of forest destined for cutting and burning and salvage what they can of the medicinal plants there. They are advised by about fifteen traditional healers, who are also paid for their work, and they solicit advice from many more. Some plants are sent to New York, while others are kept for nurseries of endangered medicinal plants at Ix Chel and a nearby college. The healers come from an eclectic tradition of folk medicine. Besides three types of Mayan Indians in Belize, there is an East Indian community whose forebears were brought over by the British from India when Belize was a British colony. There is also a Mennonite community, a Spanish community, and the Garifuna, people of African descent with their own language and customs — all in a country the size of Massachusetts with a population of 180,000.

Belize possesses about five thousand species of native plants. "The Mayans had about four hundred generations to become trial-and-error experimenters about this environment," Balick says. "That is all being lost in this generation because none of it is written down. Our work is a race against time." Don Eligio has been the key contributor to that effort, and Balick is one of his most ardent admirers. "Don Eligio says to me, 'Look, the Maya have been forgotten. They treat the old people as if we're devils. Civilization has crushed us. But if I can build a bridge between Mayan medical knowledge and western medicine, then the Maya will become immortal.' When I first met Don Eligio he said he'd give us six months and then, he said, he would die and join his wife. He was very lonely. That six months has turned into about five years."

When Balick talks about "our work," he means preserving cultures as much as an individual's knowledge. The money he puts into Ix Chel (now called the Ix Chel Tropical Research Foundation, a nonprofit foundation) helps pay for seminars in which Don Eligio and other healers lecture scientists and other visitors from abroad, who sit side by side with Belizean farmers and schoolchildren. Many from both groups remain skeptical. Some scientists do not believe that herbal cures have much to offer, and even in Don Eligio's family, two hundred strong, no one has taken up his practice. Ultimately, Belizeans will decide for themselves whether to let old customs die. In the meantime, Balick, Arvigo, and Shropshire hope to record whatever they can.

In a paper published in the journal *Conservation Biology*, Balick has shown that harvesting medicinal plants in Belizean forests could earn more income than growing traditional crops. He and his Belizean co-workers harvested seven different medicinal plants from two small plots, about one-quarter of a hectare apiece. These included gumbo-limbo (*Bursera simaruba*), used locally to stop itching, for stomach cramps and kidney infections, and as a diuretic; contribo (*Aristolochia trilobata*), for flu, colds, constipation, fevers, indigestion, and parasites; and *cocomecca* (various species of *Dioscorea*), for urinary tract ailments, bladder infection, coughs, fevers, and something Belizeans call "kidney sluggishness." After labor costs, the net value of these plants on the local markets came to $564 per hectare for one plot and $3,054 per hectare for the other. Rotating harvests so that the plants in each plot can regenerate would keep them going for decades. Meanwhile, estimates for income from corn, beans, and squash in similar Central and South American forest plots range from only $288 to $339 per hectare.

Balick also has caused a stir among plant-hunters with a study of Belizean plants and the AIDS virus. Of twenty plants in Don Eligio's practice that the curandero described as "powerful," five, or 20 percent, were in some way active against the AIDS virus in the test tube (although none has yet been tested on humans). That compares with one hit in eighteen Central American plants collected at random and tested against the virus, or a 6 percent rate. Balick acknowledges that his sample of plants is too small to serve as scientific proof of ethnobotanical superiority. Moreover, while a curandero's plant may have some medical benefit, it may not be the right kind. Drug companies are very specific about what they want; if a company is looking for something to reduce cholesterol, a plant that soothes an itch would not be of interest. Or a plant medicine may work by virtue of a well-known compound. Cancer researchers in particular are bored with these; they want novel compounds that have never been seen before. Nonetheless, Balick argues that his preliminary findings suggest that medicine-hunters would do well to look first at traditional folk medicines for new leads.

The debate over folk medicines is rather distant for Arvigo and Shropshire. They are organic farmers, vegetarians, and small-scale utopians who believe most twentieth-century science and technology has gone dangerously awry, filling food with chemicals and the air with hazardous radiation. Here, among the mahogany, palm, and fruit trees, where the air is filled with the calls of keel-billed toucans, parrots, and hummingbirds, they carry on what Arvigo calls "Don Eligio's lamp of knowledge." They also educate. On a typical day, Arvigo leads tourists (for a fee of five dollars each, but free for Belizeans) along the Panti Trail, a well-worn path through the forest where about three dozen medicinal plants and trees are marked. She points out *pimienta gorda*, known to science as *Pimenta officinalis*, a source of allspice (the species name *officinalis* denotes that a plant provides food or medicine). This genus produces not only allspice but clove oil used as an anti-inflammatory and antiseptic, and bellyache medicine is made from the leaves. Arvigo stops by a tree from the genus *Strychnos*, one that provided South American Indians with arrow poisons. Its branches are opposite, each pair forming the sign of the cross with the main stem. Local curanderos associate the cross with "powerful" or toxic plant species in what ethnobotanists call the traditional "doctrine of signatures" — heart-shaped leaves are thought to be good for heart ailments, kidney-shaped ones for kidney disease, and so on. Farther on, there is a stunted, bulbous *Dioscorea* bush, used by Aztec women for birth control, and the plant that rendered the hormones for the first birth control pills. There are also trees here for building, thatch, food, varnish, and incense.

While Arvigo speaks for Ix Chel, her husband spends most of his time keeping the farm running. He is an industrious, taciturn man with a rose tattoo on his left forearm and a self-styled uniform of a work-shirt over a T-shirt and a bandanna around his neck. Skeptical of outsiders, he prefers to build or fix rather than mix with the public. His biggest project is a small factory for the herbal medicines that Ix Chel manufactures. The largest structure on the Ix Chel farm, it bears a sign above the threshold, "Stand Up For Your Roots." It will house their one-year-old company, called Rainforest Remedies, whose products are mostly tinctures made from traditional Belizean and Mayan herbs steeped in alcohol. These include "Travelers' Tonic" for diarrhea, "Male Tonic" for impotence, "Female Tonic" for painful cramps, "Jackass Bitters" for gastritis, an insect repellant called "Jungle Salve," as well as raw herbs such as Billy Webb bark for making medicinal teas. It is a sustainable industry whose profits are shared with its Belizean employees, says Arvigo. "We don't claim to cure cancer or anything," she tells tourists, who comprise a large part of her clientele. "Traditional medicine is mostly primary care."

Conventional medicine would almost certainly regard Ix Chel and its owners as a superstitious curiosity. At the Ix Chel farm, for example, Arvigo has built a Mayan healer's hut in which she occasionally conducts a Mayan mass, or *premisia*. She burns sacred copal wood, leads a chant to honor Mayan spirits and invite them into the hut, and prays for the welfare of those in need, whose photographs or personal effects are laid out on a table during the ceremony. When she describes the Mayan cosmology of the underworld, the upper world, the cycles of world strife and renewal, and the intervention of spirits in human life, it is unclear whether she believes these myths or whether she is merely recounting them as interesting anthropology. She supports the unconventional, like bush doctor Leopoldo Romero, a grizzled forty-nine-year-old with few teeth and a taste for beer at breakfast-time. Romero says he can cure most diseases in a matter of days with a pharmacopoeia of about twenty-odd plants, many of which are prescribed along with drafts of rum, and some of which require special measures, such as avoiding at all costs the gaze of a pregnant woman when snake-bitten.

Yet Arvigo and Shropshire have aided science by providing NCI with lots of plants, some of which have been used to heal Central Americans since the Maya civilization arose three thousand years ago. Any of them could prove to be a treatment for cancer or AIDS. Arvigo and Shropshire also have helped introduce the idea of intellectual property rights to the healers and community health workers who work

beside them in the bush. After three conferences with traditional healers in Belize, it was determined by vote that any share of profits from
a drug discovery would not go to individual healers, most of whom are
over seventy years old, but to a healer's association Arvigo helped set
up to pay for seminars on healing practices, trips to study practices in
other countries, and preservation of the raw materials — the forest
itself.

The odds for finding a new drug from Belizean forests are long.
Even if one is found, NCI had no formal agreement for profit-sharing
with the Belizean government as of early 1993. Balick has pressed NCI
and drug companies to formally promise a share of royalties to source
countries, either to their governments or to organizations like the healer's association. NCI officials say they will try to persuade drug companies to share royalties, but that may not satisfy Belizeans. Already,
members of Don Eligio's family suspect that the North Americans are
planning to get rich off of traditional Belizean medicine. Arvigo replies
that she and Shropshire are only paid a salary for collecting and are
doing this mostly to record Mayan medicine. Says Arvigo, "I feel that
what Don Eligio has and what I have been able to capture is a world
heritage. As an herbalist and traditional healer myself, I just could not
stand by and watch it die."

Schultes's disciples have been fanning out for almost four decades now,
trying to make ethnobotany matter to the rest of the world. Their styles
differ. Mark Plotkin of Conservation International is a popularizer and
showman, regaling audiences with stories of exploits among South
American forest dwellers and photos of himself, bare-chested and
painted with *achiote* designs, snorting hallucinogenic snuff from *Virola*
resin. He describes the Schultes technique for winning information
from shamans: collecting plants and telling the brujos that they are
used by white people for some imaginary disease until, in disbelief at
such stupidity, the brujos tell him what the plants are *really* useful for.
Like Schultes, Plotkin has concentrated on one geographic region, the
forests of Suriname and the Tirió people, and he returns regularly to
maintain a close relationship with his Tirió informants. He is media-
savvy and knows that a catchy name will garner attention, thus his
"Sorcerer's Apprentice" program at Conservation International, which
is aimed in part at helping shamans pass on their knowledge before
they die. "We need people who can straddle different cultures," he says
of ethnobotany, "people who are at home in the forest as well as the

halls of Congress." Some fellow ethnobotanists are ruffled by his high profile and jocose manner, and complain that they rarely see him published in the trenches, in the peer-reviewed scientific journals. However, Plotkin's enthusiasm has helped bring this obscure science to the public's attention.

Another of Schultes's students, Wade Davis, spent years studying the customs and plants of cultures ranging from the Waorani in Ecuador's Amazon to the Athabascans of Canada. "Eventually, I got extremely frustrated by what I saw of ethnobotany, you know, sort of collecting grocery lists," Davis says. "Going into the 'booga booga' and just recording the plants indigenous people use isn't very satisfying. There's no intellectual content to it." Davis wanted to put more anthropology into ethnobotany, and his work in South America and Haiti (the latter the basis of his book *The Serpent and the Rainbow*, about the practice and pharmacology of voodoo) are as much about cultures as about plants and medicines. Yet for Davis, working with remote indigenous people had a certain futility to it. When people live in deep isolation, the notion that they have a culture apart from others, or the idea that their culture is being lost, has little meaning. It takes a certain amount of education from the outside for people to see that their customs are slipping away. Then, says Davis, it is too late. "By that point the only people who want to live the old ways are those who never knew them."

Some of Schultes's students have stayed in academia, such as Djaja D. Soejarto, originally from Indonesia and now an economic botanist at the University of Illinois. Another of Schultes's students, Calvin Sperling, struck a compromise between the classroom and the outside world at the U.S. Agricultural Research Service, where he labors at the less glamorous task of preserving unique crops from around the world before they are wiped out by development. He began a project to establish a "living nursery" in a national park in Ecuador where rare Andean crop plants will be preserved in a natural forest setting.

All of Schultes's disciples are quick to quash any notion that any of their number will play Aristotle to Schultes's Plato. "There will be no 'new' Schultes," says Mike Balick. "I think too much of him to believe there could be someone amongst his students or peers who would replace him. It's just too early for that." One man who might have assumed the Schultes mantle was Timothy Plowman, whom Schultes and many of his students considered perhaps the master's best pupil. Plowman's work on the coca plant and its uses remains, by consensus, among the discipline's finest, and for years Plowman was, in effect,

Schultes's "sorcerer's apprentice." Plowman died of AIDS in 1988.

With no clear leader, the ethnobotanical community has been struggling for a new definition of its methods and goals. It is a discipline with only a handful of practitioners vying for a small pot of money and the attention of a public that is hypnotized with the glitter of the space shuttle and supercolliders and the drama of killer viruses spread by sex. Meanwhile, ethnobotany's fuel, as it were, the indigenous peoples of the world, are decamping from their lands, abandoning their traditions, and moving into cities like Lima, Djakarta, Vancouver, Lagos, and Bangkok. As in any small professional community in such a situation, competition for scarce resources and attention crackles behind the sheen of professional collegiality.

Balick is now the closest thing to an ethnobotanical standard-bearer. At his office in the Bronx, a sort of cultural flea market where botany and chemistry texts sit side by side with rainforest herbs and salves ("I've taken most of them," he notes, "except the ones for female problems"), Balick argues that Western science and native healing are elements along a single continuum whose ends are starting to curl back toward each other. Every week now he gets an inquiry from someone who wants to invest in rainforest exploration. Most callers, however, still don't understand what ethnobotany, or at least the kind Balick is pushing, is all about. They have money and want to make more, and of course they plan to help people with new products along the way. But they rarely are willing to guarantee much in return to the people in the rainforest, not enough in any case to earn Balick's cooperation. He and his colleagues at the Garden are trying to change these attitudes. They have pushed the National Cancer Institute and drug companies, for example, to put such guarantees in writing before sending Balick's crew off to a new destination. Balick's colleague Brian Boom also has been encouraging the academic societies in anthropology and botany to adopt a code of ethics that would end what Boom calls the "dark side of botany," the old practice of collecting in tropical countries for a drug company while advertising oneself as just a harmless academic.

So ethnobotany's resurgence comes with a modern new look, one with ethics codes, royalties for indigenous peoples, and allegiances to conservation groups. And it has crossed over into an open partnership with drug companies, a move considered by purists as akin to inviting art thieves to guard the Louvre. But there is little if any alternative. Soon the world's great tropical forests and their cultures will be gone. To slow or stop their destruction, someone must prove they are valuable as they stand — soon. With help, ethnobotanists could do it. "Finding one drug from the rainforest that will save lives," says Balick, "would be worth more than all the lectures by famous people and all the rock concerts. If you can just hold up *one plant.* My mission in life is to find such a plant."

5

Biophilia

By the 1980s, ethnobotanists had found allies among biologists and conservationists who also believed that sustainable products like medicines could forestall tropical deforestation. Many of these people, however, claimed a somewhat different philosophy about prospecting in the rainforest. They called themselves "eco-rationalists." It was a term that irked some ethnobotanists, with its implication that everyone else was somehow not quite as "rational" as the eco-rationalists. What it actually meant was this: Learning from native healers is all well and good, but it is not the best way to find chemically potent substances in tropical forests. Native medicines are often cure-alls, nonspecific medicines, the equivalent of aspirin. Modern medicine needs ultra-specific compounds for special tasks. Moreover, native healers have only scratched the surface of what grows in rainforests with their trial-and-error methods. The best way to look for new chemicals is to examine the forest itself, to watch how its plants and animals behave, and to unravel its ecological processes. Parasitism, chemical defense, reproduction processes, plant distribution, symbiosis, decay — these are the clues to unlocking the forest's chemistry.

To understand the eco-rationalist approach, one must first understand something about tropical forests and what is happening to them. Tropical rainforest is a habitat with a relatively tight or closed canopy of mostly broad-leaved evergreen trees that grow where at least a meter of rain falls every year. When Western scientists first began to study these forests in Africa, Asia, and especially the New World, their size, and the diversity of life within them, seemed almost immeasurable. "The largest river in the world runs through the largest forest," Spruce wrote of the Amazon. "By little and little, I began to comprehend that in a forest which is practically unlimited . . . clad with trees and little else but trees, and where the natives think no more of destroying the noblest trees, when they stand in their way, than we the vilest weed, a single tree cut down makes no greater a gap, and is no more missed, than when one pulls up a stalk of groundsel or a poppy in an English cornfield."

Spruce could not know that in fact the world's tropical forests contain half the world's known species of flora and fauna. It has taken a century since Spruce for tropical biologists, informed by sweaty experience more than by leaps of insight and theory, to arrive at these numbers. Over the past decade, ingenious new tools have been invented that have boosted exploration almost as much as the seaplane and the outboard motor. In Panama, the Smithsonian Institution built a construction crane to carry scientists up into the treetops. In Peru, another group from the Smithsonian, led by Terry Erwin, used pesticide foggers to bring insects down from the trees and into waiting nets. And French scientists invented an inflated doughnut-like platform with a net stretched across its hole that they lay down over the treetops. These inventions have put biologists up into the last unexplored part of the rainforest, the tree canopy, where so many new organisms, especially insects, have recently been discovered.

Why is tropical forest, especially rainforest, so much more diverse than all other habitats? Biologists still do not know for sure. Harvard's Edward O. Wilson votes for something called the Energy-Stability-Area Theory of Biodiversity, or ESA theory. "In a nutshell," he says, "the more solar energy, the greater the diversity; the more stable the climate, both from season to season and from year to year, the greater the diversity; finally, the larger the area, the greater the diversity." Hot, wet places, if enough nutrients are available, tend to produce more biomass and animal tissue, which in turn provides for more species. Although nutrients are in fact scarce in most acidic tropical soils, and rarely descend farther down than two inches, the forest neatly circumvents this by living on itself. Every living thing, from mite to mahogany, is recycled as soon as it dies (if not sooner, as anyone with flesh and blood can attest after a day shared with tropical insects).

If the tropics promote productivity, however, what is to prevent one species, superbly adapted, from taking over an entire habitat the way conifers do in northern climates? The answer probably lies with the environment. In temperate zones, plants must endure extremes in temperature and precipitation — hot summers, cold winters, dry spells, or wet northeasters. They acquire mechanisms to tolerate these extremes, like shedding leaves during winter, or in the case of animals, hibernating, burrowing, or migrating. If organisms adapt to a variety of environments, they often can survive in wider geographical ranges; if a moth can survive winter in northern Florida, it probably can also handle spring in New England. In short, they become generalists and spread out quite easily.

Stable climates with barely noticeable seasonal changes encourage competition for the same space. Animals and plants must vie for narrower niches within the habitat, and species eventually are packed tight, like electronic junctions on a computer chip. A specialist, like a worm underneath a submerged rock in a chilly stream in the Andean foothills, or a mite nestled in the oily secretions under the green feathers of a Mexican parrot, can wrest more out of a small piece of real estate than a generalist. Specialization can reach bizarre extremes. Wilson describes the parasitic mites that live aboard one of the forest's most voracious animals, the army ant. "While sucking the blood of the ants, [the mites] allow themselves to be used as artificial feet; the ants walk on the bodies of the parasites with no sign of discomfort on either side. The mite covers the claws of the ant by which the ant hangs while nesting and renders it useless, but no matter: the mite has curved hind legs the size of the claws, and the ant uses them instead."

The benign tropical climate also permits some organisms to grow very large, and they become the foundations on which other organisms can live. Big trees in the rainforest, for example, support piggyback organisms like orchids, bromeliads, and philodendrons. These in turn support insects and other invertebrates, and so on down the line. Large, relatively undisturbed areas also favor diversity. As a rule of thumb, a tenfold increase in area results in a doubling of the number of species. Tropical forests are indeed large, spreading wide the protective wing of climate and constancy. Yet they contain many different "microhabitats" — mountain slopes and mesas, lakes, swamps, impassable rivers — where species can arise, specialize, and find refuge. The more complex the environment, the more niches available for species to inhabit.

How these phenomena work together is not simple, nor are many of the principles proposed to explain them firm enough to merit consensus. For example, the idea that the unvarying conditions of tropical rainforests act like a benign hand over the birth of new species is a matter of debate. It is now thought that the *destabilizing* events in the forest are what primes the pump of speciation. Some evidence for this comes from ancient pollen samples, which suggest that there may have been some retreat by the forests, due to drought during glaciation, into pockets that biologists sometimes call *refugia*. These redoubts of richness — the Chocó in southern Colombia is thought by some to be the remnant of such a refuge — then reseeded the tropics when the climate grew wet and warm again.

Modern, smaller-scale disturbances are abundant. Storms, for example, or unusual flooding, or even the hand of man disturb the rainforest with regularity, each time upsetting the apple cart and allowing new arrangements as life seeks to move back in the direction of equilibrium. Indeed, ecologists now say that when a habitat actually arrives at equilibrium, it supports less diversity than when the struggle for order is in full swing. And some argue that even before that most interfering of creatures, man, came on the scene, disturbances were so frequent that the natural world has always been in a state of rebuilding. Thus the gradual rise over the aeons in biodiversity.

Whether periodically pumped with diversity or gradually accreting species like barnacles on an abandoned boat, the tropics, to borrow from the seventeenth-century poet Andrew Marvell's entreaty to his coy mistress, have had world enough and time that their "vegetable love should grow/ Vaster than empires, and more slow." But the empires of tropical life are now crumbling. Spruce could never have imagined how much of what he explored would be cut down over the next one hundred years. In fact, it was not until the 1980s that large numbers of scientists began to comprehend and speak out against the continuing deforestation of the tropics and the man-made extinction of species. Among the first was Stanford University biologist Paul Ehrlich. He pursued the unpopular notion that it was not the loss of cuddly pandas and magnificent whales that mattered so much as it was the loss of plant and insect species that typically have done so much to sustain our own species for millions of years. Ehrlich's British colleague, Norman Myers, described what humans were doing as an "extinction spasm" unlike any the Earth had experienced in six hundred million years.

Ehrlich and Myers won a few converts and many critics. The latter labeled them as Cassandras. Extinction was nothing new, the critics said, it was normal, a codicil of life. Over the previous six hundred million years, extinctions had taken place at a rate of about one species every year or so.

What was the extinction rate now? No one knew then or now. It was like the much-parodied, Zen-like question: If a tree falls in the forest and no one is there to hear it, does it make a sound? No one was present to record the death of the last Madagascar elephant bird, the last Mexican imperial woodpecker, the last Centinelan butterflies on the mountain ridges of Ecuador. Even if witnesses had been there, they would have missed the passing of more numerous insects, fungi, and the bacteria that disappear every time a forest tract is destroyed. So biologists can only make educated guesses at the current extinction rate. These are chilling. One estimate, just for the world's rainforests, is twenty-seven *thousand* species extinguished every year.

That is seventy-four species per day.

Three every hour.

Biologists grew alarmed and angry at what was happening and frustrated with their inability to do much about it. So they convened a remarkable meeting in Washington, D.C., on September 21, 1986. For four days, at the Smithsonian Institution's Museum of Natural History, biologists, economists, philosophers, and others concerned about what was being flushed down the planet's drain debated about what they could do.

Talk, it seemed at first, was about all. Yet the meeting brought forth a new word, and new words have power in a society hip-deep in sterile information. The word was *biodiversity* (its invention has been attributed to Walt Rosen, an organizer of the meeting). Now, at least, there was a label for this slippery concept, a verbal grip on the public's lapels. That year also saw the creation of the Society for Conservation Biology, dedicated to the study of how to conserve the world's natural resources, as well as numerous informal groups with the same goal. And perhaps most important, an idea was taking shape. The idea was that if people realized they had more to gain by *keeping* the forest rather than replacing it, the fire aboard Earth's ark could be put out.

There were few ethnobotanists at the Smithsonian meeting. Instead, most were the hard core of modern zoology and botany — tax-onomists, botanists, entomologists, and most of all ecologists. Their interests lay mainly with the ecological; that is, with the processes that govern organisms as well as the organisms themselves. They were not especially interested in humans. In fact, a few had a certain animosity toward them, for it was Homo sapiens who was tearing up their play-ground.

Lest their sound and fury signify nothing more than a four-day whine, the conferees chose one of their most articulate spokesmen to carry the message to the public. They picked a man who was and remains as much the intellectual pilot of the biodiversity movement's ecological wing as anyone. To find him, one need only walk down one flight of those stairs that Schultes ascends to his office, past the intri-cately crafted glass flowers in their wooden cases, and into the adjoin-ing Museum of Comparative Zoology. Pass by the dioramas of skeletal saber-toothed tigers and stuffed black bears and around a catwalk sus-pended above arching dolphins and saucer-eyed emus, and you will enter the realm of the insect. Specifically, the ant.

In Edward O. Wilson's office, the ants outnumber the professor several thousand to one, crawling throughout a plastic ant-city the size of a doghouse he has built for them. Ants are his favorite subject and his life's work. In 1975, however, he took some time off and rudely remade the world of biology. Wilson argued that some of human behavior is influenced by our genes, and described why in his book *Sociobiology: A New Synthesis*. He wrote several more books, including a Pulitzer prize winner, *On Human Nature*, to fill in the cracks of his theory, then moved on to a subject he now considers more pressing — biodiversity.

Biodiversity is a big idea. It encompasses Colorado aspens and Costa Rica's poison frogs, coral reef parrotfish and arctic lichen, sulfur-loving bacteria in deep-sea vents and African elephants. Wilson feels wonder in that variety of life-forms, but he understands that most people do not think much about it. So he has created the speech. It is essentially the same whether delivered at the Carnegie Institution in Washington, D.C., at a hearing room in Congress, or over a bag lunch with a visitor in his ant-ridden laboratory. The voice is soft, the ca-dences as flat as the vaguely midwestern accent, and the arguments roll out with the eurythmic flow of scientific, and especially ecological, reasoning: C is due to B, B depends on A, and A of course rests on C. While Wilson does not exhort, he bends his listeners to his quiet will with his most salient trait: sincerity.

In the speech, Wilson says, deforesting the tropics "is like burning a Renaissance painting to cook dinner." Recent estimates calculate that sixty thousand higher plants could disappear from the planet over the next sixty years. That would be one of every four higher-plant species on the Earth. If the destruction of the great library of Alexandria over two thousand years ago set back human knowledge by centuries, he asks, what does the loss of this genetic library bode for humanity? "The sixth great extinction spasm of geological time is upon us, grace of mankind," Wilson says with almost biblical sweep. "Earth has at last acquired a force that can break the crucible of biodiversity." Is humanity suicidal? he asks his audiences. "Perhaps a law of evolution is that intelligence usually extinguishes itself."

If the words sound apocalyptic, it is because biodiversity and its preservation might as well be Wilson's religion. Born in Alabama in 1929 into a churchgoing southern Baptist family, he was raised in a South that rested comfortably on the pillars of the church, the sermon, and the tent revival. Religion, Wilson says, is to our species something like what gravity is to the planets. He suspects that humans may be genetically inclined toward certain aspects of religion, such as the transformational experience of conversion and trance-like states. For Wilson, however, it was the grandeur of Darwinian theory that transformed him.

After studying biology at the University of Alabama, Wilson followed a friend's advice and moved to Harvard in the early 1950s. He got his doctorate there in 1955, became a professor of biology, and eventually was named Curator in Entomology at the Museum of Comparative Zoology and Frank B. Baird Professor of Science. From the beginning, he was as interested in what insects say about all life as he was in their peculiarities. Discovering the chemical, called a pheromone, that fire ants use to keep their brethren in line when they forage, for example, was more to Wilson than just a publishable observation in an obscure journal. These and other genetically determined phenomena that he observed among primitive organisms led to his theories of sociobiology. He stitched Darwinian-driven genetics and behavior, especially human behavior and culture, into a quilt of ideas explaining why humans act the way we do. It became sociobiology, a theory of the biological basis of social behavior in animals. Sociobiology irked social scientists who believed that human behavior is strictly the product of society and that unpleasant human behavior — lying, violence, selfishness — could be fixed if only society would make the effort. Wilson, heretically, appeared to be saying that we could behave as we wanted and blame it on our genes, that we lacked free will, that we should live by the rule of "survival of the fittest." He meant nothing of the sort, only that *some* behaviors are without doubt influenced by inborn traits, and that behaviors that confer success to individuals can act to select certain genetic traits much the way the environment does in classical Darwinism. Nonetheless, the battle over sociobiology still rages.

Wilson eventually went back to his ants and, finally, on to biodiversity. By the time he was called upon to speak for the movement in 1986, the ground was well-furrowed with numbers: rates of deforestation, numbers of species extinguished, acres of habitat lost — numbers that to the average person had all the emotive force of the Dow-Jones average. Intricate explanations of life's variety and complexity were little better. Money moved people, Wilson knew. But sometimes so did the spiritual and the humane.

The worlds of the spiritual and the scientific have in the Western mind grown apart. The romanticists of the nineteenth century balked at the eighteenth-century Enlightenment's philosophy that all things, including nature, were ultimately knowable through reason and scientific study. Poet Alfred, Lord Tennyson spoke for generations of Westerners when he wrote that "science grows and beauty dwindles." William Butler Yeats carried the sentiment into the twentieth century, lamenting that the world's "antique joy" was gone and "Gray Truth is now her painted toy." It was, he said, a world where "the ceremony of innocence is drowned."

Wilson had crossed the divide between science and the humanities, however, by mixing biology and genetics with behavior and its manifestations, be they the customs of tool-making or high art. The possibility of a similar union between biodiversity and behavior was provocative. "Human beings," Wilson says, "have a deep and complex, innate propensity to enjoy and affiliate with a wide diversity of life forms . . . in the midst of which the human species has evolved over millions of years." This he calls his "biophilia hypothesis." One way this innate urge to "affiliate" with nature manifests itself is in a sort of habitat selection. For animals, habitat selection is the first order of the day for survival. The first thing a blind, newborn kangaroo does after climbing out of its mother's genital opening is to cross her belly and find her pouch, where the nipples are. Trout seek out overhanging rocks under which to hide, while the alder flycatcher will choose only swampland for nests.

Humans, of course, have learned to live almost anywhere. Yet there is a consistency to the habitats that we prefer. In his book *Biophilia*, Wilson says, "It seems that whenever people are given a free choice, they move to open, tree-studded land on prominences overlooking water. This worldwide tendency is no longer dictated by the hard necessities of hunter-gatherer life. It has become largely aesthetic, a spur to art and landscaping." We see biophilia in miniature gardens in Japanese teahouses that create the trompe l'oeil of distance and running water. It is echoed in the landscaping of trees, shrubs, pools, and fountains in the buried villas and gardens of the Romans' Pompeii as well as the monuments and tree-lined reflecting pool of Washington's Mall. Everywhere, we yearn for and recreate contact with some copy of the ideal natural world.

How did these habitat preferences come about? After we dropped from the trees and learned to love the feel of Miocene mud between our toes, we spent a few million years in the tropical savannah. It was a landscape of grassy, rolling plains overlooking water, stands of trees, and perhaps a few cliffs where one could watch for predators or find shelter in a cave. It was biodiverse, rich in plants and animals, and thus a good source of shelter and food. Hunter-gatherers on the move learned to choose such a habitat whenever possible.

Now peoples' preferences in landscapes seem so obvious that they are rarely questioned. Just look at real estate prices for that "wooded lot" or "river view." Gordon H. Orians, a zoologist at the University of Washington, from whom Wilson drew some of his thinking on the subject of biodiversity and behavior, points out that the values of a society that nobody questions are the ones that reveal the most about a culture. They are the ones most likely to be "evolutionarily programmed," Orians says.

Here then was the eye-catching centerpiece around which the eco-rationalists could arrange their less user-friendly data — the notion that, as Wilson described it, humans retain "a deep genetic memory of mankind's optimal environment," an environment that is rich in biodiversity. It is not a great leap to surmise that all of us still need biological diversity, not just because it is pretty, but because we evolved in its midst; it is as much part of the human condition as the need for love or the urge to reproduce. If we wipe out biodiversity, says Wilson, "we may be tampering with a part of our environment that future generations will discover to have been very important for the full development of the human psyche, as a spirit."

How could biophilia be so fundamental to the human spirit? One explanation lies in sociobiological theory. Sociobiology employs a cultural currency that Wilson calls a *culturgen*. Such a unit of culture might be as rudimentary as the way a hominid made a stone ax or as complex as a style of music or clothing. The choice of one culturgen over another is influenced, though not absolutely determined, by the way one's brain is put together. Brains are constructed, in turn, according to a set of "epigenetic rules" that are written in groups of genes. No one gene controls any one set of behaviors, yet one type of brain may be more likely to prefer one culturgen over another. Natural selection then sets to work on this construct, say Wilson and his coauthor Charles Lumsden in their books *Genes, Mind, and Culture* and *Promethean Fire: Reflections on the Origin of Mind*. A culturgen that favors survival and reproduction — perhaps a better way to make or use an ax — will be reinforced, along with the epigenetic rules that fostered it.

So is biophilia such a culturgen that favors survival? Wilson is not ready to go that far. Yet he notes, "Human beings tend to develop along certain lines automatically and not along other lines, and the intellect and emotions can flower much more readily in certain environments than others." Philosophy and religion tend to undervalue biophilia, Wilson says, even though "our existence depends on this propensity, our spirit is woven from it, hope rises on its currents."

"We live," Wilson is fond of saying, "in an unexplored world." It is a world that he has searched through on his hands and knees, watching it breathe, eat, reproduce, and decay. It is a world that Schultes explored with Indian shamans. In this, the two men independently have arrived at the same place. Both are now spending the remaining years of their lives on a final, desperate gambit: the valuation of the tropical forest as a means to save it.

Wilson has helped rally his colleagues in a multitiered effort to identify "hot spots," areas of unusually high biodiversity that are threatened with destruction. The next step is to dispatch an army of biologists to thoroughly map several large "warm" spots, regions of the world with high biological endemism, that is, places that contain many species not found anywhere else. Finally, a fifty-year effort would finish the job — a total biotic survey of the planet.

Biodiversity surveys do not feed hungry children, however. Saving biodiversity looks a lot like giving up something else, such as pasture for cattle or fields for crops — in short, wealth, food, comfort. "That's the awful symmetry of the planet," Wilson says. "The financially wealthy countries are poor in biological wealth, and the biologically wealthy countries are poor in money." As the eco-rationalist medicine-hunters have invoked Wilsonian theory, so he now counts himself among their number. It is time, he says, to inventory the vast biological wealth of the rainforest with calculator and spreadsheet in hand, bearing in mind that the people who live there must profit along with the pharmaceutical industry in order to protect the resource. The task will require risk-taking, entrepreneurship, and the creation of new markets by the industrialized world. "But that's what we're supposed to be very good at," says Wilson, "isn't it?"

6

Biodiversity Prospecting

Between 1980 and 1990, the rate at which tropical forests were being cut down rose from thirty million acres a year to forty million. For comparison, all the forest cut down in the United States in a year for agriculture, housing, factories, and shopping malls added up to roughly one-thousandth of that amount.

Nothing galvanizes quite as well as fear. In this case, the threat was mass extinction. Environmental groups like The Nature Conservancy and the World Wildlife Fund tried brokering "debt-for-nature" swaps, in which they persuaded wealthy northern donors to pay off Third World debt if the debtors promised to preserve some rainforest in return. These were but a few straws snatched from the fire, however. Countries with rainforest desperately needed land for pasture, for crops, and timber for export, while the developed world's appetite for beef and timber grown in the tropics showed no sign of satiation. Protests from the worried wealthy, the trust-fund backpackers, the spectacled butterfly-catchers, and the plant-hunters smacked of neo-colonialist patronizing by the well-fed. Biodiversity was cheap.

So debt-swaps were augmented with eco-tourism. Tourists—"eco-cattle," as one biologist described them—could sometimes earn more money per acre for a tropical landowner than hamburgers on the hoof. In places like Costa Rica, eco-tourism became a big industry. For countries in relative chaos, like Peru, it was more difficult. And in any event, eco-tourism was still not enough.

Then came what is commonly called "sustainable development." Sustainable development meant extracting raw materials like wood, oils, fibers, pigments, and vegetable products in such a way that the natural resource is not significantly drawn down or permanently diminished. Forests and other natural land put aside for such development are called "extractive reserves." Francisco "Chico" Mendes, the martyred Brazilian activist murdered by ranchers, put the idea into practice by helping colonists in the Amazon tap rubber trees and sell the product. Conservation International midwifed a rainforest renewable product, tagua nuts (vegetable ivory), for the button market. Sustainable development was applied to timber-cutting as well, whereby strips of rainforest could be cut alternately up hillsides in such a way that the cut land could be naturally reseeded and would regrow quickly.

But could such enterprises actually make money? On June 29, 1989, three North American scientists published a modest, two-page paper in the British journal *Nature* that finally applied hard numbers to the sustainability equations. The paper, "Valuation of an Amazonian Rainforest," by Charles M. Peters, Alwyn H. Gentry, and Robert O. Mendelsohn, assessed the value of trees in a hectare of forest along the Río Nanay, thirty kilometers southwest of Iquitos, Peru. The area was typical of the eastern Andes. Rainy most of the year, its white-sand soil relatively infertile, it nonetheless supported a mix of colonial and indigenous people who made their living fishing, cultivating a few staple crops, and selling a variety of forest products in the markets of Iquitos.

The scientists found 842 individual trees, representing 275 species, on their small site. Of those, 72 species and 350 individuals yielded products with some market value in Iquitos. These included timber species, fruit-bearing trees, rubber trees, medicinal plants, and oil-bearing palms. The scientists calculated the amount of labor needed to harvest these products, the productivity of the plants, transportation costs, and market prices for each good. Finally, they determined the net present value of these renewable resources.

They found that fruit and rubber latex alone would return a value of $6,330 per hectare. Selective timbering that would not exceed the speed at which the forest regenerated would add another $490 per hectare. Income from medicinal plants, small palms, and lianas was not added in, yet the total was still twice the proceeds from a one-time timber harvest of the most popular local hardwood, *Gmelina arborea*, which would clear only $3,184. Pastureland for cattle compared even less favorably, earning only $2,960, and that was without adding the costs of weeding, fencing, and animal care.

So why was the renewable worth of the forests being overlooked? "We believe the problem lies not in the actual value of these resources," said Peters and his colleagues, "but in the failure of public policy to recognize it." Timber is sold internationally and reaps valuable foreign exchange for debt-ridden developing countries. The "non-wood" products, Peters noted, are small scale, the stuff of subsistence farmers, shop-owners, middlemen, and indigenous people. They live far from the cities and the glitter of the marketplace, the marbled banks, and the pillared centers of commerce and government. Nor were there proven markets, especially international markets, for renewable goods — yet.

Environmentalists and rainforest conservationists treated the Peters paper as if it were a missing page from the Dead Sea Scrolls, citing it everywhere from foreign aid hearings in the U.S. Congress to open-air classrooms at research stations in the rainforest. Admittedly, it was preliminary and flawed even in the view of its authors. How, for example, would prices for such goods stay up if extractive reserves succeeded and the supply of the products rose? Moreover, circumstances in Peru were different from those in other countries. Nonetheless, the paper propelled the biodiversity movement forward. Other scientists started examining rainforests more closely for renewable products. Among the leaders were members of Cultural Survival, in Cambridge, Massachusetts, an organization that tries to help indigenous cultures deal with encroaching modernization. Its executive director, Jason Clay, was a big, florid, and enthusiastic anthropologist who had lived with indigenous groups in South America. Clay had long argued that capitalism with a human face was probably the only way to keep the Amazon's forests and its cultures from being reduced to ash and memories. Clay set up an operation within Cultural Survival to market renewable products to North American and European companies. He required companies to set aside one percent or so of sales to be returned to Cultural Survival and thence to the local producers, usually small collectives of Amazonian colonists or indigenous groups. Ben & Jerry's Ice Cream was an early collaborator, putting Brazil nuts from the Amazon into premium products like "Rainforest Crunch" ice cream for the yuppie market. The Body Shop, a chain of cosmetic stores that wrapped itself in the green flag by selling all types of body ornamentation with some sort of natural constituent or connection, also signed on the Clay plan, and more green capitalists followed.

Finally, pharmaceutical companies began to see the value in the green label. As it happened, their synthetic chemists were not turning out many new drugs. "The synthetic chemists had made the easy molecules," observes Charles D. McChesney, a phytochemist at the University of Mississippi who is organizing a multimillion-dollar project there to search for new plant-based drugs. "In terms of new discoveries, synthetic chemistry is now a game of diminishing returns." Perhaps Mother Nature, with millions of years at her disposal, really was more creative than synthetic chemists, having manufactured not only compounds too numerous to count but the very chemists themselves. At the very least, tropical plant compounds could serve as starting points for new synthetics, just as the coca plant became cocaine and then procaine, and poppies became morphine and finally hydromorphine.

In addition, medical scientists and biochemists knew more than before. The decade of the 1980s was for bioscience what the 1930s and 1940s were to physics. Great leaps were being made in understanding the mechanism of diseases like cancer, heart disease, arthritis, and mental illness, while new viral diseases like AIDS and maladies of aging like Parkinson's disease were demanding attention and generating lots of money for research. As the mechanisms of disease became clearer, medical scientists developed a new approach to scan the near-infinite number of compounds for likely drugs to confound those mechanisms. They called it "mechanism-based screening."

It used to be that if a new chemical compound did not kill one kind of cancer cell or cure a diseased laboratory rat, it was thrown out. Now medical scientists had learned to trace the course of an illness through the body as one might track a metal ball through a pinball machine. Each turn of the disease and the body's response to it involves a reaction with some type of biochemical. Like pinball flippers, these reactions keep the disease rolling. Because they now understand the machine's layout better, scientists can look for some chemical that will inactivate any one of its flippers, robbing the illness of its momentum. In medical terminology, the flippers might be the enzymes that make chemical reactions happen, or they might be receptors, lock-and-key mechanisms that allow access to cells. For example, scientists at the drug company Smith, Kline and Beecham in New Jersey have modeled the multistep process by which constriction of the blood vessels increases blood pressure. They have zeroed in on a key enzyme in the process and are now looking for natural compounds that will block the cellular receptors for just that enzyme and short-circuit the whole process.

With the drug companies in the game, money for plant-hunting started to materialize. The National Cancer Institute, which had abandoned plant-hunting in 1982, decided to spend almost $5 million dredging for new plants from the rainforests. The institute took an eclectic approach. It funded the ethnobotanists, who advocated learning from traditional healers, at Mike Balick's shop at the New York Botanical Garden. It also funded the eco-rationalists, those who favored using clues from the forests' organisms to track down drug candidates, from the Missouri Botanical Garden in St. Louis. A third group, at the University of Illinois, fell somewhere in between the ethnobotanists and the eco-rationalists. The three groups were to spend five years in Central and South America, Africa, and Asia, respectively, searching for new drugs from plants. In addition, NCI paid several marine biologists to start looking for new compounds from the ocean, from coral reefs to windrows of seaweed on remote beaches. At the same time, drug companies like Merck & Company, Monsanto, and Smith, Kline refinanced their plant chemistry departments and started sending botanists back out into the forests.

What had begun in the mid-1980s as an exasperated cry of warning from a handful of biologists had swelled to a full-throated oratorio. The effort to wring value from rainforests now had enough urgency and emotional heft to move public opinion, and enough field data had been gathered to suggest that sustainable harvesting might even pay. Those few who knew medicinal botany's past certainly had reason for hope. One-quarter of all prescription drugs in fact contain a useful plant ingredient. Around the world, 121 prescription drugs are made from higher plants (and that does not include antibiotics from microorganisms). Almost half of the plants in these medicines come from the tropics. And 74 percent of these were discovered by following up native folklore claims.

And now there were hard-nosed businesspeople and government bureaucrats who were risking relatively large sums of money to try out this idea. But it still needed a name, something that captured the essence of rainforest exploration and medicine-hunting for profit as well as the need for conservation. The whole thing was like prospecting, really, part educated guess and part gamble, with an overtone of rugged outdoor romance. Some people started calling it *chemical prospecting*, a term entomologist Thomas Eisner at Cornell used. Others preferred *biodiversity prospecting*. But prospecting it was. The prospectors were biologists and anthropologists, and instead of dark pits in the earth, they would mine tropical forests. And in less time than they imagined, they would strike a vein of green ore.

7

From Osa to New Jersey

From the start, the race for rainforest medicines looked to outsiders to be a kind of relay event run by scientists and conservationists, each handing off the baton to the next runner, with the forces of deforestation as the opponent. In fact, there was more than one team running, and plenty of internal competition. Denying their differences publicly, the ethnobotanists and the eco-rationalists each vied to be first, not just for themselves, but for their different philosophies. In science, you fight not just for yourself, but for your way of thinking.

Schultes and his students stood as ethnobotany's coach emeritus and team members, with Mike Balick's various enterprises around the world being the most visible entrants. As for the eco-rational approach, Wilson was perhaps the most quoted theoretician. But the man who was first to put principle to practice was Daniel H. Janzen.

Janzen is Central America's most famous ecologist: a field scientist, a preserver of forests, a fund-raiser, an arm-twister, and a biological visionary. In 1984 he won biology's version of the Nobel Prize, the Crafoord Award, and in 1989 he was awarded a MacArthur Fellowship, popularly known as the "genius" award. Many who know the man call him arrogant and abrasive, yet all who know his work agree that he is brilliant.

Janzen was and is the most inside of outsiders in Costa Rica, a slip of a country in Central America that nonetheless hosts a huge variety of tropical environments. By the late 1980s, Janzen had worked in the country almost twenty years and written over 250 scientific papers, most on how tropical forests work. There is whimsy in his work. "Why Tropical Trees Have Rotten Cores" is his treatise suggesting that hollowed-out tree boles are good at attracting animals that then defecate nutrients directly where the tree can use them. "Why Food Rots" is an explanation of how microbes have evolved to work quickly before animals get to the food. For fun, Janzen once weighed carob seeds, the original standard for the carat, and found that only three times out of four did the prescribed amount actually weigh one carat.

Janzen lives a nomadic life, split between a patch of wilderness traditionally known as Santa Rosa National Park in northwest Costa Rica and his faculty job at the University of Pennsylvania. To say that he is committed to tropical biology would be an understatement. He once let warble-fly larvae grow out of his skin to better understand their life cycle. Overcoming what he describes as his "fecal phobia," he picked through horse manure to see how the big seeds of the guanacaste tree in Costa Rica are dispersed. He concluded that since all the large herbivores native to Central America are extinct, horses and cattle now do the job, leading Janzen to suggest that livestock may not be such a bad thing for some types of tropical forest, a very contrary notion for tropical biology.

Next to contrariness, Janzen enjoys the convolutedness of nature. Among his most famous projects was tracing the life cycle of the tropical fig wasp, *Blastophaga*, and the fig tree, *Ficus*, a coevolution of two organisms with a plot line as complex as an Homeric epic. Janzen observed that the female wasp enters a hole in the immature, hollow fig, which looks like a bulbous green fruit but is actually a gourd-like flower. Inside are hundreds of florets, some male, some female, some sterile. The female wasp deposits pollen in the female florets' ovaries and her own eggs inside the sterile florets, and then dies. After about one month, wingless young male wasps crawl out of their florets and either fight and kill one another or, preferably, find a female counterpart still encapsulated inside a floret. Those lucky males who succeed bore a hole through the floret, insert an extendable abdomen, and inseminate the females. Shortly thereafter, two things happen. The newly mated females emerge from their florets just when the male florets mature and bear pollen. The timing is impeccable — the females immediately ingest the pollen. Meanwhile, the inseminating male wasps, in a gesture of sacrifice worthy of the defeated Trojan Hector, cut an exit hole in the wall of the fruit and die. The females use the hole to make their exit and fly off to find new fruit, leaving their home to ripen and be eaten by vertebrate animals with simpler lifestyles and tastes.

Piecing together such biological puzzles takes a lifetime of living close to nature. Janzen started young. Born in 1939, he grew up in a time when living on the edge of town meant that the woods began at the back door and the city at the front. "I shot my first deer from my back steps," Janzen recalls of his youth. The same day, he walked out the front door, got on a bus, and went to the Minneapolis public library, his favorite place inside four walls. "I was completely anti-social," Janzen says of his youth. "People just didn't exist." His mother had to offer him ten dollars to go out with a girl on a date. She and his father, a regional director for the old Bureau of Biological Survey (later to become the Fish and Wildlife Service), thought Danny was weird, maybe gay, although people did not talk about that sort of thing in those days in a middle-class Minnesota household. Neither money nor love got Danny's blood racing. "I went with one girl on one date in high school. I took her to a basketball game." It was not a success. "My response was, 'What the hell did girls have to offer?' "

What pointed Janzen onto the track his life was to follow was a trip to Mexico during the summer of his first year in high school. He discovered insects, especially butterflies, the likes of which he had never imagined. Danny was hooked. The following year the family went again, this time all the way to Guatemala. By now, the skinny kid with the butterfly collection was earning a reputation in Minneapolis. He happened to be a paperboy, and the local newspaper, the *Minneapolis Star Tribune*, carried a story about this kid with his international collection of bugs. The advertising department photographed the paperboy among his butterflies, and used it in national advertisements. Danny became the first poster boy for biodiversity.

The publicity ended up intriguing a member of the Disney family, who offered to fly the boy to Mexico for a summer. When Janzen was seventeen, he arrived in Mexico City, "where I see in retrospect they wanted me to be this little toy" for publicity. He insisted on going into the country, and, after some conflict, he was given his freedom to roam for the summer. "I rode all over Mexico for two months on a motorbike, collecting butterflies. I nearly killed myself three times in accidents . . . but I learned a lot about Mexico."

This single-mindedness intensified as Janzen got older. "I was very unconscious, I think that's the right way to put it, all the way through my undergraduate years. To me classes, studying, the subject was absolutely everything. Things like tuition, where you live, they just did not exist in my mind . . . and of course I am still that way." After graduating from the University of Minnesota, Janzen pursued his doctorate at the University of California at Berkeley, where he was told that he would focus on insects in California. He wanted Mexico. "I said, 'Look, you guys, I can collect more insects in two months than you guys get in one of your expeditions with twenty people.' " He got his way, and eventually earned his degree studying the Mexican insects he knew and loved so well. His world was now an interior one of books and "the exterior," an intricate puzzle where the living pieces lay about along forest paths, in treetops, under rotting logs, or hugging the bottoms of leaves, all waiting for someone with a thousand years to patch them together. Janzen knew he did not have a thousand years to spend. So he lived as if he only had one.

In 1988, after cataloging a large chunk of Costa Rica's flora and fauna, Janzen decided to do more than just study ecology. He started to *create* it. The undertaking was the restoration of a tropical dry forest, the type that holds the dubious honor of being the most endangered of tropical forests. When the Spaniards arrived in the New World, there was enough dry forest — relatively open-canopied, deciduous, and without rain for months at a time — in Central America alone to cover France. There is now less than two hundred square miles left, most of it in the northwestern corner of Costa Rica. It is almost as rich in species as rainforest. Yet many of the species within are "living dead," says Janzen. If they flower, they do not set seed for lack of pollinators. If they set seed, the seeds are not dispersed for lack of dispersers. Saving species is not enough; whole habitats have to be restored. That is what Janzen is trying to do — regrow a tropical dry forest of 120,000 acres. You do not just go out and *plant* such a forest. You stop fires and the invasion of grasses and let nature take it back. You let pristine areas "inoculate" those that have been destroyed. You might even introduce cattle to trample and eat unwanted grasses that have pushed out the native species. You lay down seed from native plants, in the dung of cattle if that is what the seeds prefer. And most especially, you win over the local people to the cause. In Santa Rosa's case, Janzen hired some as live-in managers, and he got the government to buy parcels of their land to add it to the park, now called Guanacaste National Park. "He protected the farmers, and that was smart," notes a local environmentalist. The reforestation of Guanacaste will take, by Janzen's estimate, about a thousand years. It does not matter to Janzen that he will be long dead before results materialize. "The battle for mesoamerican tropical dry forest conservation should have been fought in the year 1800," he says with typical use of combat metaphor. "Don't wait until the year 2000 to begin to fumble with the rainforest pieces worth restoration."

In the course of trying to stave off biological extinctions, Janzen came around to the idea that commercializing endangered biodiversity, and especially its chemicals, might be useful. But his methods for finding medicines in tropical forests are as different from the ethnobotanists' as surgery is from psychiatry. "I can tell more about a plant's chemical toxicity from what a bunch of ants on the forest floor eat or don't eat than a native healer," says Janzen. To see what he means, you have to go south, to the dry, windblown forests along the Gulf of Papagayo.

Along the slender tendon of land that connects the two continents of the New World runs a single vein of concrete, forty feet wide: the Pan-American Highway. A stretch of this highway rides the rise and fall of mountain and valley through central Costa Rica, through forests of ceiba and fig trees, plantations of mango, steep hillsides stitched with rows of coffee plants, and finally down into the plains of Guanacaste Province, named after the country's most famous tree. Here the wind blows like sandpaper over the flat, brown land. Villages give way to barbed-wire fences and cattle ranches, then all signs of habitation melt away, leaving the sun-baked land to the insects, lizards, snakes, and birds that own this corner of the Earth. Near the Nicaraguan border there is a narrow turnoff, marked by a single wooden sign that reads "The forest is the fountain of life and development." The red-pitch road leads the traveler into the Santa Rosa forest and to its protector.

Bearded, naked to the waist, Janzen sits sweaty and loose-limbed astride a rude wooden bench in his block-and-stucco bungalow. All around and above him, in bottles, boxes, cartons, and plastic bags clipped to clotheslines strung from wall to wall, are dried insects, pickled snakes, animal parts, spongy clumps of fungus, and leaves and flowers from scores of plants. A sign over the front door says "Closed for Inventory." Janzen is fifty-two years old and has spent the better part of a ninety-six-degree day collecting plants and insects in this rarest of habitats, the dry tropical forest. At least half the year, he can be found here, usually with his companion and fellow biologist Winnie Hallwachs, living and working in the kind of conditions he thrives on: primitive.

A biologist who once worked with Janzen in the field likened him to Henry IV urging his men on at Agincourt. Another described him as a short-tempered Patton. Unquestionably, he radiates confidence. "Modern medicine is turning back to nature," he declares. "Getting drugs from plants has been going on for centuries. But this time, we are going to make the forest pay for itself." The wind whistles outside and a branch smacks the tin roof like a bass drum. A startled bat rockets out of Janzen's bedroom, and the connection between the world of brain scans, heart transplants, and designer drugs and the baked wilderness outside is murky at best.

Janzen explains. He has just returned to Costa Rica from Philadelphia, where he has been helping with the final wording of an agreement between a Costa Rican organization called the National Institute of Biodiversity (INBio) and the world's largest pharmaceutical manufacturer, Merck & Company in Rahway, New Jersey. The agreement is the first of its kind. Costa Rica will give Merck controlled access to the country's flora and fauna in return for cash up front, technical assistance and education, and a cut of royalties on any drugs the company develops from Costa Rican plants. And for the first time, insects will be part of a major drug company's systematic search for new medicines. Insects, says Janzen, who was trained as an entomologist, are an almost untapped resource of novel chemicals.

"Nothing like this has been done before," Janzen says. "The sign in front of this park says 'The forest is the fountain of life and *development.'* What it has cost in dollars and human energy to add that one word to a national park entrance sign, you cannot imagine." The idea that a biological reserve, a park, a wildlife refuge is actually a commodity, Janzen predicts, "is going to make for some unhappy people." He seems to relish the idea of annoying academics in the lecture halls he has left behind. "Biologists have had a free ride. Those that have been working in Latin America and not turning anything back into the system have been off-base." He leans over and pushes a bowl toward his household pet, Flatface the opossum, who snuffles contentedly and digs into what appear to be ants. "Termites," Janzen curtly corrects.

"The irony of it all," he continues, "is that if people say 'biodiversity has value' . . . then it will fall under the social rules that all other things that have value do. You bargain for it, you hide it, you steal it, you put it in the bank." He pauses, searching his mind for the right apothegm, and finally intones, "Biodiversity is no longer the toy of the English rich." Happy with that, he strides to his workbench to sort through his day's collection. It is May of 1991, another year of deforestation, another tick of the clock. Whoever scores the first big hit in the search for green medicines will slow that clock. Janzen would like to see it happen here, in the trammeled forests of Costa Rica.

The idea that a country's entire biological identity, all its plants and animals, could be inventoried and marketed first began to take shape in 1988 in San José, the nondescript capital of an otherwise remarkable Central American country, Costa Rica. At the time, Costa Rica was riding high on the fame awarded its president, Oscar Arias Sánchez, who had just won the Nobel Peace Prize for his efforts in bringing warring factions in El Salvador and Nicaragua to the negotiating table. Costa Rica had abolished its army almost forty years before, had the highest literacy rate in Central America, and enjoyed one of the highest standards of living in the Americas.

So idyllic was Costa Rica's reputation compared to its neighbors that it was sometimes mocked as the continent's Disneyland. Indeed, the government had put aside about one-quarter of its territory for national parks, reserves, and other forms of protected land. In a country the size of West Virginia, that is more protected real estate — at least on the books — than any country in the world. Every day jumbo jets rolled up to the airport in San José and disgorged battalions of tourists. Retired schoolteachers could double their life lists of birds and retire to air-conditioned hotels amid the montane forests of Monteverde, while young backpackers could pitch their tents along lemon-wedge beaches that curved beneath towering rainforests at Corcovado. Tourism had become the second-leading source of income in Costa Rica, next to bananas.

Costa Rica's wildlands were far from secure, however. Over the previous three decades, the country had in fact been one of the most furious deforesters in the region, a time during which one of the nation's popular mottos was "Be a patriot, cut a tree." Outside of the parks and reserves, Costa Rica's original forests had been almost entirely cut.

Some Costa Ricans believed that the wealth gained by cutting down forests would be short-lived. Among them was Rodrigo Gámez, an environmental adviser to President Arias. He had studied plants most of his adult life, especially their diseases and predators, which are myriad in the tropics. Educated partly in the United States, Gámez had witnessed the rising tide of environmentalism in the North and had heard the term biodiversity bandied about. He knew what it was, living as he did in a land that had as many habitats as all of the United States and

Canada combined, and he had no quarrel with those who wanted to preserve it. Yet as usual, it was northerners who were imposing their views on the South, where poverty and hunger dictated a different set of compromises. He believed Costa Ricans could look after themselves, and their wealth of biodiversity, if the will and money could be found.

An amiable, round-faced man whose tanned, smooth pate and twinkling eyes give him the look of a cerebral priest, Gámez was not politically inclined. He could dream up ways to use and preserve biodiversity, but he could not put them into practice by himself. He did have access to Costa Rica's leadership, however. So in October 1988 he helped get the country's ministers of natural resources, agriculture, and the environment, and the directors of the national museum and the nation's largest university, to meet in San José to discuss the yawning gap between what they wanted to do to preserve biodiversity and what they could afford.

According to an observer at the meeting, it was mostly a gripe session. That observer was Janzen. The biologist had just returned from a trip to what he calls the "outside" — the United States — looking for money to support his work in Costa Rica. He knew the equation: money in the North but little biodiversity; diversity in Costa Rica but little money. "I told Rodrigo," Janzen recalls, "that what I hear on the outside world is, if you guys would just put your hand up and say, 'Hey, we're going to do something specific with our biodiversity,' then those guys would pay, because it would be the first example of a concrete thing they could land on." Four months later, a meeting of about two hundred Costa Rican leaders was held at the national insurance building in San José, a place considered neutral territory. The minister of natural resources, Álvaro Umaña, suggested a national commission be formed to come up with a plan. The commission was formed almost immediately, and in June 1989 it gave birth to a unique species in the world of biology, the National Institute of Biodiversity, or INBio. No institution like it existed in the world.

INBio started small as a seed: a white stucco building planted across from a coffee plantation in a crowded suburb outside San José, in the country's cool central highlands, with a small staff scavenged mostly from universities. There was an air of defiance among those first enlistees. "We wanted to show the world that we, Costa Ricans, could capitalize on our rich natural resources, not just multinational companies and universities from the North," Gámez recalls. He smiles as he remembers their enthusiasm. Don Rodrigo, as his staff calls him, is a soft-spoken man who rests his hand on your shoulder as he talks, and the language of confrontation makes him self-conscious.

Janzen was right; the money came. The MacArthur Foundation, the U.S. National Science Foundation, the Pew Memorial Trust, the W. Alton Jones Foundation, the government of Sweden, and environmental groups like the Conservation Foundation started writing checks. With a fair-sized chunk of money, it was time for INBio to produce. But what exactly *was* INBio to produce?

According to Janzen and Gámez, three things had to be done with biodiversity: save it, identify it, and use it. This became the organization's unofficial motto. While government had put a large part of the country out of bounds of traditional agricultural uses, getting something valuable out of it was, Janzen says, "like fishing in a black box." In 1989, INBio began to identify what it had by inventorying its entire flora and fauna. That meant at least one sample of everything that lives. The goal was to do it in ten years, at a cost of as much as $70 million.

No other tropical country had ever undertaken such a thing. Hundreds of thousands of species lay in wait, from algae on the bed of the Rio Sarapiquí that flows down from the central cordillera, to the mites on the back of a rattlesnake in Guanacaste's jiragua grass, to the flowers atop the two-meter-thick *Terminalia amazonia* trees in the depths of Talamanca's lowland rainforests. There are more species of birds in Costa Rica than in the entire United States, more species of butterflies than in all of Europe, and ten times the number of plant species in all of China. In all, there are thought to be half a million species of organisms in Costa Rica, including more than ten thousand higher plants and three hundred thousand insects. Together they represent as much as 7 percent of the world's biodiversity. Only a fraction of these species had been collected and described by the late 1980s. If the remainder were divided by the number of staff at INBio, each person would be responsible for collecting hundreds every day in the field. It was like some impossible task handed down from Olympus to test the devotion of mortals.

The people at INBio put their heads together and came up with a unique solution: the parataxonomist.

Rodolfo Zuñiga is a parataxonomist. A lanky, broad-shouldered man of twenty-nine, Zuñiga spends much of each day in a two-room field station at the edge of the Carara Biosphere Reserve, a patch of rainforest midway down the Pacific coast of Costa Rica. Less than 150 miles southeast of Janzen's Santa Rosa redoubt, it is a day's winding trip by car through dry coastal plains, mist-covered mountain forests, and cool, vernal valleys. The road running by the station is well-traveled, carrying tourists down to swank hotels and beaches to the south and goods from the highland *fincas*, or farms, to villages along the seashore. Few travelers give a second thought to Zuñiga's shack, which sits dwarfed like a dollhouse in the shadow of a wall of great trees.

The station is a portal into the depths of biodiversity, and Zuñiga is one of its keepers. "My job during the day is to carry a car battery in a sling up into the forest," he explains on a steamy afternoon as he prepares for just such a trip. "I go different places on different days. Some times of the month, for example, when the moon is low, are busier than others. I also carry a fluorescent light, which is powered by the battery. Next to the light, I hang a white sheet. I turn on the light, then I come back here and wait." What Zuñiga builds in the forest is a light trap. Insects that fly, especially moths, are attracted to the glow of the fifteen-watt light on the sheet, and cling to the sheet as if it were a lifeboat in an empty sea. The more ultraviolet the light, the more moths. One theory holds that the insects normally locate a natural light, such as a star or the moon, and orient their flight by keeping a constant angle to it. If they choose an artificial, stationary light, however, they fly in an ever-tightening spiral until they arrive at the light and, thinking it is daylight, roost.

Zuñiga returns to the forest in the late evening to collect his captives, snaring those insects not already in his collection in a bottle laced with sodium cyanide. He makes another trip at about three in the morning, because different species of moths fly at different times. A night's work can garner scores of novel insects. When he is not collecting moths, Zuñiga might spend part of the day laying out other types of insect traps, like the veteran yellow pan trap for the small Hymenoptera, the order that includes the wasps, bees, and ants. These insects are attracted to yellow objects because their food includes the yellow droppings (entomologists perversely call it "honeydew") of aphids or lantern flies (of the insect order Homoptera). Zuñiga lays out yellow bowls filled with soapy water or alcohol, into which wasps fall, die, and achieve immortality as specimens for human examination. (They who made the bait also serve humanity. Lantern flies, according to Central American lore, will bite, and any girl so bitten must go to bed with her boyfriend within twenty-four hours or die, the insect thus serving, in its way, to help Homo sapiens proliferate.)

Zuñiga preserves his insects in naphthalene and every few weeks takes somewhere between two thousand and five thousand mounted specimens to INBio by motorbike, where they are coded and stored until they can be officially identified. Moths are of particular interest, along with certain beetles, caddis flies, dragonflies, and wasps. Next to the plants, the beetles are thought to be especially good candidates for drug compounds.

What makes Zuñiga unusual — a *para*taxonomist rather than a real taxonomist — is that even though he does the work of a scientist, he has never even been to college. "I was a park ranger for a while, and I worked as a laborer on a farm," he says. "I like the outdoor life, but it wasn't leading anywhere." So he signed up to be a parataxonomist. It was a title and a job that INBio dreamed up out of necessity; there was too little money to pay for scientists to collect specimens, so INBio trained ordinary people — bus drivers, housewives, farmers, park rangers, cooks, any of the working class who could live in primitive conditions and were curious about basic biology — to do the job. Like the so-called "ninety day wonders," the pilots given minimal training during the worst days of World War II, parataxonomists were not experts, but they got the job done.

Janzen started the first classes for parataxonomists in 1989, and botanist Barry Hammell of the Missouri Botanical Garden and visiting scientists from the United States, Great Britain, and Europe helped train the first students. The six-month course, with regular refresher sessions, has graduated several dozen parataxonomists, and most were still in the field in 1993. "One of the best things about the parataxonomist idea is that not only are they preserving Costa Rican biota, but they are learning to appreciate their own wildlands," says Rodrigo Gámez. "Many live right next to these wildlands. They were raised to see the forest as something to be pushed back. Now they are becoming biologically literate, learning how to use the forest, and educating others." The waiting list of applicants is long.

INBio also dislodged a brick from the wall of Latin patriarchy and enrolled an all-female class of parataxonomists in 1992 to train at Janzen's camp at Guanacaste. Within a week, INBio got a desperate phone call from Janzen, long past his diapering-daddy days, who blurted into the phone, "More toys! Send more toys!" Janzen eventually had the women playing soccer with the male members of the Guanacaste staff, a breakthrough by Costa Rican rules of behavior, and most of the women went on to become successful parataxonomists. INBio also created a similarly recruited and trained team of curators to prepare and mount specimens collected by the parataxonomists. They label the insects with bar codes on tiny slips of paper, an idea that

occurred to Janzen's companion and fellow biologist Winnie Hallwachs as she stood in line at a North American checkout counter.
Janzen has also begun training para-ecologists as well, people a step
more sophisticated than parataxonomists, with enough knowledge of
forest ecology to seek out special plants and insects for study and pharmaceutical testing.

With the saving and identifying of Costa Rica's biological wealth
begun, there remained the final commandment of biodiversity — use it.
How would INBio make any money from the boxes of beetles and
stacks of dried leaves piling up in the corners of its little warehouse by
the coffee plantation? Tropical biologists had always loved coming to
friendly Costa Rica to collect exotic organisms and would even pay for
samples — from five to fifty dollars each. That was hardly fair return.
INBio wanted Costa Rica to be more than just a wholesaler of biological
goods that were treated like rumpled seconds in some thrift store. The
likeliest way to make real money, INBio's directors agreed, was from
new pharmaceuticals derived from Costa Rica's biodiversity. "But we
wanted to be perceived as partners," Gámez says, "not as a resource
that could continue to be exploited."

Finding that partner was INBio's most difficult and controversial
move. The outcome, still to be determined, is one that the Third World,
now locked into a debate with the North over the rights to its genetic
resources, watches in anticipation. INBio's efforts could be a victory for
the biota-rich, cash-poor countries of the world. Or it could be a sellout
that will sink INBio into the familiar mire of handouts and loans from
the North, proving once again that he who pays the piper calls the tune.

Daniel Janzen may have been the most unlikely businessman ever to
walk through the wide glass doors at corporate headquarters of Merck
& Company. The man lived most of the time in a three-room bungalow
in a tropical forest with bottled gas for cooking, bats in his rafters, and
homemade furniture. He cared little what he ate, where he slept, or the
state of his clothes, and it showed. He knew more about the social
behavior of wasps and ants than he did about corporate America, and
that showed too.

"They had their own culture," he recalls of his first meetings with
Merck executives. "It was like meeting people from Malaysia." His
clunky black glasses, electrified white beard, and nonexistent haircut
screamed, "I am not like you and I don't want to be." Yet there was a
certain logic to this man coming to the industrial megalopolis in Rahway, New Jersey, and presuming to tell Merck a few things it did not

know. For Janzen did know more about the "goods" that Costa Rica had for sale than anyone. And he also had good connections.

One of those connections was Thomas Eisner. Eisner was another of what Janzen calls biology's "silverbacks," a reference to the dominant, mature males of the mountain gorilla. Eisner's background was as different from Janzen's as two lives could be. Born in 1929 in Germany, Eisner's father was a Berlin chemist, his mother an artist. The Jewish family fled Germany in 1933 and moved to Spain, which soon was embroiled in its civil war. The family moved again, to Paris, where children taunted the boy and his sister for being German. The family decided to quit Europe altogether and sailed for South America, first to Brazil, then south to Uruguay, where they settled.

Like so many wanderers, Eisner learned to depend on himself for entertainment. His parents encouraged him to play the piano (Eisner still plays and even has a piano in his laboratory), but it was nature, unquestioning and, in Uruguay, more various and novel than anything Europe had offered, that drew him most. He would leave Uruguay at seventeen when the family emigrated a final time, coming to rest in the United States. Eisner went to Harvard and studied biology, and is now a professor at Cornell, where he has become what his friend Edward O. Wilson calls the "pointillist" of biology, a man with an eye for the novelties of insect behavior and physiology, whose remarkable discoveries are each like a daub of paint on the canvas of life.

Eisner believed that pharmaceutical companies had overlooked a huge, underground reservoir of potential drugs — insects. To tap that reservoir, scientists required a special knowledge, a sort of chemical map, one that Eisner had spent his professional life drawing. That map depicted the world of chemoecology.

Chemoecology is the study of how plants, animals, and especially insects interact chemically in nature to serve their needs. Many insect messages, like "I want your body" or "Keep away from me," are communicated with chemicals such as pheromones or benzoquinones that insects exude. Eisner found the study of these messages to be a little like sampling the perfumes made by his father, whom he credits as the probable source of his skill at sniffing out interesting chemicals.

Eisner's gaunt frame, deeply lined face, and severe, metal-framed glasses belie the childlike playfulness with which he illustrates the potential of chemoecology. Consider the story of the legionnaires, the frogs, and the beetles. Eisner once came across an obscure report in a French journal of military medicine dating back to 1861. A physician identified as M. Vézien had discovered a unit of French legionnaires whose members had a peculiar complaint: *"Erections douloureuses et prolongues"* — technically called priapism or, simply, persistent erections. "The account stayed in the back of my mind for years," Eisner says. "I imagined these guys lying in bed on their backs singing the Marseillaise." Vézien suspected cantharidin, known then and now as the infamous aphrodisiac Spanish fly, and made from the dried bodies of meloid beetles. The legionnaires denied taking aphrodisiacs, but, being Frenchmen, they could not resist an item of the local cuisine — frogs' legs. Vézien tracked down the pond where the frogs had been caught, cut open a few of them, and found they had gorged on meloid beetles.

If a frog could be turned into a prince, why not into an aphrodisiac? After twenty years of pondering this account, Eisner decided to try to verify it. The story was puzzling, Eisner says, "because cantharidin is about as concentrated as any animal toxin." A tenth of a milligram can blister the skin, and the lethal internal dose for a human is less than a tenth of a gram. It had a colorful history in the annals of sex and death. "The Marquis de Sade experimented with it," Eisner notes, "and the Roman Lucretius supposedly died of an overdose." So Eisner fed live meloid beetles, which are quite common, to leopard frogs. The frogs enjoyed them thoroughly; one ate ninety-five of them. The toxin turned up in their slime, feces, and leg muscles, but did them no apparent harm (nor, apparently, did it give them erections). If the beetles did not harm the frogs, Eisner reasoned, perhaps they conferred some kind of protection to them. So he offered cantharidin-stuffed frogs to water snakes. "Without undue delay, as is usually the case, they ate them," Eisner reports, and survived none the worse. Perhaps snakes just did not know any better. How about leeches? Eisner thought. He attached some to more frogs' hind legs. To keep the frogs from dislodging them, he cut off the receptacle ends of condoms and slipped them over each frog's front legs and torso. The leeches suffered no lack of appetite for cantharidin-rich frogs' blood. "I don't want to make too much of this," Eisner says of his experiment, but the upshot, he adds with some degree of seriousness, is that if one fancies frogs' legs, it might be best not to gather them from the wild.

These and other experiments, many with his Cornell colleague, chemist Jerrold Meinwald, are part of Eisner's effort to show that chemistry can indeed be destiny. They have shown how the caterpillar *Utetheisa ornatrix* eats poisonous pea plants to make itself so chemically repellant that even when it becomes a moth, spiders will cut the creature out of their webs rather than eat it. The toxin doubles as a sexual attractant to female moths. Perhaps the scientists' most famous discovery was of the remarkable "bombardier" beetle's ability to defend itself with a spray of boiling, bitter chemical. Visitors to Eisner's lab are invited to give these beetles a poke to experience their pulsed-jet defense (which Eisner says he discovered when, his hands occupied, he put a bombardier in his mouth for safekeeping). When the beetle mixes different benzoquinones in a sort of reaction chamber in its gut, the reaction makes them boil and spurt out of a nozzle at the back of the abdomen in pulses of several hundred per second. The setup is not unlike the German V-1 rocket, and Eisner's photographs of the beetle blasting away with its miniature gun turret have become a classic of entomology.

"Chemical communication," Eisner explains, "is the oldest and most basic way of getting messages across." He believed that biodiversity prospecting — he calls it chemical prospecting — would have a good chance at INBio if wealthy partners could pay some of the cost. Eisner channeled some of his own grant money through Cornell to INBio. Gámez, meanwhile, had contributions from the Swedish government and from various foundations. He also helped engineer a debt-for-nature swap from the Swedish government that wiped out more than $27 million worth of Costa Rican foreign debt in return for a government promise to preserve a portion of its tropical forests. By the middle of 1991, INBio had almost $6 million in donations for its ten-year inventory, along with a staff of twenty-two full-time employees, eleven consultants, and thirty-one parataxonomists in the field. For a two-year-old environmental experiment, it was a formidable accomplishment, but not enough to finish the job.

Merck & Company was known as one of the few large drug companies that had kept up its natural products division during the 1980s. The company had struck pay dirt, quite literally, with its drug Mevacor, which lowers cholesterol. It came from a soil fungus, *Aspergillis*, and it earned Merck $735 million in sales in 1990. Natural products also had produced the antibiotics Mefoxin and Primaxin and the antiparasitic Avermectin, which was discovered in a soil sample taken from a golf course in Japan. And other drug companies had had some lucky strikes too. Sandoz, for example, discovered the immunosuppressant cyclosporine, used to keep transplant patients from rejecting donor organs, in a fungus (it was first screened as an antibiotic and almost discarded because it did not work well as such). Six years after it was marketed, sales had reached almost $100 million.

Granted, all these agents had been discovered at least a decade before INBio appeared. But Merck still had a few natural products with potential. One was physostigmine, from the tropical plant *Physostigma venenosum*. The chemical and a synthetic version had been used for certain kinds of glaucoma, but Merck believed it might help people afflicted with Alzheimer's disease. One theory holds that the disease is caused by a lack of the neurotransmitter acetylcholine, and physostigmine seemed to increase levels of it. Another promising compound was zaragozic acid, produced by a microorganism in leaf litter in pristine pine forest in North Carolina. It was found that zaragozic acid inhibited a key enzyme in the cholesterol biosynthetic pathway, and could be used to treat people at risk of vascular and heart disease from high cholesterol.

It was Eisner and Meinwald who got INBio its chance with Merck. Meinwald remembered a former graduate student of his, Paul Anderson, who had risen within the Merck organization to become senior vice president for medical chemistry. When Eisner and Meinwald told him in October 1990 about what INBio was doing in Costa Rica's rainforests, Anderson was interested. With a door partway open, INBio needed someone to put a foot into it. Who better than Janzen?

The Cornell group brought Janzen and Gámez up from Costa Rica and invited Anderson and a few other industry scientists in for a presentation. Anderson fondly remembered his days with the Cornell group. "They had me work on cockroaches," he recalls with a laugh. "The cockroaches would squirt materials, quinones, on themselves to ward off predators." Anderson was impressed with Gámez and Janzen. "I liked the objective — doing something for the environment — and I liked the people," Anderson says. Trust was not immediately mutual, however. Janzen and Gámez were leery of the drug industry. "They were concerned that a company would come in and rip them off," says Anderson. Yet the Costa Ricans were very serious about their plan, and Janzen's scientific presentation was convincing. Anderson said he would see if he could get Merck interested.

He faced plenty of skeptics at the drug company. Some biologists were doubtful that anything new was left to find. Moreover, plants often were too much of a good thing. That is, they could produce so many closely related compounds and so many hits on preliminary assays that no one could follow up on all of them. Many of these, like tannins, were useless as drugs anyway. Getting resupplied was always a worry too. On the other hand, Anderson argued, this was no slick venture capital group trying to sell a chemical pig in a poke. Janzen and Eisner, meanwhile, were adamant that new drugs could be found.

"Why," Eisner insisted, "should we rely solely on our own powers of imagination and inventiveness when millions of other species have been working out [chemical] solutions for hundreds of millions of years?" And no one, Eisner pressed the Merck scientists, had ever looked at the *insects* out there.

At the time, Merck was spending about $1 billion a year on research, about as much as Costa Rica's annual government budget. Only a small part of that was reserved for natural products, but what INBio needed would barely register. Or so INBio believed. Merck executives were not so sure. While many thought it an intriguing way to get new molecular leads, no one wanted to pay for it. Microorganisms from soil samples were easier to work with and grow in large batches than plants or insects. Then there was public opinion in the developing world, where multinationals might as well have been tapeworms in the breakfast sausage. Indeed, such hostility was running high as the 1992 quincentennial of Columbus's arrival in — and exploitation of — the New World neared.

Anderson found an ally at Merck in the person of Lynn Caporale, a biochemist and director of scientific evaluation. Caporale was at the time preparing to spend a vacation in Costa Rica. She had long wanted to visit this country of rare orchids, exotic birds, and galleries of centuries-old trees. She had read much about its wildlife and also about its history. "For one thing," she recalls, "Costa Rica had abolished its military years ago. I found that very impressive. There was history of peaceful conflict resolution, and the population was well-educated." Caporale liked INBio's idea.

Janzen flew back and forth between Costa Rica and Merck's research headquarters. "I couldn't stand it," he recalls now. "It was like going to a dance in high school." He found that lawyers and businesspeople did not have the same notion of truth he had. "The Merck lawyer would say one thing one day, a different thing the next. . . . It was a constantly shifting thing, no *absolute truth*," he says. But Janzen also knew that the green label now carried clout in the marketplace. "I said, 'Let's cut the bullshit. . . . You wanna be the good guys? Or do you want to be forced to that position? If you are the good guys, you are first in line and you get to set things up the way that serves you well.' " That kind of attitude did not always charm Merck executives. Nor did INBio's initial proposal that it should share patent rights on discoveries made with Costa Rican organisms. Moreover, INBio wanted a larger cut of the profits than Merck was prepared to give. Drug companies generally compensate collaborators involved at the front end of drug development, such as university researchers, at somewhere between 2 and 5 percent, according to Merck and other industry officials.

After almost a year of negotiating, the chemical prospectors persuaded Merck to take a stab at their proposition. Merck, meanwhile, convinced INBio to accept the company's position on patents and royalties. On September 20, 1991, Merck, Cornell University, and INBio announced a deal. Merck would pay INBio $1 million in advance to collect almost a thousand species of plants, insects, and soil samples for microorganisms, and would throw in another $135,000 worth of equipment to help INBio and the University of Costa Rica set up an extraction laboratory. There the plants and insects would be dried, macerated, and turned into liquid extracts. These would be sent to Merck laboratories for screening. For its part, INBio would be free to pursue similar arrangements with other institutions or companies, so long as it sent them different sets of organisms (if after two years Merck did not opt to develop anything from the samples it got, INBio could sell these elsewhere as well). Cornell would help train INBio staff. Most important, and most tantalizing, were the royalties from net sales that INBio would receive if Merck found something hot and turned it into a drug. Even if a Costa Rican bug or plant only served as a starting point for a synthetic process, INBio would get its royalty. While neither party has revealed that royalty percentage, Merck officials say it is "consistent with that in other similar agreements," such as contracts with academics.

INBio did not "own" the raw materials it would provide, of course. They belonged to Costa Rica, its people, and their government. INBio finessed this point by promising 10 percent of its $1 million to the Costa Rican park system (the first payment went for a reserve on Coco Island, off Costa Rica's Pacific coast). And if any of the samples ever becomes a moneymaking product, INBio must put half of its royalty payments into Costa Rica's parks and reserves.

INBio finally was in business, literally. Granted, what Merck paid for its share was small beer for a $10 billion-a-year company, although Merck officials insist that it is a significant chunk of their research and licensing budgets. On the other hand, INBio got far more than any developing country had ever received for what has essentially been a free good. Most important, it established a principle that was lost on neither northern corporations nor fellow developing countries. "What we did," says Gámez, "is show that a developing country owns its biota, its genetic resources, just as it owns its oil or minerals." Now it was time to find out if the prize was worth the running.

*   *   *

It is January 21, 1993, the day a new path is to be opened between the green hills surrounding the town of Golfito on Costa Rica's southwestern Osa Peninsula and a jungle of smokestacks and factories at Merck's labs in New Jersey. Osa's rainforest is dense, the kind you see on the "save the rainforest" posters and nature programs on television, with spectacular buttressed tree trunks, cords of woody lianas entwined as tightly as wet knots, and arcades of pendulous leaves. This place is well-watered, with up to four meters of rain a year, and it has the wet rainforest's egalitarianism, where no single species dominates. No other forest like this still stands here on the Pacific side of Central America. And this one probably will not stand much longer.

The town of Golfito is an odd place. A fishing village until the early part of this century, it was remade by the United Fruit Company, the granddaddy of multinationals working in Central America. If you like bananas or pineapples, you can thank United Fruit for putting them on your table. If you are a Central American, you may curse them for running the region for decades as if it were its own orchard. United Fruit is gone from Golfito now, replaced by lesser North American companies that take a lower profile. You can see the blond children of the company executives bicycling through the streets during the day, or at night mingling with Costa Rican schoolmates or the occasional ecotourist at the bustling outdoor restaurants that all seem to specialize in grilled chicken. Golfito is a good place for the two cultures to meet, for the Americans are not too terribly rich, nor the locals too poor. Most of the Costa Ricans in Golfito farm, work the port and fruit processing plants, or tend to rainforest-seeking tourists. They also run a frenetic free port, to which Costa Rican shoppers flock like migrating birds each weekend to buy truckloads of discounted refrigerators, VCRs, stoves, and liquor. The town has a quaint architecture all its own, another legacy of the fruit companies: rectangular, two-story bungalows in splashy bright colors, with red tile roofs spreading cool shadows, with their wide-hipped eaves, wrap-around verandas, and rows of shuttered windows. Formerly the houses of the fruit barons, many have been converted to cheap hotels, where you can get a room for less than the cost of breakfast if you are willing to share it four ways and shower in cold water at the end of the hall.

In one such room on this humid, stagnant day, a team of workers spreads out a vanful of equipment on the floor in preparation for an expedition into the forest. There is a clutch of aluminum poles, one of which is crowned with a hinged, curved blade controlled by a long snatch line, that when engaged could slice off a finger. In a heap lie orange-handled clippers, hunting knives of all sizes, a hatchet, and, in leather scabbards, darkly stained machetes sharp enough to part a sheet of notepaper. There are butane tanks and burners set in a cage-like contraption, tubs of alcohol, and several pairs of snake boots, thick leather shin-guards that lace to the knee like the buskins of Roman legionnaires. The place looks like a staging area for a small insurrection. In fact, one would be hard pressed to find a gentler group of people in this town than these who now strap on their machetes like gunslingers. They are plant-hunters. Their deadliest armament is the insect repellent they smear on every spot of exposed skin they can find, for the implacable enemies they face are inhuman — fleas, wasps, mosquitos, and chiggers.

A half hour's ride out of town, the plant-hunters pile out of their convoy of a Toyota Land Cruiser and a refrigerated truck, fall in behind their leader, and head up an unmarked path in the forest behind him. Nelson Zamora is a botanist in his mid-thirties with the pale skin, fine features, and charcoal-black beard of the Spaniards from whom he is descended. He has led this team for nine months now, since his first collecting trip in May 1992 for INBio, his employer, on behalf of Merck. He has walked and watched these forests since childhood. Following this steeply dipping path, hemmed in with walls of trees so numerous and varied that just naming those captured in a single photograph would take half an hour, he can pick out the species on sight. There is the heavyset tree whose massive trunk disappears up into the canopy, *Terminalia amazonia*, its height of forty-odd meters worthy of its name; the hanging vine *Anomospermum reticulatim*, draped like bunting from branch to branch; the bushy little *Gonzalagunia rudis*, with its tiny leaves, small white flowers, and delicate white fruits the size of baby peas; the thick, furry leaves of *Episcea*, their mid-ribs lime-colored and their inviting flowers a striking vermilion, carpeting the path; or the *Anonna pittieri* tree, whose flowers grow directly out of its trunk, looking as if they have been glued on by some prankster.

What runs through Zamora's mind as he walks, eyes upward and feet somehow sensing where to overstep the roots that scallop the path, is an extension of what is in his pocket. Therein is folded a piece of paper with a long list of plant species that Merck scientists suspect are good candidates for new medicines. They were drawn from a list of thousands that Zamora and INBio considered relatively easy to find in Costa Rica and not endangered with extinction. Merck's wish list covers plants from many families, such as Araceae, which includes philodendrons, the ornamental diefenbachia, and a host of genera with alkaloids and cardiac glycosides; Piperaceae, the pepper family, with many aromatic species popular among indigenous peoples as medicines and stimulants; Moraceae, the fig and mulberry family, members of which contain alkaloids, sterols, triterpenes, coumarins, and flavonoids, and which includes a fig tree whose latex is used against intestinal worms and a fruit that some Brazilians believe is an aphrodisiac; Myrtaceae, the myrtle family that produces cloves and eucalyptus; and Menispermaceae, the moonseed family, also with many alkaloids and other bioactive compounds, including the genus *Chondodendron*, the woody vine from which the arrow poison and muscle relaxant curare is made.

Zamora must keep a mental list of these and dozens more families to be tracked down as he scans the woods. As the tip of Merck's Costa Rican supply line, he has a million-dollar pair of eyes. He has far more than that, however. He has a multimillion-year-old skill, one that kept humans alive for aeons: the ability to read the geometry of nature. It is not the "carpentered" geometry of angles, rectangles, and corners that most of us now are accustomed to in our houses, offices, and cityscapes. Nature's geometry is far more complex, and the rainforest is the most irregular of its myriad forms. Zamora is one of the few who can differentiate among these shapes and shades. He knows, as early humans knew, that distinguishing lines and shapes can reflect the chemistry within the plant.

Janzen, who also has learned, or relearned, this skill, calls it an instrument of the "human-to-the-predictable-world interaction." It is something that humans developed to accomplish the complex tasks of hunting, fishing, growing food, building shelter, treating disease, and otherwise interacting with the more predictable parts of the environment. Those skills stand apart from mental capacities needed for human-to-human interactions, such as the innate ability to understand language, and those needed for the human-to-unpredictable world, such as the predilection for religion. For the predictable world, humans need the mental capacity, the "hard-wiring," to do things like see and discriminate among colors and shapes, to hear different tones, or to manipulate objects. The motor skills needed to drive a car are the same that were first naturally selected so that Homo sapiens could run down prey, climb trees, or jump over a creek. "We invented the car," says Janzen, "to match this hand-eye coordination." Survival also depended on recognizing nature's patterns. Nature was diverse, the most diverse thing our species ever experienced, so the skills needed to deal with it had to be diverse. One can still see those skills at work even in someone who could not tell a fern from a fig tree. "A lawyer in New York City may know three thousand people, with a little 'natural history trail' behind each one of them," says Janzen. "What he is doing is applying that form recognition. If you look at evolutionary history, in the village his ancestors once lived in with six families and thirty-one people, they didn't need to recognize three thousand people. That ability was not evolved to recognize people. It was evolved to recognize a complex natural environment, to recognize three thousand kinds of *plants!* And *birds!* And *insects!*"

Zamora, staring up into the forest in the Osa Peninsula, is activating that ancient, atavistic mental program, like an archaeologist practicing some forgotten metallurgy of an extinct civilization. He says he does not think of what he does this way but simply as his personal passion for science. But he is absorbed in the forest in a way most people cannot fathom, as if he were being drawn physically up through his binoculars into the canopy. Even the most modest flower that has fallen along the trail stops him, drawing from him a smile. "Lovely, isn't it?" he will say of the plainest blossom. He seems quite unaware much of the time that four assistants trail along behind him, waiting for the word.

When the word comes — "There," he says, pointing up into the pinpoints of light that pierce the canopy like sunshine through a muslin cloth — the crew members drop their knapsacks and water bottles. Somehow he has spotted a spray of small green fruit up in the tree's top branches (tropical trees generally do not start branching until near the top). In the brush by the path, illuminated by a patchwork of light, he retrieves a piece of vital evidence. It is a huge calyx, the part of a flower's sepals that shroud and protect the young bud. It is light and spongy, about the size and color of a well-done pancake, and it confirms his suspicion, that looming above is a rare tree from the genus *Chaunochiton*, found only in moist tropical forests and, in Costa Rica, probably only in this region.

The team must get a small quantity of leaves, woody stems, bark, and new green stems from each plant they seek. With smaller plants, they also get roots. Any seeds and flowers they find will be bagged as well. Zamora's right-hand woman, forester Nora Martin, also keeps a separate batch of samples that will be tested for hitchhiking microorganisms.

Besides his brain, Zamora's most important asset is a slingshot, a formidable weapon with an aluminum brace that rests against one's forearm to add steadiness and power to each shot. Through his binoculars Zamora searches the crown of the *Chaunochiton* and finds his target, a branch that stands free of encumbrances. He places a lead fishing weight that is attached to a spool of fishing line in the sling. Meanwhile, Victor Hugo Ramirez, the team's burly, mustached driver and strongman, plows through the thickets like a two-armed backhoe to the far side of the tree. Zamora aims his slingshot toward the sky, squints at his target, and draws the rubber sling back to its limit, his left arm trembling with the strain. "Cuidado," he calls out. With a snap and zing he releases, and the weight soars up into the treetops, the fishing line singing with the stringy whine that fishermen love to hear.

After about a dozen attempts, Zamora gets the weight to soar just over his branch but no others. "This is usually the *easiest* part of the job," Zamora says as he pays out line until the lead shot drops into Ramirez's waiting hands. Ramirez detaches the weight and ties a thicker nylon line to the fishing line, which Zamora smoothly retrieves, back over the branch and to his feet. They repeat the process in reverse, Ramirez drawing toward him an even thicker line, in the middle of which is a six-foot length of double-edged chainsaw blade. Zamora hands his end of the line to Eduardo Lepiz, a ponytailed string bean of a man in his mid-twenties who is the team's droll wit and tree-climber, and directs his two assistants. "Dele," he shouts. "Give it to him." Ramirez yanks, and from above they hear the saw's teeth set. "Dele, Lepiz," he says, and Lepiz yanks back with all his weight. Leaves rattle and fall from above, accompanied by the throaty sound of blade cutting through wood. After a few strokes, though, the blade sticks. Zamora adds his weight to Lepiz's, while the youngest member of the team, Esteban Ureña, joins Ramirez. "It's very hard wood, this tree," Zamora grunts as he grips the line. They throw their weight backward, grunting, their heels dug into the soft earth, until they are almost parallel to the ground. The blade refuses to move.

It is agreed that they are too close to the tree and the angle of force is too vertical, which pulls the saw blade down instead of across the tree limb. Holding the ends of the rope, the team crashes through the bush with a remarkable nonchalance; the forests around Golfito are notorious for harboring the deadly fer-de-lance, and in fact an hour before the team had frozen in midstep along the path where a young fer-de-lance had coiled itself half underneath a large leaf, its diamond pattern of cinnamons, chocolates, pale yellows, and blacks all but invisible in the litter. Ureña flicked it out of the path with the end of a machete. "I hope your mother is not nearby, little one," Lepiz called after it. The team's leather snake boots, meanwhile, lie back on the floor of the

Toyota. "I never use those things," Zamora says blandly. "They are too hot and uncomfortable, especially when they are wet."

After a great deal of maneuvering, arguing, and pulling, the team frees up the blade and resets it. With a dozen more strokes, they are rewarded with a loud crack, a swishing of leaves and branches, and an earthen thud. There is much satisfied shouting. Ramirez, first to reach it, bolts upright, takes a half-dozen steps, then stops dead still and grimaces. "Wasps," he mutters through clenched teeth, waving off the others. Eventually, the wasps fly off, leaving Ramirez's neck with a rainforest tattoo.

Within half an hour, four plastic bags have been stuffed, weighed, labeled, and placed by the side of the trail, to be picked up on the walk back. Zamora checks off another species from his list and gives the scientific name to his crew. Lepiz, a forestry student who hopes to make a career working in the rainforests, and Ramirez keep their own records of the plants they have seen and sampled. Martin, who has a degree in silviculture, knows mostly commercial tree species, so she is getting an on-the-spot education in forest ecology as well. When she is not in the field, she is studying English so she can read the scientific literature. "Social life?" she laughs. "Someday, maybe." Overcoming her fear of snakes has been the most difficult thing for her. The very word makes her moan.

Zamora is happy with this sample. "That was a rare tree, difficult to find," he says, adding that the tree will no more miss its limb than a blood donor a pint or so. The team members rest on a fallen log and pull their lunches from their backpacks. A patch of sunlight across the path attracts butterflies that put on a spiraling performance. Cicadas, as if by musical score, begin a chorale so loud it makes the ears ring, then stop suddenly, to be replaced by the intermittent buzz of individual insects that swoop in and out of earshot with a dizzying Doppler effect. A single large, succulent leaf catches a rivulet of breeze and flutters comically, as if someone hidden below were shaking its stem. Zamora, finishing his lunch with some condensed milk poured over saltine crackers, looks across into a thicket of small trees and laughs. He points to a small tree. "It is another *Chaunochiton*." It is a young tree, with branches and leaves within arm's reach of the path. The team members groan. "Ah, well," Zamora says, "at least the one we got had flowers."

By the end of the day, the team has gathered about eight species. They vary from herbs of the genus *Diplasia*, which burst from the ground in two-meter-long linear leaves the color of new grass and margins sharp enough to leave the hands bloody with invisible cuts, to a huge tree, *Endlicheria*, another rare find with wood so hard the saw rope snapped, sending Lepiz and Ureña tumbling ten feet ass over elbow down an embankment. It took three hours to get that sample, but the effort was worth it, Zamora says, for the tree was the only individual of the species that he had seen in the forests around Golfito. The tree limb almost claimed the chain saw, which stuck again, but Lepiz shinnied sixty feet up a double helix of entwined vines hanging from the canopy and hacked off the limb with his machete. He stayed to admire the view and, laughing like a schoolboy, hurled epiphytes and epithets at his colleagues below, but then descended suddenly, cursing, and arrived with his face and arms covered with the bites of a nasty swarming insect called the *purruja*.

The trek back to the vehicles is brutal. Each collector carries a good forty pounds of plant material, in addition to the collecting gear, over a series of knife ridges that undulate like the corrugated tin roofing that covers most of Golfito. The path is strewn with roots, the soil crumbles beneath the feet, and razor grass and tree trunks speckled with sharp spines line the way. The parked trucks hove into view just before dark, and the exhausted plant-hunters pile their cargo into the refrigerated truck (alcohol or preservatives would alter the chemicals in the plants that Merck is interested in, so they are chilled instead) and collapse. The silence is broken only by the distant whine of chain saws, working on until the sun sets.

As the white sky over the Dulce Gulf turns to rose, the team drives home down the rutted, red-dirt road. Zamora, however, is still enraptured. He leans out the passenger window with his binoculars glued to his eyes, using the last bit of crepuscular light for a final review of the gallery as it wraps itself in darkness.

When Zamora's bulk samples reach INBio, they are frozen to kill insects and other organisms and then dried. Next, they go through a grinding machine that chops them up like so much ground beef. Insects, which are collected by Janzen and his assistants, are frozen and eventually macerated into a soup with a solvent. The samples then go to the University of Costa Rica and the cramped laboratory of Gabriella Rossi, a young chemist who, under instructions from Merck, mixes samples with different solvents. Each solvent separates out different types of compound from the parent sample so that unwanted materials, like fats, can be removed. Hydroxylated and nitrogenous compounds are of most interest, while the plant compounds most people are familiar with, the tannins, carbohydrates, proteins, sugars, and starches, are not. When the fluids are boiled off, what remains of each sample is a sticky residue like glue, usually green but sometimes yellow, red, or orange, that fills about one-quarter of what looks like a nail-polish bottle. This is then dried.

The lab turns out extracts from about twenty to thirty plant species a month. Insects go through a slightly different series of separations. "There is very little experience in making insect extracts," Rossi says; Merck had to devise a protocol from scratch. The lab expects to deliver about one hundred species of insect extracts a year. "We did some horrible cockroaches," Rossi recalls. "Also big orange grasshoppers, lots of butterflies, and caterpillars, some in their cocoons." She says INBio and Merck have high hopes for insects. "They usually have some toxic or biologically active molecule as a defense mechanism. Sometimes you find that the nuclear part of a molecule taken from an insect comes from a plant that it eats, so you want to catch some insects when you know what they've been eating. Or pheromones change their chemistry, so you try to catch them just before or after their reproductive period."

From Rossi's laboratory, the green pipeline runs to the Costa Rican division of Merck, which ships the samples to Merck's labs. Environmental samples go to Spain, plant extracts to Rahway, New Jersey, and insect extracts to West Point, Pennsylvania. That is where they are put through their first tests. Exactly what kinds of tests, or "assays," Merck uses on these new plant and insect extracts is a closely held secret. Most of their techniques, however, are brand-new, because they rely on knowledge only recently acquired about the human body and the diseases that afflict it.

Robert Borris is a Merck phytochemist who helped put together the company's plant shopping list. Though his office is closet-sized, it affords a view of woods, a rarity in the brickwork city that is Merck's research laboratory headquarters in Rahway. Borris remembers the days when natural products were tested first on live animals. Now, instead of rabbits and mice, he tests them on between forty and a hundred biochemical targets or assays. An assay can be a crucial working part of a bacterium, a parasite, or a fungus that Merck would like to knock out. Or it could be an enzyme that controls the way the AIDS virus reproduces or a cancer cell divides. Or it could be a cloned version of a receptor in the brain that goes haywire in people with Alzheimer's disease. The revolution in biotechnology during the 1980s created the tools with which scientists can design genes to mass-produce such biological assays almost like yeast turning malt into beer. Testing chemical compounds against these screens is now close to a production-line operation. Merck, Borris says confidently, can test several hundred candidate compounds in the time it once took to do a half-dozen in animals.

Borris is an eco-rationalist when it comes to plant-hunting. That does not mean throwing new compounds blindly into the maw of Merck's massive screening system, however. "I don't believe in random screening," he says. "That is what the National Cancer Institute did for twenty years." A true chemical detective applies new knowledge about humans to what ecologists and phytochemists already know about plants. For example, a receptor that enables a cell to communicate chemically with other cells may form a chemical link only with molecules with a special structure, say, an indole nucleus. Indole nuclei occur in all sorts of natural substances, from coal tar to orange blossoms. So to find something in nature that would interact with that receptor, it makes sense to look for indoles. "We know from thousands of reports in literature that the family Apocynaceae [which includes the poisonous oleander and the snakeroot plant, *Rauwolfia*] is a really rich source of indole alkaloids," Borris says. So that would be a good place to start looking.

If an extract "rings all the bells," that is, reacts with most or all the assays, it is normally discarded. It probably is just too toxic, or simply interferes with the assay in some mechanical, blunt-force way that would be inappropriate for a drug. If it rings one or a few bells, the extract, which may contain a hundred or more constituent compounds, is broken into its individual chemical parts, or fractions. Each fraction is tested against the bank of assays. When Borris finds the one that works, technicians then characterize its structure.

If tropical plants are an unfinished chapter in pharmacognosy, insects and spiders are a barely opened book. Many spiders, for example, have unusual poisons. "If you want to kill something quickly," explains Merck's Caporale, "one easy way to do it is to disrupt all the electrical activity and muscular activity, so the animal can't run, can't breathe." In 1982, Japanese scientists discovered that some spider poisons seemed to block the action of one of the body's many neurotransmitters, glutamate. Soon scientists at the drug company Pfizer found the exact mechanism: the poisons gum up ion channels, canals through which cells communicate by exchanging electrically charged atoms. Apparently, only those channels switched on and off by glutamate were affected. That is important because too much glutamate is believed to contribute to cell death after a stroke, and to some types of epileptic seizure. Then there are tropical microorganisms, another unread volume. A handful of detritus from the jungle floor harbors hundreds of species, and Merck is prospecting for them in Costa Rica, especially in tree bark, roots, insects, fungi, and aquatic plants and animals. Such a microorganism could well be Costa Rica's first hit, for their chemical armamentarium is large and, because they are the source of antibiotics, their behavior is fairly well understood.

Merck scientists say they are prepared for a long walk through the rainforest; Caporale says the company plans to screen a huge swath of the planet's flora. Without doubt, organic molecules never seen before will turn up. Then comes the toughest part: making them work for humans.

Costa Rica can be seen as a corporation, with its population of about three million being the shareholders and caretakers. They own about 19,500 square miles of land, of which about one-quarter is a greenhouse. In the greenhouse reside the assets: some 470,000 species of arthropods and other insects; 35,000 bacteria and viruses; 10,000 higher plants; 2,500 fungi; and 1,500 mammals, lizards, birds, and other vertebrates. This is how Janzen, now quit of corporate meeting rooms and back among his parataxonomists at INBio's new boarding-house behind its headquarters, describes his adopted country. Biodiversity prospecting has already begun to change the nature of conservation, he says. It started when biodiversity was seen as a resource to enrich the country, like its water, soil, or schools. Its first tangible products, its "livestock," Janzen likes to say, were eco-tourists, who "stand in the hot sun, pay three hundred dollars a day, and take pictures of termite nests." The next products will be chemicals and genes. "We are in *kindergarten* now as far as knowing how to use wildlands, while traditional agriculture has had tens of thousands of years of practice. We're just beginning to learn." Eventually, says Janzen, biodiversity will become "socially embedded" in the minds of the public as a source of national wealth, while the original goal of INBio and its backers, conservation, in effect becomes a by-product. "Soon big lumps of society will applaud INBio who couldn't care less about conservation," Janzen predicts.

So far, INBio is simply foraging for plants on Merck's list. In its way, the search has been based on eco-rational principles: Solanaceae has been good to humans, for example, so look for more Solanaceae. But at Cornell, Eisner says that true chemical prospecting requires people to go further, to actually read nature's clues to buried chemical treasures. "Look for signs of 'chemical promise,' " advises Eisner, master of chemical sleuthing in the insect world. "A leaf on the forest floor that remains uncovered by mold may be the source of new antibiotics, as may certain insect eggs that remain untouched by microbes as long as the mother administers her salivary fluids. Or a plant that is untouched by insect pests may contain a useful insect repellant." Even things like the color red are signs; natural selection has chosen red as a common advertisement that its wearer is poisonous. This, says Eisner, is the truly eco-rational approach to prospecting. And it is one that INBio is still learning.

There are some who feel that INBio has been shamefully presumptuous, that it has sold Costa Rica short. An articulate spokesman for that point of view is lawyer Mario Carazo, an urbane Costa Rican with a philosophical bent and a keen sense of history. Carazo is not like other lawyers in San José. Besides running a commercial law practice in San José, he is codirector of Fundación Ambio, a small environmental group dedicated to promoting what he calls "environmental awareness and responsibility" in Costa Rica. He also has family ties that extend deep into Costa Rican politics and science: his father, Rodrigo Carazo, was president of Costa Rica from 1978 to 1982, and his wife is director of the National Museum of Costa Rica.

Sitting in the sunny lounge of a San José health spa where he jogs most afternoons, Carazo lays out his objections. "INBio's technical goals are very altruistic," he says. "The problem is the way it was done." INBio was created as a private, albeit nonprofit, company by Gámez, former President Oscar Arias, and his minister of natural resources, Álvaro Umaña, during a time when privatizing government-run industry had become, Carazo explains, "the 'in' thing to do." "Then INBio called itself 'national' and used the country's national herbarium, one hundred and five years of Costa Rican work, to get money from the rest of the world. You cannot do that. They are a closed club, and they cannot sell the national patrimony." Merck's million-dollar advance payment "is like the little mirrors the Spanish gave to the Indians," he says, while the promise of royalties is just that, a promise, and the history of Latin America is littered with the broken promises of multinational companies.

One might note that these things are nonetheless far more than any developing country has ever won in return for plants and animals generally regarded as obstacles to be ploughed under to pave the way for development. What INBio has done is put value on things that heretofore had almost none locally and had been available to anyone, scientist, collector, or medicine-hunter, with a fistful of twenty-dollar bills. Carazo's square, handsome face creases into a half-smile, half-grimace. "This is not a nice comparison to make, I know," he says, "but really, that's like saying to the Bosnian women who have been raped, 'Here, we'll give you a dollar.' "

Carazo is only one of several influential people in San José who have taken this line of argument. Some are motivated by jealousy or overwrought nationalism, say Costa Ricans who have watched INBio's rise, others by memories of Central America's long exploitation at the hands of the United States. A few in the national legislature tried to block the Merck arrangement with a law stating that all of Costa Rica's flora and fauna were the country's "national patrimony" and could not be bought and sold by "private citizens," meaning INBio. It was pointed out that the law might forbid farmers from cutting down trees or selling their fruit, or fishermen from netting the country's "patrimony" from the sea. By October 1992, a revised bill passed that created a special niche for INBio to carry on its business as a licensed organization of the government, much as mining and timber companies get concessions to trade in national resources.

Umaña, as much responsible for INBio's birth as anyone, now heads his own environmental group — along with expedition outfitters, environmental activism is a booming business in Costa Rica — called the Center for Environmental Study. It is a small, bustling operation housed in a stately residence in an upscale neighborhood of San José. Umaña, with a thick head of tousled black hair, dense thickets for eyebrows, and a door-wide, six-foot-three-inch frame, radiates confidence in the choices he made. "It was an unusual thing, to form a private organization like INBio," he acknowledges. "But there was no mood for creating new government ministries. We thought the scientists should be in control. . . . If it had been a government body, it would have been tied to government procedures, and salaries, and strictures, which would have slowed its effectiveness." Yes, he agrees, $1 million is petty cash. "But it's a start. We are capturing rent on our biodiversity." That is a concept he believes can be taken still further. He leans forward heavily on his desk and explains with enthusiasm. "There are one hundred million tons of carbon stored in Costa Rican forests. At ten dollars a ton, as a 'tax' for storing carbon, that is one billion dollars . . . something worth thinking about."

The debate in Costa Rica over INBio's right to sell Merck a slice of the country's wildlife can be expected to boil up again. "I come from a family of politicians," says Carazo, "and someday I hope to be one." He will make a good candidate; he is attractive, well-educated, and an adroit spinner of metaphor who can draw on Cervantes and Shakespeare in the same breath. He realizes, like any would-be officeholder, that today's rhetoric is tomorrow's campaign slogan.

History favors Carazo's arguments. Brazil, where natural rubber in the nineteenth century made hundreds of men millionaires almost overnight, lost what had been 98 percent of the world market when the seedlings of the *Hevea* rubber tree were stolen by the Briton Henry Wickham in 1872 and planted in Malaysia. The Andean countries of South America had been the source of cinchona bark for centuries until the British and Dutch took the seeds of their best trees. Diosgenin from yams harvested by Syntex started the steroid and birth control industry, then North Americans bought the business and took it north. Curare never made money for either the indigenous people of Ecuador and Peru who first discovered it or for the governments of those Andean countries. Nor has *any* of these plants proven reason enough to slow the deforestation of the forests from whence they came.

Even if INBio hits the jackpot with a plant or insect, it could be too late. "Deforestation continues," Gámez acknowledges. "There is an expectation in this society to generate quick, easy money. The question of value — that it is more valuable to keep the forest than cut it — remains to be confronted." Gámez knows, for example, that the chance of finding one compound for a specific disease is something like one in ten thousand, a figure quoted by many natural products experts. If a supplier in the tropics is lucky enough to score a hit, there is then perhaps a one-in-four chance that the compound will prove safe and effective and become a commercial product. It would take ten years and about $230 million (widely accepted industry figures) to bring that product to market. After applying a discount rate to the investment and covering the drug company's costs, a drug that nets, say, $10 million a year would return an annual income, assuming a 3-percent royalty rate, of only about $50,000.

There are reasons to be hopeful, however. Drug companies now have dozens of screens for various diseases and medical conditions, which raises the odds. And given feverish demand for drugs against AIDS, cancer, and common viruses like herpes, a hit could easily become a billion-dollar drug, which would return tens of millions of dollars to the source institution. Moreover, many in the pharmaceutical industry are beginning to view rainforest collaborations with favor, as are several Third World tropical countries. "At first," says Gámez, who now spends much of his time flying to foreign capitals to give lectures, "they thought we were being ripped off. Now they are beginning to believe us." Indonesia and Mexico are planning to create organizations patterned after INBio, and both have signed agreements allowing them to visit and study the Costa Rican operation. Kenya is on the verge of a similar agreement.

With drug companies and foreign delegations at its doorstep, INBio has clearly discovered a formula that seems to appeal to both buyers and sellers of biodiversity — even before it has delivered a real product. True, it is an untested formula and fraught with questionable assumptions. Skeptics like Carazo and historical precedent are not encouraging. But the experiment is being watched by a host of people with reason to keep close track of how INBio fares and how it is treated by its corporate partners: Third World governments looking for new revenue ideas, First World aid agencies, conservationists in search of sustainable resource successes, and crusading biologists. And profits or no, INBio already has made a certain kind of history. It has given that orphan concept biodiversity a name and a face. For the first time, someone is trying to bag it, mount it, record it for history, and show that if our species insists other forms of life must pay their way, they can — first-class.

8

Shamans, Profits, and Ethics

Plant-hunting for medicines might seem the kind of earthly enterprise that would strike a favorable chord in the ecologically aware 1990s. On closer inspection, however, it is splintered with controversy.

The cracks are visible on a January afternoon in 1992 as an argument winds around a large, baize-covered conference table in a basement room at Rockefeller University in Manhattan. First one, then another person is struggling with a fundamental question: Who owns the planet's biodiversity? On the floor around them, cross-legged and shoulder-to-shoulder, sit several dozen listeners, most uniformly in blue jeans, sweatshirts, and hiking boots with the occasional woven, talismanic wristband worn as ornamentation.

At the table, a woman in a business suit, Merck's Lynn Caporale, is defending the point of view that biodiversity can be bought and sold. Merck's pact with INBio has been under a magnifying glass since the deal's announcement, and the questioning today has been especially heated. Many people in this room are angry about the Merck/INBio contract. They are from environmental groups, university faculties, and student groups — anthropologists, socialist sociologists, and young activists who are suspicious of big business and its patriarch, "big" Western culture. They want to know why Merck and INBio have not included indigenous peoples in the deal. They wonder whether, if a plant used by the Bri-Bri people of Costa Rica becomes a cure for cancer or AIDS, the Bri-Bri will share in the profits, and if so, to what extent. What about the farmers who live on the land taken for natural reserves and then explored for potential pharmaceuticals? And who gave INBio the right to sell the country's biota? Will the flora and fauna of Costa Rica be locked up, held secret? And why can't the public see the contract INBio signed with Merck?

There is a tightness behind Caporale's even voice, and her eyes have begun to reflect a frayed, trapped look. She explains that Merck prefers to look for interesting organisms using *ecological* clues rather than investigating the folk remedies of indigenous peoples. While many traditional medicines do actually work, most tend to have the same biochemical mechanism of action. Merck, like other drug companies, wants diverse compounds with unusual activity, chemicals the likes of which scientists — or even shamans — have never seen before.

A woman from Brazil points out that northern industrial concerns have profited from the biological wealth of Latin American countries for centuries. Corn, potatoes, rubber, coca . . . the list of products is long, but the ledger of profit to the South is short. Latin American governments in turn have exploited and robbed their own indigenous peoples. The Brazilian is Elaine Elisabetsky, a Brazilian pharmacologist and anthropologist who has lived with and now champions indigenous peoples in the Amazon rainforests. The fatigue in her voice is not lag due to the nine-hour flight from Rio but despair at having seen too many native cultures consumed. Merck should realize, she insists in a syrupy Portuguese accent, that the indigenous peoples of Latin America have spent hundreds of years learning the medical secrets of the forests. Their knowledge, and their husbandry of the rainforest over centuries, will help Merck. Will Merck's money help them? "Maybe ethnobotanical leads are not in your screening process because you would have to share royalties?" she suggests accusingly. The audience on the floor applauds. The mood is shifting from debate toward confrontation.

At the table, a gray-suited executive from another large drug company, here to see how Merck's experiment plays with the "save-the-rainforest" community, whispers in a colleague's ear. Merck may be taking a beating here, he says with a smirk, but it has wrung a good $10 million worth of good press out of a mere $1-million gamble. Indeed, despite the scene at the university, the Merck/INBio deal has won the company much favorable attention, as well as imitators — several pharmaceutical companies have begun investigating new drug leads from natural products again. Even some conservation groups that normally treat multinational corporations like paroled convicts have cautiously approved the initiative.

Yet doubters suspect it is business as usual. The secrecy surrounding the royalty arrangement has raised suspicions, and the nagging question remains, Is Costa Rica getting a fair return for its natural resources? And who owns those resources? No one has resolved such questions, nor do answers appear at hand.

INBio's Ana Sittenfeld, a microbiologist and head of the venture's biodiversity prospecting program, hunches over the conference-room table as if she is about to climb onto it. Her salt-and-pepper hair is close-cropped and her jaw is square and, at the moment, clenched. The few remaining indigenous people in her country, she explains, are largely acculturated. The old ways are mostly forgotten. Now biodiversity belongs to *all* Costa Ricans. She leans back in her chair but tosses out a challenge. "Secret?" she asks. "Yes, our biodiversity can be secret. What's the difference between a tree in Costa Rica and chip in Silicon Valley?"

Sittenfeld and others at INBio are insulted by the notion that the "poor little Costa Ricans" could never have driven a fair bargain with an American multinational company. Privately, they blame much of the criticism on Costa Ricans who are simply jealous of INBio's success. They are jealous that INBio hired some of the country's best scientists away from the local universities, and they are embarrassed at their own failure to capitalize on the country's biological mother lode. Some are jealous that INBio got custody of the country's largest botanical collection. Some are jealous of the attention INBio is getting from the world press. Petty squabbles in Costa Rica, INBio's executives have begun to think, are playing out in the North as if there were a national uprising on the streets of San José.

A weathered brown man in denims and red calfskin boots stands up at one end of the table. He wears a bolo necktie with a chunk of turquoise in it, and his dense black hair is tied back in a ponytail. The argument at the other end of the table trails off into silence. He speaks, and his words have the sharp, clean edges of the southwestern desert, with their hard r's and the o's held long in the back of the mouth. "My name is Richard Deertrack. I am from the Pueblo of Taos. I want to suggest something about the notion of wealth in western society. Take water. Water is the lifeblood of our Mother Earth. No one can put value on it. No one has a right to own it or control it. You will find with indigenous people that this is their concept. No one here has considered the spiritual connection of the people to what you are asking for. It's their life. How are you going to put a value on their life in all this?"

A scientist from Merck, George Albers-Schonberg, has been quietly grinding his teeth throughout the debate. He is well-acquainted with the arguments, being the company's director of natural product chemistry. "With all due respect," he interjects, "if what you respect is going up in flames, something has to be done. And it cannot be done for free."

For Deertrack, these arguments miss the point. He explains. "When you begin to get medical herbs, you begin to tamper with the spiritual connection between people and those herbs. Can we put a monetary value on that? If you go to a doctor, you expect to pay him. But if you go to a shaman to be healed, you may give him a horse, or you may just say, 'Thank you, may you live a long life.' How do you put value on that? That is all I ask."

Clashes between conservationists and the business community are as common as tavern brawls. As the renaissance in plant-hunting for medicines begins to take shape, however, some of the combatants believe it might serve as a unifying enterprise. With the drug industry's monetary might and the conservation movement's dogged idealism, perhaps the unlikely union of profit and preservation in the rainforest might work.

The meeting at Rockefeller University has been organized by an environmental group, Rainforest Alliance, with help from the New York Botanical Garden's Mike Balick and his Institute of Economic Botany, in an attempt to clear the air of rumor and let the former enemies get to know each other. As the basement tête-à-tête showed, however, the two groups, almost too comfortable in their long-standing rivalry, are still edgy and suspicious. Hovering somewhere in the middle are the tropical biologists. For them, the influx of interest in rainforest research looks like the British ships arriving at the beach at Dunkirk. If they are skeptical of the drug industry's promises, they are nonetheless happy to see fresh money for their cause. Many academics have in fact been quietly taking money for decades from drug companies in return for botanical samples they bring back from the tropics. Botanists do not discuss the practice outside the profession, but it has always gone on. Most academics, observes one well-known ethnobotanist in an ungenerous moment, "are whores."

The second day of the meeting at Rockefeller proves to be a repeat of the first, writ large. Several hundred people sit in steeply raked rows of seats in the semi-darkness of a university lecture hall as a procession of anthropologists, sociologists, botanists, political activists, drug company executives, chemists, and conservationists make their cases. A recurring theme is the alleged rip-off of the people of Madagascar, source of the rosy periwinkle that generated huge profits for the drug manufacturer Eli Lilly & Company. The Lilly scientist who made the discovery in the early 1950s stands and defends the company, pointing out that the species of periwinkle in question grew in many parts of the tropics, and no more "belonged" to Madagascar than pine trees belong to the Cheyenne. Next, the National Cancer Institute is accused of having once ripped up an African country's entire population of a rare plant in its search for a new cancer drug. There are also stories circulating here that a small plant "brokerage" is capitalizing on the new frenzy for plant-drugs by grabbing plants in herbaria and reserves from Central America to Indonesia and selling them to big drug companies without compensating source countries. And Merck comes in for more criticism. While the company is claiming that folk remedies are not on its collecting agenda, it is accused of having recently experimented with an Amazonian Indian arrow poison called *tike-uba* for use as an anticoagulant.

One drug company, however, silences the critics. Even the company's name advertises its cultural correctness: Shaman Pharmaceuticals. Shaman is a small but growing company with headquarters in San Carlos, California, that in 1992 is barely two years old. It calls itself an ethnobotanical enterprise, the only drug company that searches for pharmaceutical leads primarily from traditional practices by indigenous peoples, mostly those who live in tropical forests.

The company was started by a confident young investment analyst, Lisa R. Conte. Just thirty-one when she put the idea together, Conte specialized in high-technology venture capital deals. She got the idea for Shaman after reading a magazine article about the cultural traditions that were disappearing along with the world's rainforests. She did not know what an ethnobotanist was, but she spent six months finding out. She then got a collection of scientific luminaries to sign on as official advisers: Nobel laureate physician Baruch S. Blumberg, pharmacognocist Norman Farnsworth of the University of Illinois; the skeptical former plant-hunter Robert Raffauf of Northeastern University; Elaine Elisabetsky, the Brazilian ethnopharmacologist; Schultes's students Balick, Mark Plotkin, and Djaja Soejarto; and even Schultes himself.

Conte knew a small company could not hope to compete against the large drug manufacturers in screening huge quantities of plants for new compounds. So she chose an "ethnobotanical screen," in which her advisers pinpointed plants they knew of from remote areas that had not been investigated thoroughly. At the same time, Conte canvassed the world of environmentally friendly investors. She ran into a lot of disbelievers who thought she was peddling healing crystals. "It's not voodoo medicine," she told them over and over. "It's serious stuff." The novelty of the idea eventually helped as much as hindered. Newspapers doted on the story, casting Conte as a female Don Quixote tilting against the big drug companies while saving the rainforests. With her scientific advisory board lending gravity and her own knack for persuasiveness, Conte got enough backing to hire a few scientists and start testing plants. Her chief plant-hunter was Steven A. King. King had lived among the Secoya people of the western Amazon forests and was regarded in the profession as one of the real McCoys, a muddy-boots field scientist.

While Conte raised money, King made the rounds at scientific meetings, within environmental groups, and among the policy-makers in Washington, D.C. With his spiky blond hair, his penchant for pastel designer suits, and his rapid-fire speechmaking, King might as well have been a tropical toucan dropping in on the gray pigeons. He would make the slide projector hum with images of the biological wealth of the Central and South American tropics, and dazzle listeners with data about what the tropics have given the North and how little has been returned. Potatoes, maize, cassava, quinine, drugs for cancer and motion sickness, cacao for chocolate — the list would be long and go by quickly. Then slides of local people — the Secoya, the Quichua, the Waorani, the Kuna, harvesting their biological wealth in a sustainable, environmentally friendly way, as they have done for centuries. King would call them his collaborators; they are the people from whom Shaman Pharmaceuticals would learn. And they would be compensated. "Any agenda to try and manage resources will have to include the human beings that live in the forest," he would say. "They are often left out of the picture." They might get money, they might get medicine. "Often indigenous forest people say they need help in access to modern medicines, modern drugs, for things they *cannot* cure." After a half hour of this, King's listeners usually left intrigued, sometimes convinced, and generally exhausted. At the very least, they could see this was no ordinary business operation.

Conte has been asked to speak at the Rainforest Alliance meeting, and she chooses the event to announce the company's first success. Statuesque, with shining black hair pulled back into professional neatness and a bright red dress worthy of a fashion show, Conte lights up the stage like a basketful of geraniums. "This is probably one of the few groups I talk to where I don't have to define the word *shaman*," she begins. She explains that more or less random sweeps of tropical plants yield "hits," or potentially useful compounds, less than one percent of the time. "But we get about a *fifty* percent hit rate in initial activity," she says. Shaman, in less than two years' time, already has three pure compounds in development as drugs. Seventy more extracts are in the pipeline from over one hundred plants that Shaman's collectors have brought in.

"Our lead product is termed SP-303," Conte announces. "It's an antiviral agent that targets respiratory diseases. This is a great disease market in every single culture and every single country, each year affecting anywhere from twenty to forty percent of the population. Available treatment in the United States is not adequate. . . . This is potentially a blockbuster market with a drug of the right characteristics." Conte's enthusiasm is more than hype. The compound is in fact quite remarkable. A topical formulation of it also seems to work against the herpes virus, another huge market. "I can't describe it too clearly or somebody here will figure out what the plant is," Conte continues. She says it grows wild, like a weed, and can be found in Ecuador, Peru, Paraguay, Colombia, and Mexico.

Exactly where and how Shaman gets the plants is described only vaguely, however. Shaman "works with organizations of cooperatives as well as government organizations," Conte explains. She assures her listeners that the company pays a premium price for the plants, with the understanding that Shaman will do the necessary research to ensure that a long-term, sustainable harvesting of the plant is feasible. Moreover, Conte says, the company is creating income and jobs in Latin America.

One thing about Shaman's mysterious plant is clear: it has a long history of traditional use as a wound-healer in Latin America and probably elsewhere, first by indigenous groups and now by rural settlers as well. Conte promises that those who help Shaman, be they cooperatives of landowners and farmers, indigenous groups, or government organizations, will get a share of profits if the drugs make it to market.

In the meantime, Shaman is helping rainforest people in other ways. Ethnobotanist King recently has gone looking for a source of SP-303 among the Waorani people in Ecuador. He showed their shamans photographs of oral herpes lesions, and the healers pointed him to the plant they used to treat it. It was the same plant Shaman had been investigating. King was accompanied by a doctor who then spent several days treating the Waorani for various illnesses, including an outbreak of whooping cough, as compensation for their help. In the future, Conte says, a foundation the company had started, the Healing Forest Conservancy, will try to help indigenous forest people in similar ways.

By the end of the conference, Conte and King have stolen the show. Eager students approach them asking if they can sign on, and conservationists in the crowd applaud this novel enterprise. Clearly, the rules of botanical engagement have changed. It is no longer acceptable for drug developers to march into the jungle with a handful of gimme and a mouthful of much obliged, and with the ethnobotanists and the ecologists as partners, at least a few in the industry appear ready to embrace the new ethic.

But until a new drug is actually created, promises to share the real spoils remain to be tested. Whether medicine-hunters actually follow the new rules is something that will be judged not in executive suites and university lecture halls in North America but along the unnamed tracks and remote rivers of the tropical forests. The witnesses will be the world's forest peoples, the Waorani and Quichua of Ecuador, the Huambisa of Peru, the Yanomamo of Venezuela, the hill tribes of Thailand, the healers of Cameroon and Malaysia, and the rest of the world's forgotten people, the first owners of our earthly goods.

Part
2

Rainforest Rx

9

Blood of the Dragon

Knowledge, like virtue, may be its own reward, but it's likewise true that even the most arcane expertise sooner or later finds a buyer. Outside of the people who live in the Amazon's rainforests, who but a few academics would have cared which species of the tree *Osteophloeum* contains the most powerful alkaloids, which of the *Brugmansia* plants the Quichua shamans prefer for religious ceremonies, or how the Shuar people use the *Piper* plant to treat pulmonary hemorrhages? Yet now the answers to these questions are important enough to have launched new expeditions into the most remote reaches of the western Amazon.

More than knowledge of plants is required to mount such an expedition. It takes knowing where to find export permits for plants, how to stroke the right officials to get them, how to negotiate with truck drivers and native shamans, even how to get traveler's checks cashed on a Sunday. The few who know the territory now find themselves in demand, and have become the small end of a huge funnel extending from the tropics to the laboratories of industry.

Among those experts is Bradley C. Bennett, an ethnobotanist who has spent a large part of the last five years living in the western Amazon. No longer just a collector of academic minutiae, Bennett now is part conservationist, teaching forest peoples principles of sustainable development for the likes of palm oil or unusual fruit. He is part marketer, having been hired by an international consortium to help indigenous Amazonians find income from their traditional products, be they woven baskets or medicinal plants. The New York Botanical Garden, agent of the National Cancer Institute, is another of his employers. And Shaman Pharmaceuticals has hired him to find out more about the secret plant from which it gets its new drug, SP-303. Like so many of his fellow plant-hunters who have long tread those paths so rarely taken, he is bemused by the sudden parade but willing to serve as guide, as the world hurries to see what it might have been missing for so long.

One axiom of working in the rainforest is that getting there is usually the hardest part. My trip down the eastern slope of the Ecuadorean Andes to find Brad Bennett and the source of SP-303 is no exception. It begins at five A.M. at the Quito bus terminal, a concrete labyrinth of shadowy recesses where the predawn transactions of the city's poorest take place: begging by the weak, hustling by the young and strong, drinking by those who have given up. It's a place where the traveler had best try to blend in with the surroundings.

By the time the sun's rays have reached across the Amazon Basin to warm the wall of the Andes, my ranchero, as the buses are called here, is wheezing out of the terminal, packed like a sausage skin: dogs, sacks of potatoes, Quichua travelers, trussed chickens, tanks of propane, mestizo settlers, plastic jugs stinking of gasoline, fifty-pound bunches of plantains, and crates of Bibles bound for missionaries. The people pay, the dogs ride free on the roof. Otherwise, all contents are accorded roughly equal treatment. Its destination is Tena, a steamy lowland river town 125 miles east of Quito, and almost ten thousand feet closer to sea level. Tena lies amid the rainforests of the Oriente, home of a fractious mix of Indians, colonists, and Ecuador's oil industry. The trip will take five hours, perhaps eight, or maybe more. Schedules are loose on the lip of the Amazon Basin.

Ranchero rule-of-the-road number one states that a seat directly over an axle is to be avoided, for the ride there tends toward the vertical. Long legs are also to be discouraged, since the seats, the size of orange crates, leave less legroom than a soapbox go-cart. The blood in the lower extremities stops circulating after an hour squeezed next to a bound rooster and two somnolent homesteaders. In the aisle, passengers stand hip-to-hip in stoic silence. There is a gripping view outside, however, startling enough at times to get the blood flowing back to the legs. A few feet away, the road's edge gives way to sheer cliffs and yawning, misty gorges that plunge down into river valleys. It's clear why many of the corkscrew turns in the road, little more than an intaglio cut along the rock face, are graced with statues of Virgin Mary and hand-hewn crosses plunged into crevasses. Older passengers cross themselves as the ranchero, its driver grappling the gearshift like a post-hole digger, edges out over the lip of each new grade.

Much of the time, however, clouds obscure everything but the gravelly road, and soon sleepy passengers' heads slump against the windows and their chins drop to their chests. It's a good time to organize my thoughts about Ecuador, and why plant-hunters are flocking here again.

Ecuador is a pocket-sized country tucked below Colombia and above Peru on the Pacific coast of northwestern South America. It's famous as the owner of the Galápagos Islands, lovingly described by Charles Darwin and now a must-see on the itinerary of well-heeled eco-tourists. The Andes, where most people live, split the country north to south, with the east covered mostly in rainforest and the western coastal plains devoted primarily to agriculture, the port of Guayaquil, one of the oldest cities on the continent, its urban center.

Like so many Latin American countries, Ecuador skirts the edge of financial woe. With a population of eight and a half million people that is growing by almost 3 percent yearly, Ecuador needs to find ways for its people to make a living. The government has kept the wolf from the door largely with oil, which has been flowing since 1972, when a pipeline was laid from wells in the Oriente across the Andes. Exports of fruit, coffee, and seafood have helped the economy as well. But the slump in oil prices during the 1980s partly deflated Ecuador's bubble of prosperity, and the government realizes that oil won't last forever. Cattle, timber, and farming have become the present as well as the future promise for prosperity. Only the rainforests stand in the way, along with the people who traditionally live in them.

About half of Ecuador is covered with either primary or secondary (disturbed) forest. Every year, about 2.3 percent of that forest, or some 840,000 acres, is cut down. If the United States were covered with forest, that would be like cutting down all the trees in Utah in one year. Typically, logging companies move in and cut the prime timber for export, then settlers stream along the roads the loggers built. These colonists spread themselves out into parcels called *respaldos,* rectangles of land that abut the roads, farming the parcel parallel to the road before selling or leasing it and moving out to the adjacent parcel, and so on. Ecuadorean law requires that colonists put 80 percent of their land into production of some sort within two years of acquiring it or risk foreclosure on the property. So it's either cut or move.

What rainforest colonists are doing is no different from what North American pioneers did. Yet as they push back nature like so much dirt before a bulldozer, they are displacing perhaps the most diverse collection of organisms in the world. Ecuador possesses twenty-five life zones overgrown with more than twenty thousand vascular plant species. Vascular plants are those we usually think of as higher plants; unlike mosses and liverworts, the vascular plants have evolved two separate circulatory systems to carry water and nutrients throughout the plant, as well as a waxy outer layer, or cuticle, to prevent desiccation. By comparison, all of North America, from British Columbia's ferns and firs to the mangroves of Florida, possess only 17,000 vascular species. Up in all those Ecuadorean trees are 1,550 bird species, twice as many as are present in the continental United States. Terrestrial vertebrate species are thought to number 2,440. That includes 280 mammals, 345 reptiles, and 358 amphibians. The species count keeps growing as scientists reach parts of the country that heretofore have remained unexplored. Within these near-impassable tracts, millions of years of speciation have given birth to organisms that tumble over one another like waves on a green ocean. Many of them are endemic; that is, they are not found anywhere else. Only Brazil, thirty times Ecuador's size, has a greater number of vertebrate animal endemics. As for the plants, one of the world's foremost tropical botanists, Alwyn H. Gentry of the Missouri Botanical Garden, estimates that of Ecuador's vascular plant species, about 20 percent, or roughly 4,000, are endemic. This is one reason why medicine-hunters are coming to Ecuador, where undiscovered species lie literally around the next bend in the road.

In a land of high endemism, each swath of forest burned probably carries a species with it into extinction. The story of the Río Palenque mahogany is an illustration of how close to the edge many species are. Before Christopher Columbus rowed ashore to what his people called the New World, the Río Palenque mahogany was much prized by the indigenous people of Ecuador's Guayas River basin for its resistance to rot. It was especially valuable in making posts for their homes, which then as now are built off the ground to keep the moisture as well as the many-legged and the slithery at arm's length. The value of the wood was not lost on the Spanish, who cut and shipped it from northwestern

Ecuador back to Europe in huge numbers. By 1970, no one could find any more of these trees. The species had been an endemic; gone from Ecuador meant gone from the planet. Whatever it was about that mahogany that made it so durable would never be known.

During the 1970s, however, botanists found a new tree in northwestern Ecuador, one they had not seen before but thought to be a new member of the genus *Persea*, from the avocado family. They were wrong. It was a Río Palenque mahogany. They found eleven more of them, all on a small patch of land that had been reserved as a science center. Had the trees been on nearby government land, they would have been cut along with all the other large trees in the area. The old, primary forest at the Palenque science center in which they survived is a single square kilometer. Alongside the mahogany grow about twelve hundred other plant species, one-quarter of them endemic to Ecuador and as many as one hundred of them new to science. The reappearance of the Río Palenque mahogany was a close call; unfortunately, most endangered Amazonian species will not leave behind pockets of survivors. And the line of these species at the graveyard gate is very long. According to the World Resources Institute, over half of Ecuador's endemic plant species are at extreme risk of becoming extinct before the turn of the century. That's two thousand plants.

The ranchero trip from Quito to Tena is a good way to see what is at stake here. Between the two towns, the traveler passes through seven life zones. The start is in Quito's montane zone, where the summer air is fossil-dry and so thin that tourists sometimes faint and bleed from the nose. The hillsides there are rocky and support few large trees, mostly acacia, eucalyptus, and some exotic pines, many replacements from abroad for native species that were cut down long ago. An hour into the trip, the bus coasts through U-shaped valleys scoured by ancient glaciers. Some of these valleys contain alpine, tundra-like vegetation, while in others the climate is humid and wet, with twisted "elfinwood," trees that grow only to six feet or so, and bands of olive shrubbery, the herbaceous *Polylepis*, that gird each mountain's midriff like a tweed waistcoat. Patches of startling yellow blossoms, a tropical relative of the snapdragon, daub the cordgrass with color. A blink of the eye and a little imagination and this could be a Colorado postcard.

Two hours from Quito, the ranchero descends into moist montane forest, also called cloud forest. Mist and drizzle dampen the windows and the ascending humidity has a tranquilizing effect on travelers. Mosses and recumbent shrubbery cover the ground, punctuated here and there by the high stalks of *puya*, a bromeliad and a relative of the pineapple, that burst from the undergrowth like pilings in a choppy harbor, their minute flowers a favorite of hummingbirds. Another remarkable species, the *Gunnera* plant, is carried by Quichua travelers walking alongside the road. A single peltate leaf (one in which the stem attaches near the center of the leaf) is the size of a manhole cover and serves, as it has for centuries, as a makeshift umbrella, pulled as needed from the roadside.

As the terrain begins to level out, the scattered copses of trees and the mossy sponginess of the montane forests eventually give way to banks of tall premontane and lowland forest, while the silvery, braided streams rushing alongside the road widen and darken into muddy torrents. The largest of them is the Río Napo, which flows eastward through some of the most impenetrable territory in South America before it finally loses itself in the greater grandeur of the Amazon River. Along the way, it passes just south of the village of Tena, where the ranchero rumbles to a halt. The passengers uncoil themselves and file out, blinking, into the bright afternoon sun, stretching and stamping their feet to get the tingling out and the feeling back in.

Tena and nearby Archidona are languid places where slim young men in loafers and shirts unbuttoned to the waist idle at corner kiosks, smoking and waiting for something to happen. Women nurse babies, snap the dust out of laundry, or simply sit in doorways and watch street traffic. The children, barefoot, muddy, curious, and energetic, seem the only ones immune to the tropical torpor that envelops the place like green aspic. The splayed, makeshift look of Tena and its neighbor Archidona belies their longevity, however; they were established before Lewis and Clark trekked across the American West to the Pacific. In the mid-seventeen hundreds, the Spanish explorers Don George Juan and Don Antonio de Ulloa passed through here on their way down the Río Napo. "The houses are of wood," they wrote of the towns, "covered with straw, and the whole number of its inhabitants is reckoned at betwixt 650 and 700, consisting of Spaniards, Indians, Mestizos and Mulattoes; but it has only one priest. . . ." Apart from motor vehicles in the street, electricity, and tin roofs, Tena and Archidona are much the way Juan and Ulloa described them, although more priests have moved in.

The final leg of my journey is a bone-jarring, two-hour ride on the roof of a truck that serves as public transportation along the Campa Cocha road, the last road east of Tena along the Napo. When not dodging two propane gas tanks that roll like ninepins atop the truck, I try to take in the roadside attractions. This is humid tropical forest, the product of about four meters of rain a year, and is spectacularly lush: in a survey in 1987, local botanists found that 10 percent of the trees here were new to Western science. Here and there, human encroachment has changed the forest, encouraging a mix of useful species like palm and balsa. The Quichua and settlers — the latter known as *colones* — plant *chacras*, or wild gardens, with sweet manioc, plantain, papayas, sweet potato, oranges and lemons, peach-palm, and some pineapple. They grow coffee for cash, as well as cacao, whose bulbous fruits congeal right on the trunk of the gnarled little tree, a trick of nature called cauliflory. Amid the trees, the scattered settlers' houses teeter on stilts like ostriches, the heat shimmering off their corrugated tin roofs and their unshuttered windows open to catch the syrupy breeze off the Napo.

The truck halts suddenly, and in the gloom along the gallery of trees I can see a narrow path. My rooftop companions, young Quichua men on their way home from Tena's market, toss my bag over the side, and the truck is rolling as soon as I plant one foot on solid ground. In seconds it's gone, and utter silence returns. A small sign nailed to a post beckons, however. "Jatun Sacha," it says, pointing up the trail. It's slippery, even a month before the rainy season begins, and ascending is less like hiking than climbing a greased pole. In twenty minutes, however, a small encampment of tin-roofed huts materializes. In the center of the clearing a small group of people surrounds a bearded, bespectacled young man who is holding something in his hand. On closer inspection, the thing in his hand resolves into a tarantula as big as his palm, hairy and black as coal. He holds it gingerly between thumb and index finger and strokes its legs. "It's not angry, you see?" the tarantula-man explains. "The forelegs are not up in a fighting position."

Entertainment in Jatun Sacha is where you can find it. Freiden Schankal, the young man with the tarantula, discovered his eight-legged version of fun in a pipe in the latrine, a three-holer that is luxurious by the standards of rainforest research camps. Schankal learned about tarantulas and other forest creatures growing up a few miles away in his family's hotel, called Alinahui, or "good view," in Quechua. He is here now with about a dozen other Ecuadoreans to learn about potential rainforest products. Schankal also is shopping for a wife, however, and the arachnid lesson seems largely aimed at a young lady from Quito, Isabel Játiva. Still holding his pet, he wraps an arm around the young woman and asks me to take their photograph. They make a handsome trio.

Jatun Sacha is one of the most sought-after destinations for tropical biologists in South America, being the only research site in the western Amazon within a day's travel of a major city yet still relatively untouched by development. The camp sits on a hill that, if the forest were not there, would afford a nice view of the Río Napo. It was created in 1986 by an American botanist, David Neill, who bought this land with some help from American and Ecuadorean backers and kept much of it pristine. The reserve has grown to just over one thousand acres and has been deeded to an Ecuadorean foundation, although Neill still manages it. The station consists of five open-sided buildings made of rough-hewn planks, adequate to keep the rain off and at least some of the terrestrial insects out. Three buildings contain double bunks in barracks style, another a small storeroom and library, and the largest, the *reunion* house, a kitchen and dining room that doubles as a lecture hall. Standing in any one of them, you can reach out and literally touch the forest. Lighting is by candle, lantern, or flashlight, the generator being saved for emergencies and special occasions. Bathing is done a half hour's walk down a muddy path, in the Napo, though the walk back up tends to undo the effort. There is also a bar within ten minutes' walk, in a lone house inhabited by a colonist and his wife, two dogs, a transistor radio, and a pig, all of which appear to be at the edge of exhaustion. Almost-cold beer and the cool dryness of a shaded cement floor can be had there, and sometimes the dubious thrill of witnessing a cockfight.

Scientists come to Jatun Sacha for its astounding diversity of life. There are about 120 species of reptiles and amphibians living here, 450 species of birds, and at least 1,400 vascular plant species. These are remarkable numbers, and the camp guest book is filled with superlatives left by visiting biologists, although their comments might not work in a tourist brochure. "Great place for bugs," says one. "Keeps the lights on at night!"

Brad Bennett is chief plant-hunter at Jatun Sacha for the moment. "Come on over in the shade," he suggests in a high, dry tenor, offering a canteen of water with the flat, metallic flavor of recent boiling. He is a pale man, just over six feet tall, beefy but not soft. He moves without haste, part deference to the climate and part simply the outcome of the kind of youth where good days were spent dangling a fishing line in a Florida lake full of bass. Though he is thirty-five, there is still a boyish truancy in the tangle of his brown hair and the wispiness of the mustache that clings above his upper lip, and his easy smile and Everglades drawl put people at ease. People call him Brad from the moment they meet him.

Brad got his doctorate in botany at the University of North Carolina, earning money to pay for it by working part-time as a homebuilder, a trade he loves almost as much as botany. His first ethnobotanical job was a plum, one of only a handful that exist in the field, at the Institute of Economic Botany at the New York Botanical Garden. He is now an assistant professor at Florida International University (FIU), which hired him with plans to establish a world-class tropical biology department. With him here at Jatun Sacha are a crew of graduate students from Yale University and FIU, some Peace Corps volunteers who want to add some economic botany to their repertoire, and Ecuadorean students with similar interests.

"The forest here needs to be seen as a thing of value for it to be saved," Brad explains as he starts his afternoon lecture in the reunion hut. "It's a source of renewable products. Pasture or crops don't usually last. The Quichua know this, they just need help in figuring out how to make it pay." The Quichua have learned to trust Brad, largely due to the good word of Rocío Alarcón. Alarcón is an Ecuadorean ethnobotanist who knows more about the indigenous population of the country than most anyone in Ecuador. She is petite and delicately pretty, with a disarming smile and a self-effacing manner that disguises a rugged constitution and determination that has earned her the respect of the Quichua. Despite being in her eighth month of pregnancy, she is here to help with the teaching and plant collecting.

Brad makes an unlikely-looking professor, standing in flip-flops and muddy trousers hung with clinging burrs like Christmas ornaments on a tree. The look and setting are right for the topic of sustainable development, however. Absentmindedly scratching his insect bites, Brad explains the abstractions of current value, cost versus price ratios, yields per growing season, and other business argot that economic botanists are trying to apply to the rainforest. "What we want," he says, "is to try to make the link between indigenous use of a plant and a *product*. It's easy to find uses but it's very difficult to make the connection between a product, whether it's a medicine, thatch on a roof, or paint used on pottery, and the actual plant. So that's what ethnobotany is, at least to me. We are also looking at the economics, but eventually I run out of my expertise. I can provide this information, I can point to products that have potential, but I'm not a business person, and I can't turn it into a cosmetic or antibiotics. What I think is important is that whatever happens, we promote products that have a use first at the local level."

One such product from Ecuador is *tagua*. Tagua is a nut whose endocarp — the inner layer of the wall of a ripe fruit — is as hard and white as ivory. The U.S. environmental group Conservation International has engineered a trade boomlet in tagua buttons by encouraging clothing manufacturers to capitalize on its green cachet. It's a renewable product because taking the nut doesn't destroy the tree, and it's harvested from the rainforest, often by collectives of indigenous people and colonists. "I'm not sure how much difference buttons and nuts are going to make," Brad says, "but they have value in raising people's awareness. If people say, 'Well, if I wear this button made out of tagua, that's not going to save the forest, but at least I'm thinking about it, I can promote it and spread the gospel of sustainable use,' then in that aspect it's important."

The day's classroom exercises require the students to calculate comparative market values for potential forest products that grow near Jatun Sacha. Some, like the palm *ungurahau*, are already used by local people, while others are experimental. After the costs of managing, harvesting, and transporting forest products to market are calculated, profits are compared to those to be made selling the timber — a one-time gain — and then raising cattle on the cleared land. The numbers are encouraging; one two-and-a-half-acre plot Brad inventoried would yield over eleven hundred dollars. So long as no one gets too greedy and market prices don't shift too much, renewable harvesting could succeed here.

Lunch is served to the sound of shuffling feet on the gritty platform floor, bringing to mind summer-camp lodges. The diet here is spartan, featuring the palate-numbing staple, manioc, something like a potato served before its time, along with plantains, the wicked stepsisters of the banana that American consumers know. Papayas and oranges are the highlights of every meal. The diners tend to separate themselves linguistically; most of the North Americans speak little Spanish and only a couple of the Ecuadoreans have much command of English. Conversation revolves around insects and their various bites, what grows on damp laundry, various ways to dress up manioc, and deadly snakes. Besides students from Ecuador and the United States, there are a few of what one might call "jungle wanderers," people like hollow-cheeked, bandannaed Bryan Hayum, a Peace Corps volunteer from Boston, here to learn something about sustainable development before heading upriver for an assignment in the town of Coca. Hayum's in-

troduction to the rainforest was a little ruder than most. He was let off
at the trail head by a Quichua canoeman. He had no idea where he
was, it was getting dark, and of course it was raining. "They say you
shouldn't walk alone at night on these trails, because of the snakes," he
says, flicking cigarette ashes over the railing into the wet earth. "Like,
they're not going to bite if there's two of you, right? Well, I ended up
walking back to the river where I got left off, and I spent the night
sitting up against a tree in the rain. The mosquitoes weren't so bad, it
was the moths that kept me awake, batting me in the face. At dawn I
had bites all over me. I got the hell out of there and finally found my
way here. As it turned out, the night before I had come within three
hundred meters of the camp." He pauses to stamp out his smoke. "It
sucked, really," he says with a sardonic smile. "Just your basic Peace
Corps experience."

Hayum's destination, Coca, may prove drier than Jatun Sacha, but
it is certainly less serene. Coca is an oil town and is also an aptly named
way station for drug dealers on the way north. Coca is actually short-
hand for the town's official name, Puerto Francisco de Orellana, after
the famous Spanish explorer who came through here in 1540. With the
European's typical bluster, Orellana set off from Quito with Spanish
troops and Indians in search of a land rumored to be thick with
cinnamon trees. The Indians soon abandoned the venture, and the
remaining Spaniards were set upon by the Four Horsemen of the rainforest — hostile natives, disease, insects, and hunger. The expedition
finally came upon the Napo and built a crude brigantine on its banks,
in which Orellana and a few men sailed downriver in search of food to
bring back to the main party. They never came back. The Napo carried
Orellana and his men 375 miles and spit them into a huge river. From
there it was the ride of their lives. During the voyage, according to the
expedition's chronicler, Padre Gaspar de Carvajal, the Spaniards were
harried by one especially persistent group who, wrote Carvajal, were
the subjects of women warriors called the Amazons. A band of these
Amazons and their men attacked the Spaniards near the confluence of
this great river and the Rio Trombetas. "These women," wrote Carvajal, "are very white and tall and have hair very long and braided and
wound about the head . . . they are very robust and go naked save their
privy parts are covered; with their bows and arrows in their hands
doing as much fighting as ten Indian men. . . ." When Orellana reached
Spain and told the court of Charles V about his battle with the Amazons, he was ridiculed; tales of sea serpents and lakes filled with gold
may have been believable, but fighting women just could not be. Be-

sides, the legend was hoary, women warriors called Amazons having been part of ancient Greek mythology. However, the world's greatest river at least got a name worthy of its own legendary majesty.

The Napo that carried Orellana into history is Jatun Sacha's bathtub and laundry. After the afternoon lecture, some of Bennett's crew follow Alicia Grimes, a forester from Yale who is here for her second season, down for a swim. The forest ends abruptly about thirty feet from the river and opens to a rocky, breezy bank. The Napo's surface has a silvery, smooth surface that is deceptive. "You can't go in beyond a few feet," Grimes warns. Indeed, the current is so strong it could knock over a steer. Grimes dunks a pair of denims and scrubs them on a granite boulder worn round and smooth as a soccer ball. Except for her blond hair, she might be one of the Quichua women who come here to bathe (in groups, and fully dressed) and to pound their clothes clean.

There are no caimans to pounce on the unwary this far upriver, she assures, though they can be found farther downriver near Coca. "But there might be dick-fish," she warns with a smile. The dick-fish, as she calls them, are the *candirú* of Brazil, or the *carnero* here in the Spanish-speaking Amazon. Jungle trekkers, usually with a casual air meant to impress the listener with the depth of the horrors they have endured, love to talk about this diabolical fish. No longer than an aquarium guppy but as thin as a catheter, it's attracted to body fluids and is said to swim up any warm orifice, especially the urethra or vagina, and therein establish itself permanently by spreading a set of spines, causing severe pain and necessitating surgery to get the thing out.

Apparently the explorer K. F. P. von Martius was the first to write about the fish. His account in 1829 says that Amazonian men would tie up their foreskins with a string before bathing in rivers, and they never urinated in the water. If penetrated by the fish, they would treat themselves by drinking the fresh juice of a plant known as *xagua*. In 1930, E. W. Gudger of the American Museum of Natural History collected specimens and concluded that the fish was a bloodsucker. He called it *Vandellia cirrhosa*, and described it as scaleless and slimy, with a torpedo-like body and a spiny head, catlike teeth, and a suction cup for a mouth. Gudger said the fish is apparently attracted to most any body secretion, including urine. He even found a statement by a U.S. naval surgeon who said he had surgically removed the fish from the urethras of three men.

An American physician, John R. Herman, found reports that the green fruit of the *jagua* tree, *Genipa americana,* was the only way to get it out. The fruit is also known in Brazil as the *buitach* apple, and looks like breadfruit. The juice is drunk very hot like a tea and is said to dissolve the fish's skeleton. Chemical analysis of the fruit shows that it's full of citric acid, which indeed dissolves calcium. As for the name dick-fish, its unofficial, having been coined ad hoc by Grimes because of the way men in particular view this loathsome creature's genito-philia.

Back at the camp, I have time after dinner to dwell on the apparent inexhaustibility of the Ecuadorean rainforest's richness. Orellana came here four centuries ago looking for wealth from cinnamon trees. Now botanical treasure-hunters are back again, this time on the trail of valuable new drugs. And they're onto something already. Somewhere near here grows a healing plant little known to Western science but used for centuries by the Quichua living in these forests. Rumor and a little botanical research suggest that in fact this ancient cure may be the source of Shaman Pharmaceuticals' secret new drug, SP-303.

A yellowish morning seeps down through the canopy, as if breathed into being by the hidden birds cooing and sighing their languid "Sleepers Awake" to mark the slow shift in the forest continuum from darkness into light. At Jatun Sacha, sleepers lie in their bunks like lizards in a terrarium until the rude clang of a machete striking the stove's propane tank breaks the spell. Breakfast is ready.

While the camp residents straggle out into the woods or the latrine, Brad, already up for an hour, prepares his gear for a half-day expedition into the forest — a satchel for samples, a notebook and pen, a folding knife, a canteen with boiled water, and some manioc, also boiled. "Travel light in the woods," he advises. Brad's mission today is to take samples of tree sap to test for chemicals, some of which might be of commercial value.

The area around Jatun Sacha is essentially primary forest, meaning undisturbed and mature, although that is a slippery term. "It's a misnomer," Brad says as he stuffs the cuffs of his trousers into his socks before pulling on his knee-high rubber boots. "The Quichua here, and indigenous people all over Ecuador, actually manage 'primary' forest. You'll see secondary species in here, like cecropia, that tree that branches up at the crown and has the big palmate leaves. These are successional species. They fill in where fires or tree falls or cutting have opened up a hole in the canopy and let sunlight in. A lot of biologists turn up their noses at secondary forests. But I'm interested in how indigenous people *use* the forest, whether it's primary or 'disturbed' forests like this one."

Lauralyn Beaverson, the expedition's phytochemist, shows up with her assay kit stuffed with filter paper and pipettes in a backpack slung over one arm, her shoulder-length blond curls falling loosely over its green canvas top. She is in her mid-twenties, a dropout from the United States Naval Academy who transferred to FIU to learn chemistry in the out-of-doors from plants, the world's original chemists. Brad's Quichua informant, Theodoro, is coming along as well. Theodoro is in his early thirties, a stocky man wide at the cheekbones with merry eyes and skin the color and smoothness of an old violin. He lives nearby with his family, cultivating his *chacras,* hunting, fishing, and in recent years, earning money from cutting timber.

The Quichua culture is defined largely by its language, Quechua. Of Ecuador's three million indigenous people, most are highland Quichua living in the mountains. As many as ninety thousand, however, are lowland Quichua on the eastern side of the Andes. Those who live along the Napo or its tributaries are sometimes known as the Napo or Quijos Quichua, and are descendants of at least three groups: the Quichua from the highlands who migrated here, the Quijos of the Andean foothills, and the Záparo, originally a rainforest people. Theodoro, like most Quichua, speaks Spanish and wears Western clothes. Chain saws, shotguns, and Adidas shoes have replaced stone axes, blowguns, and bare feet. But these are surface effects. Theodoro still possesses a profound knowledge of the forest. His people, for example, have at least eighty different therapeutic uses for plants. Most are for treating parasitic infections, snakebite, inflammations, diarrhea, and the fungal infections so common in this wet climate. While a few of the plants have already been studied by Western scientists, many others are still unknown or poorly understood.

Theodoro is intrigued by the North Americans' interest in Quichua plants, especially medicinals. Haven't you got powerful medicines of your own? he had first asked Brad. Why would you care about *mar pindu* (a plant used to wash clothes) when you have soap in a box? Logical questions, especially after centuries of being told by Westerners that modern ways, from the Bible to brassieres, are superior. In fact, Theodoro and his family take Western medicines. Yet they still use plant medicines, along with 80 percent of the population of developing countries. Theodoro is no shaman, but he knows where most plant medicines come from, when they should be harvested, and how to prepare them. In fact, even within the boundaries of the camp, Theodoro says, there are healing plants. He points out a bushy tree about eight feet high with voluptuous, two-toned blossoms the color of fresh cream outside and salmon pink inside that hang like overturned pitchers from long, drooping stems, as if spilling out their scent. Their fragrance is potent; one of the students sleeping in the nearest bunkhouse found it so overwhelming she had to move to another hut. "We call this plant *huanduj*," says Theodoro. "You take the bark and use the water from it and drink it. It puts you to sleep. You get drunk." He smiles, the slightest curl at the corners of his wide mouth. "It is very strong. Also, you use it for sickness." What kind of sickness? He shrugs his shoulders.

"You have to live with the people first," Brad explains as we start down the trail. "People don't realize how much hard work goes into ethnobotany. You have to stay in peoples' homes, play with their kids, eat their food, drink their *chicha*." Chicha is the local equivalent to beer, made out of manioc first chewed by women and then spit into an earthenware pot to ferment. The best chicha is reputedly made by the prettiest women. "The taste isn't bad," Brad says, "but the *lumps* . . ."

Brad says the *huanduj* plant belongs to the genus *Brugmansia*, in the same family as the deadly nightshade, the potato, and the eggplant. Several species grow in the eastern Andes, from the highlands down to the lowland jungle, and various Ecuadorean indigenous cultures use different parts for different purposes. The sap or the flowers may be applied to the skin to treat pain, while juice from the inner pulp, if ingested, is said to give visions of the future. Despite the redolent scent of the flowers, it's the leaves, bark, and seeds that manufacture the powerful tropane alkaloids that give the plant its narcotic effect. As with so many Andean plants, *Brugmansia*'s use by indigenous people was recorded by the Frenchman La Condamine in the eighteenth century, and again by von Humboldt and Bonpland in the nineteenth. Several Amazonian cultures use the leaves to treat rheumatism and even feed it to dogs to make them hunt better. Among the Shuar Indians to the south of the Napo, misbehaving children are given a drink made from the plant so that, when intoxicated, they will be admonished by the spirits of their ancestors.

Theodoro leads the way along the path, accompanied by another Quichua informant, Cesar Gabriel Grefa Mamallacta, known simply as Gabriel. Above, crowns of the tallest trees, the emergents, have burst out of the canopy and spread their branches wide like the spokes of an umbrella. The shorter understory trees reach various heights — experts say they can distinguish as many as five strata between ground and crown in the rainforest — and spread their branches and leaves in more elliptical shapes. Leaves are rarely lobed like those in temperate forests but are heart-shaped, lanceolate, or linear, and are often thick and shiny, with pointed ends, called drip tips, that encourage water to slide off. Direct sunlight reaches down in scattered shafts, and the light-starved undergrowth is spread thinly yet is of enormous variety. To the wide-eyed newcomer, the scene induces a dumbfounded inability to focus. Von Humboldt once remarked of the Ecuadorean forest, "One divines, but one does not distinguish." The rainforest's effect is more than just visual, however. It pricks the tactile senses with organic overtones of mold, slippery mud, and the unseen trickle of water. A single plant is a small planet of texture, with waxy leaf surfaces, coarse woody branches, perhaps a sheen of hairlike fibers on its stem, and tiny flowers with petals as soft as a cygnet's feather. The straight, smooth trunks of the trees lend geometry to the irregularity of the landscape. The fig trees, *Ficus*, for example, have flange-like buttress roots that radiate from their bases along the forest floor like six-foot-high medieval walls, and help support the tree. Other trees spread prop roots, less massive than buttresses, that flare like a tripod's legs.

This is fairly dynamic forest, Brad explains, with about 3 to 5 percent of it opening up every year. Termites can so weaken trees, or epiphytes make them so top-heavy, that they blow over quite easily in a windstorm, each tree taking others whose fates are tied to theirs by lianas. "Really, the most dangerous thing about being in a rainforest like this is during a windstorm when you can get hit with falling limbs or trees," Brad says. A fallen tree is a seminal event in the rainforest. Sun shines through the gap within the canopy and changes soil temperature and humidity. Within days, a green invasion of successional species takes place. These new plants are distinct and easily identified: cecropia, which invades a gap within the first year; the energetic *Trema micrantha* tree, which grows up to twenty-three feet a year; palms of several varieties; the colorful, lobster-clawed *Heliconia*, from the Greek *helios*, for the sun; and numerous vines and shrubs.

Brad stops at an especially thick tree whose bark is dark and smooth. "This is *Otoba glycycarpa*," he says, "from the family Myristicaceae. This is the kind of tree we're after." He pulls a Gerber knife from its sheath, unfolds the blade, and makes a horizontal cut in the trunk. The bark is tough and resists. "Gringo knife," Brad mutters in Spanish. The Quichua laugh; it's well-known that gringos never seem to be able to keep their knives or machetes very sharp. Finally the bark yields and a milky sap seeps from the cut. Lauralyn holds a hollow glass pipette up to the cut and snares a teardrop of sap, which she dabs onto a piece of white filter paper.

"This should give us something interesting," she says. "The Myristacaceae are full of alkaloids." It's Lauralyn's job to test samples for any of several compounds that might serve medicine or chemistry. As Lauralyn bleeds the tree, Brad asks Gabriel and Theodoro if the sap has a use. The two Quichua look closely at the tree bark, scan up to its crown, and study the sap, their brows furrowed, like jewelers examining an unfamiliar stone. "No," says Gabriel in Spanish after conferring with his partner in Quechua. "We don't think this one is used. Not by the Quichua."

We move on to other trees, make more cuts with the gringo knife, and watch them bleed. One exudes a smooth, buttery sap that is sweet to the taste. "I don't recommend sampling plants this way," Brad says as he dabs it to his tongue. Brad pronounces the tree's scientific name for the Quichua. "El nombre is *Symphonia globulifera*." Gabriel gropes beneath his T-shirt, whose front, with an illustration of a fox in sunglasses on a surfboard, proclaims him to be a "Surf Rider," and draws out a notebook to copy this down. Raised in a thatched-roof house nearby, he says he wants to be a forester, a compromise between the modernity of Tena and his traditional Quichua life. Brad asks about the tree's wood. It is nut hard, they say, grows to medium height, and is common in this region but has no local use.

We soon come upon a plant that does have a local use. Gabriel calls it *Maria panga*. The bush is from the Piperaceae family, one with some five hundred species in the Americas and two thousand worldwide. A species in the Pacific Islands is used as a sleeping potion, while another species in the northwestern Amazon, when added to tobacco and urine, makes a poultice to treat the bites of the *cungamanda* ant. We in the North have only managed to find one common use for the Piperaceae: a source of white and black pepper. The five-foot-high bush we have found, Gabriel explains, is called *candela* in Spanish after the way the small flowers are densely packed on an erect, candle-like stalk. The Quichua use it to treat headaches. Gabriel seems pleased that the group has finally found something that Brad deems worthy of writing down in his notebook.

Farther down the trail, Brad makes his own "discovery." He kneels by a knee-high shrub and, using his fingernails, gently tears open a hole in its hollow, rubbery stem. A horde of tiny ants streams out onto his fingers. "These are lemon ants. Taste just like lemon." Brad licks the ants off his finger. "They also have a nice, satisfying crunch," he mumbles, using a finger to keep the ants from escaping down his lower lip. "Those snack experts at Kraft work real hard to achieve that kind of texture."

"That's gross," Lauralyn observes.

"*Don't* try this at home, kids," Brad warns in mock television voice. In fact, the plant in which these ants live, *Duroia hirsuta,* looks very much like a shrub from the Melastomataceae that is home to a quite different ant with a nasty bite that it uses to protect its home from predators.

Theodoro draws Brad's attention to a shrub sporting four-foot, sword-shaped leaves with rose-colored borders. "This is *mar pindu,*" he says. "We cultivate it and use it to wash our clothes. It makes them very white. I learned this from my grandparents, and they from theirs. We also use it to wash our hair." Brad takes this down and gives Theodoro his word for the plant, *Cordyline fruticosa.* We move off the path, Brad barreling through the underbrush, elbows and arms held up at shoulder height like the linebacker he used to be as an undergraduate at Bucknell University. The idea seems to be that the commotion will scare off anything unsavory in the leaf litter. The silent Quichua, meanwhile, seemingly palm the ground with their bare feet, and if they find the gringo's abandon amusing, they don't let on.

"Ah, to be a botanist wandering in the jungle," Brad calls out. The lemon ants seem to have had a rapturous effect. "This forest is so *complete,*" he says, his eyes scanning the gallery above. "Two hundred and fifty types of trees in this one small plot." In describing nature, the botanical science stands second to none, yet it has no terminology to express the emotions that such a place inspires in someone whose life revolves around plants. With not ten, not one hundred, but thousands of the most exotic objets d'art hanging literally within one's reach, one thinks of the first archaeologist who crawled into Tutankhamen's tomb. And though these artworks of nature are hugely complicated, they can be understood, they can be *possessed,* if only there were enough time. How tantalizing and fragile a predicament.

After an hour's walk in the rainforest, one's eyes become accustomed to the gloom and begin to catch the small details, especially colors, that at first are lost in the wash of green. There are the burned orange bracts of heliconia plants; tiny bright blue seeds half-buried in the leaf litter underfoot, fallen from which tree neither Brad nor the Quichua know; and the delicate five-petaled flowers, yellow as kernels of corn, of the hallucinogenic liana *Banisteriopsis,* provender of the

Amazonian gods. While the colors are easy to spot, searching for a particular species, or more difficult, a new one, is an art. Edward O. Wilson, who has spent a good part of his life wandering through rainforests, offers naturalists this advice: stop and drop to your knees. "Do your exploring right then and there," he says, "without getting up off your knees through the morning." Wilson should know; he once identified forty-three species of ants in a single tree in the Peruvian Amazon, probably a world's record for ant species in one spot. He says this: "You must have the hunter's instinct and the naturalist's trance. When you go out in the forest, you have to have a special property of hunting, in that you don't know what it is you are hunting. You are prospecting." You start prospecting, he says, by narrowing your field of vision down to a few meters, then down to just one or less. Soon there comes an unhinging of the mind, a separation of the senses from all that is outside your gaze, from the sounds of your companions on the trail, even from thoughts of where you are, from the tactile pressure of the ground against your knees, from the tug of your backpack's straps over your shoulders. Stare at a rotting log and creatures begin to materialize. Spiders no bigger than the letters on a printed page leap in surprise. Feathery, steel-blue mosquitoes float in and out of view. An ungainly beetle pushes up from under a rotting leaf and struggles to secure a hold on its serrated edge. A single-minded leafcutter ant follows its colony's invisible chemical highway homeward, a fragment of lime-green leaf ten times its size raised on its back like a spinnaker on a sailboat. A black and yellow centipede undulates, wrapped in a blanket of hairy spines like a strip of Velcro. Each conducts its life according to the conditions laid down by its environment, matched by natural selection to its niche in the forest. Into what in toto seems like a biological maelstrom, each organism contributes its orderly, measured life.

What many tropical botanists like Brad are now trying to do is connect all this, the ecology of the place, with economics. Over the past three years, for example, he and Rocío Alarcón, working in plots here in Jatun Sacha, have gathered ethnobotanical information on some five hundred tree species, and sent about one hundred plant specimens to the National Cancer Institute, where about twenty have been chemically tested.

What Brad is looking for today is a tree called *Virola peruviana*, from the Myristicaceae family, one known for its alkaloids and by many Amazonian cultures as a sacred tree with healing and hallucinatory powers. He finally finds one a few meters away from the trail, a medium-sized tree, about a foot and a half in diameter, perhaps seventy feet tall. A woody tendril hangs down alongside it, seeking earth and nourishment for its owner, an aroid on a branch somewhere in the gloom above. The leaves are pinnate (leaflets arranged on either side of a common axis, like a feather) and glossy. The flowers are tiny, like so many in the rainforest, and have a pungent fragrance. Brad cuts into the bark and a pale sap runs first clear, then blood red. Gabriel and Theodoro watch silently, frowning. Brad wonders from their expressions whether he has violated some taboo. "It's the nail," Gabriel explains. Brad is confused. "The nail that holds the tag," says Gabriel. "It will kill the tree." Many trees in Jatun Sacha have had identification tags nailed into them. Apparently the Quichua believe that even a single nail in a tree eventually may kill it. "It may be true," Brad replies. "Perhaps botanists should use only aluminum nails."

Lauralyn blots four samples of sap onto filter paper and packs them away in her knapsack. Brad is happy that he has a local species of *Virola* to test, and rewards himself with a quid of Red Man chewing tobacco. The day's collecting is done. As we head back toward camp, Brad wonders aloud whether there could be enough renewable products from this reserve to keep it from being cut. "We could be lucky," he says. "There is one tree here that could make the whole region worth saving." He pauses to spit. "The Quichua have used it for generations, and it's already worth a lot of money to the local economy." I wonder if he means Shaman's plant. Before I can ask, Gabriel suddenly leaps off the trail into the bush.

"Huatin! Huatin!" he croaks in an excited whisper. Theodoro leaps after him. Assuming a predatory crouch, they vanish in two blinks of an eye. Brad and Lauralyn stand rooted.

"What is it?" Lauralyn whispers.

"I think he said 'huatin,' " Brad replies. "At least I hope he did." He starts off after the Quichua. "It's an animal," he calls out over his shoulder.

"What *kind* of animal?" Lauralyn says, staying where she is.

"Oh, kind of a big rodent," Brad says before he too disappears into the bush.

We find Gabriel and Theodoro a few meters away, crouched over a depression where the red dirt has been dug up beside the buttress root of a fig tree. At the bottom of the pit is a hole, presumably where the huatin has taken refuge. The Quichua stand over it, clucking their tongues. The huatin is closely related to the agouti, a rodent found from Mexico to the southern cone of South America, and can grow up to three feet in length, with spindly legs, a brown pelt, and a prancing gait more like a deer than a rodent. When chased, it emits a high-pitched bark. Much to the disappointment of Theodoro and Gabriel, whose machetes would have made quick work of him, this huatin won't end up on a dinner plate.

Brad offers Gabriel some chewing tobacco as consolation. "Tobacco juice is good for insect bites," he recommends. The irony of a white man offering an Indian tobacco, incidentally labeled Red Man, escapes us at the moment. Gabriel chooses instead a leaf he has plucked from a fern. He secures the leaf between his two thumbs and, pressing his palms together as if in prayer, brings this reed to his lips and blows. A dying call, like a bird's lament, fills the spaces between the trees. Gabriel turns and heads back to the trail, tooting every now and then as if to announce that the intruders are taking human time back with them and leaving the forest to its own time, time that is measured out in the tidal ebb and flow of sap and the heartbeats of a million creatures.

The laboratory at Jatun Sacha stinks of chemicals and damp cardboard. Boxes of camp supplies share the corners with the nests of wasps, iridescent green beetles, and a lantern fly that now and then spreads its two-inch wings, lifts its alligator head, and takes a spin around the room. Over the lintel of the only door, a magnificent black and yellow spider has spun a web and quietly awaits callers.

The lab has neither running water nor electricity, and Lauralyn must make do with the light that filters through the two broad windows and the open doorway. She is cutting up leaves and grinding them with mortar and pestle, adding a bit of sand to speed the process. She pours a little methanol into each bowl to break down the plant's cell walls, mashes some more, then sets the mixture aside to let the methanol evaporate. Bits of pasty extract from small glass beakers that she prepared the day before are blotted onto filter paper, then fastened on a line strung across the room to dry. Theodoro sits on the threshold alternately watching Lauralyn and the spider go about their work.

If a plant's chemistry shows nothing remarkable here, specimens will probably go no farther than a file drawer at the herbarium in Quito and the New York Botanical Garden, with a note reading something like "No. 3785, Bombacaceae, riverine, 1.5 kilometers from Jatun Sacha, June 25, 1992." But if Lauralyn finds something unusual, it may enter the pipeline to the drug industry. If a drug were actually discovered from a local plant, however, no one here at Jatun Sacha is likely to get rich. Their rarefied botanical tastes run to habitat distributions or pollination strategies rather than contracts and royalty checks. As for the Quichua, talk of patents and royalties might as well be messages written on the sands of Mars. They are a people who are struggling just to lay claim to their own land and to feed their families. No one has ever explained the notion of intellectual property. Not yet, anyway; Brad, for the moment, is working on local marketing schemes. One step at a time, he says.

Lauralyn's field assays are crude, she explains, just a quick yes or no on whether the plants contain any of the major bioactive compounds. To find an alkaloid, she adds to each blotter a chemical called the Dragendorff reagent, after the man who first applied it to this use. In another simple field assay, she applies antimony chloride to a sample on a blotter, then gently heats it over a flame. If the sample turns purple or brown, she has a different kind of hit — either cardiac glycosides or saponins. Cardiac glycosides get their name in part because they can be fatal to normal hearts. In small amounts, however, they jump-start hearts that need stimulation to keep pumping. Saponins are soap-like compounds found in many tropical plants that destroy the fatty component of the cell membrane. Poisons employed by South American Indians to kill fish in streams often contain saponins, which interfere with respiration and cause the fish to rise to the surface, where they can be netted or speared. These compounds all are well-known and many are already the basis of drugs. The point now is to find new ones with unusual molecular structures that could have heretofore unknown effects on living things.

"An *Osteophloeum* we bled yesterday scored really high," Lauralyn reports as she holds a piece of blotter paper over the blue circle of a flame from her portable gas stove. "It's got lots of alkaloids, which is what you'd expect, since it's an hallucinogen. And the mar pindu that the Quichua use to wash their clothes, that was positive for saponins." Theodoro looks up from the doorstep and smiles at the mention of mar pindu. Some of Brad's team had collected some growing at the edge of the camp and washed their clothes with the plant's blood-colored leaves, succeeding only in staining their clothes bright red. "They should have asked us how to do it first," he says. There are, he says, other powerful plants right here at Jatun Sacha. "You have to know how to look," he says with a smile but does not elaborate. But then why should the Quichua reveal their secrets? If outsiders find anything of value here, why wouldn't they simply take it, as they have done with the Quichua's land, their gold, their rubber trees, and now the very forest that sustains them? The violent history of the colonization of the

Americas hangs over the Amazon like the guilty memory of a cruelty once committed that one would rather forget.

Brad limps up to the lab carrying a plastic box, sits down heavily on the front stoop, and pulls his right knee up to his chest. Protruding from his flip-flop, his right big toe sports a deep gash and is marbled with the purplish signature of infection. "I rammed it into something in the dark, night before last," he explains. Stuffing his foot in a damp rubber boot and bounding down muddy trails has not helped it. He snaps open his field medical kit and draws out a Q-Tip, its cotton ends matted from weeks in the damp air, and a small, unlabeled glass jar filled with an ocher, resinous pool of liquid. With the Q-Tip, he spreads a dab from the jar on the cut. The liquid oozes over the toe, casting a faint but not unpleasant odor something like burned barbecue sauce. Several more applications make the whole mess look gorier than ever.

"That looks like nail polish," Lauralyn observes.

"Nail polish?" Brad replies. "I *never* wear my nail polish when I'm out in the field."

Lauralyn laughs, a breathy staccato that is more punctuation than release.

"No, it's not nail polish," Brad says. "It's very special stuff. Maybe magic, maybe medicine. If it works like they say, it'll fix this cut in no time flat. Right, Theodoro?"

Theodoro nods solemnly. "It is powerful," he says. "It is *sangre de drago.*"

"Sangre?" Lauralyn says. "That means blood. Oh! Is that Blood of the . . ."

"Yep," Brad replies. He screws the top back on the jar and holds it up on the tips of his extended fingers, as if he were displaying a Fabergé egg. "Blood of the Dragon."

The sound of packing tape being stripped off its roll can be heard from the lab, where Lauralyn is boxing up her chemicals and glassware for the trip back to Quito. It's the last day of the expedition. Camp residents collect laundry, still damp despite days of hanging out on lines, and stuff it into backpacks, chatting all the while of hot showers, flush toilets, clean clothes, and plates piled high with meat and green vegetables served on the white tablecloths of Quito's wood-paneled restaurants.

Nixon Revelo E. Atuntaqui stands in the camp's central clearing and watches the Americans' eager preparations with a sardonic smile. He is a handsome man in his early twenties, with features in sharp relief: high cheekbones, square chin, broad shoulders suspending a sinewy torso, and a head of hair that stands at attention like the bristles of a horsehair brush. He looks every bit the Inca. During Brad's stay, Nixon has played the role of camp joker, bridging the gap between the cultures with droll humor. Evenings, he would hold court at the bar down the road, the last to arrive and the last to leave, drinking beer and listening while Bryan Hayum, the Peace Corps wanderer, smoked and played pathetic songs by Leonard Cohen on a mangled old guitar.

Nixon, who is conducting research on a project he vaguely describes as "important tree work," is said to know about the Quichua medicine, sangre de drago, which certainly fits the description that Shaman's Lisa Conte revealed in New York — a wound-healer commonly used by indigenous peoples of the western Amazon. As Nixon watches the students pack up their gear, he remarks that now he can get back to his important work — tending the sangre de drago plants. "You know about this plant?" I ask. "Of course," he says. "Would you like to see some?"

Nixon leads the way down a trail, almost overgrown and unmarked, that proceeds for about half a mile before ending at a clearing about the size of a tennis court where the earth has been plowed and pushed into long hummocks. Seedlings poke up out of the dirt, their pale green leaves spattered with mud from the last rain. At one side of the field, on two makeshift tables about thirty feet long, rows of pots and dirt-filled plastic bags hold more seedlings.

"There are thousands of them here," Nixon says as he walks along the line of plants like a doctor making his rounds, pausing here and there to scrutinize a particular seedling as if to divine its special needs. Each has been germinated from seeds harvested by Nixon and the Quichua that have been hired for this job. We walk out into the field of young seedlings, their leaves shimmering in a light breeze. Nixon looks as if he is standing knee deep in an alpine stream. He bends suddenly and pinches something off a leaf. "Grasshopper," he says with contempt, and flicks it like a cigarette butt out toward the wall of trees. "They eat too much," he says. He looks around, searching for something in the air. "There," he points at a circling wasp. "They kill the grasshoppers. We need to bring them here. I wish I knew how to do that." Nixon explains that the seedlings go from the pots into the ground, eventually to be replanted in other plots near Jatun Sacha to mature into trees. The North American botanist in Quito, David Neill, is looking for land to plant them and more people to tend them. In the meantime, Nixon's work will help him get his degree from the Catholic University in Quito.

Back at the camp, the bunkhouses are mostly empty now. Satisfied that everything is in order for the next group due in tomorrow, Brad hoists his backpack. "Before we go," he says, "I'll show you something." He walks past the florid, nocturnal *Brugmansia*, its blossoms half closed against the sunlight, to a nondescript, spindly tree, about thirty feet tall, with a few rubbery-looking branches splitting off from the main trunk. Only its leaves could be called impressive; heart-shaped and lime green, they are the size of paper plates, each held high and horizontal to catch the sun's rays. The tree's bark is smooth but mottled with grayish blemishes, like age spots. Brad takes out his knife and slices off a thumbnail-sized piece. The wound shows white for a moment before bubbles of burgundy sap materialize. Up close, the stuff smells like pork barbecue. "This is *Croton*," Brad says. "That's the genus. It grows like a weed in light gaps, and this one is only about two years old. That sap is the Quichua medicine, sangre de drago." He looks down at his right foot, now encased in his mud-caked rubber boot. "I hope it works," he says.

On the drive back to Quito, Brad passes the time describing some of the high and low points of practicing economic botany. "Everybody wants to be an ethnobotanist now," he says as he swerves around the potholes of the Campa Coche road. "Some people just aren't cut out for it. There was one woman at Jatun Sacha who was real quiet, until one day at the dinner table she just covered her face and started screaming, 'I can't take it anymore. I can't take it anymore.' Scared the hell out of the rest of us." He slows the van to a crawl and creeps over a narrow bridge of freshly cut planks thrown across a rushing stream. "This bridge reminds me of one of the other hazards," Brad remarks. "The oil workers. You'll find them out here in the bush sometimes, Texans and Oklahomans flown in by helicopter to look for oil. They wear cowboy boots out here in the bush and carry bags of black-eyed peas and bottles of Jack Daniels. I was stuck once when one of these bridges washed away, so I talked some good ole boy to a couple of 'em and they jumped on a John Deere and in two hours they'd built a new bridge. But I had to keep 'em away from my female students the whole time."

The lure of Quichua hallucinogenic plants also has caused trouble at Jatun Sacha. The previous year a couple of Brad's North American students were bathing down at the Napo when a Quichua boy in a dugout canoe stopped to investigate. They asked the boy if he could sell them some ayahuasca, and pretty soon the Quichua stopped coming to the camp. "It took a while to convince them we weren't here for some kind of *luuuv*-in," he drawls. One of these Americans, Brad recalls, was decidedly weird. "He had a strange affect. He'd rock back and forth when he talked, would use exaggerated gestures. We had a radio on one night at the camp and he did this very strange dance, waving his arms all over. It scared one of our Quichua cooks, Marlena Salazar. That night, I heard her cry out from her bunk, she was sobbing uncontrollably. Rocío knows the Quichua better than anybody, and she finally calmed her down. It turned out that this guy, his whole appearance and his mannerisms, fit perfectly with a mountain spirit that the Quichua believe roams the night and rapes women.

"The next day, I was outside Marlena's cabin and I noticed that her shoes were sitting out on the steps. They were burning, smoking. I asked what was going on, but Rocío told me to be quiet, not to notice. I found out later that in her culture, it was a defense against this spirit. If she died while she was at Jatun Sacha, the spirit would follow her soul and attack her in the afterlife — forever. The only way to keep that from happening was to burn her shoes. My God, those shoes were probably worth a couple weeks' pay!"

Picking the right people for fieldwork is tricky, he says. "I try to choose people who've worked, who've had to pay their way through college, who've been on their own. The ones whose mom and dad have said, 'Hey, why don't you go to South America for the summer? Here's a check,' don't usually have the desire it takes. I like 'em hungry."

In Quito, we check into a hotel, shower, and head out for a steak dinner and a pitcherful of margaritas. We have two days of comparative luxury before we're to head northwest to the Pacific coast. Brad's mission is to travel up the Cayapas River to the last settlement of the Chachi people before the river disappears into the Cotacachi-Cayapas reserve, a tract of untouched primary forest that climbs from the humid lowlands up the western slope of the Andes.

I use the two days in Quito to find out more about sangre de drago. Rumors of North American interest in the Quichua medicine have circulated among indigenous groups in Ecuador, where it can be found in village markets in the Oriente and in the brujos' huts in the forest. But information about who's buying it up is scarce. Spanish and Swiss companies are said to be quietly buying supplies of it, and a Belgian scientist has taken samples to Antwerp for analysis. The biggest footprints on the trail, however, are those of Shaman Pharmaceuticals.

They lead to Quito's National Herbarium, a squat concrete building set on the edge of Quito's large central park, La Carolina. There, much of the knowledge of Ecuador's flora resides in the mind of the lean, bearded botanist David Neill.

Neill is a thirty-nine-year-old of very few words. He's of medium height and built thin as lattice, with an angular face squared off by a mustache-less beard that gives him the look of a young Lincoln. He works for the Missouri Botanical Garden in St. Louis, but has adopted Ecuador as his home. If not the St. Peter to Ecuador's heavenly rain-forests, he is at least their botanical pope, their ultimate interpreter. Like many botanists, Neill prefers time with his plants to conversation with strangers, the idea of which seems to strike mild panic in him. Once engaged, he seems to operate phytochemically, with a plant's sense of pacing.

Neill created Jatun Sacha in 1986 after spending several years in the Peace Corps and seeing how biological reserves worked in Costa Rica. He and a fellow North American partner spent two thousand dollars each and bought three plots of fifty hectares each along the Napo. With continued donations from Americans he eventually raised twenty-five thousand dollars to build Jatun Sacha. Now that it is run-ning relatively smoothly, Neill has turned some of his time to other pursuits, such as helping Shaman manage *Croton,* the source of sangre de drago. The company is especially interested in learning how to grow it on poor soils and land degraded by deforestation. Shaman would prefer not to create plantations but instead employ mixed agroforestry, growing *Croton* alongside other renewable commercial crops or timber as an alternative to traditional farming. Neill and Bennett are also investigating the distribution and the genetic diversity of *Croton* to see if there are other types of tree that are hardier, faster-growing, or pro-duce better medicine. In the meantime, Shaman is collecting bark by the container-load. In Ecuador alone, the company's goal for 1993 is thirty-three thousand pounds of dry bark collected from the wild. By 1996, it plans to have managed plots producing almost two million pounds of bark, rising to fourteen million pounds by 1999, and leveling off at about five and a half million pounds by the year 2000. In addition to Ecuador, Shaman is getting bark from at least one other country, Peru.

Sangre de drago's reputation in the western Amazon has only re-cently been tested scientifically. Neill says scientists have told him that they think something in the sap or resin helps transport fibroblasts to a wound to speed the healing process. It was once thought that an alkaloid in the resin called taspine was responsible. Belgian scientists have isolated another compound, however, called dimethylcedrusin, that they believe may be involved as well, especially in helping endothelial and epithelial cells grow around a new wound. They also found that taspine seemed to be active against herpes. Neither of these compounds, according to Shaman, is the source of its medicines, however.

The trail of sangre de drago also leads to a small company in Quito called DTM Inc. DTM stands for Douglas T. McMeekin, a man who might be called a tropical phenotype: a rangy, energetic American, with wisps of blond hair holding back baldness and an expressive face that emanates confidence, he has a knack for getting things done where others throw up their hands in dismay. McMeekin has adopted Ecuador and settled into a comfortable home of polished hardwood floors and Quichua artwork on a quiet street in Quito. "I would never go back to the States," he says firmly. "You can live well here without having to make a lot of money." McMeekin's curriculum vitae covers a lot of ground: coal miner and heavy-equipment operator in Kentucky, where he grew up; environmental consultant for oil and timber interests working in Ecuador; and general man-with-the-answer for people who want to do business in Ecuador's tropical wilderness.

"I believe in sangre," McMeekin says, an easygoing twang in his voice. "I use the stuff. I once had a couple of fever blisters on the inside of my mouth, so I got a toothpick and put a dab here, a dab there, and presto — the next day, they were gone. My mother comes here every year, and she used it on some kind of lesion she had on her forehead. It wasn't malignant, but she couldn't get rid of it. She put some sangre de drago on it, it got all red, and the next day it disappeared. I use the pure stuff. The stuff you buy in the markets is cut with alcohol because the pure compound has to be refrigerated. I tell you, with the worldwide interest in natural medicines . . . Well, I'm enough of an entrepreneur, I might just start bottling the stuff myself."

McMeekin does not bottle sangre (an Ecuadorean company called Renase, or Natural Forest Remedies, does, however). Instead, he supplies bark and resin from Ecuadorean *Croton* to Shaman. His first shipment, of raw latex, was held up by Ecuadorean officials for over a year. "It wasn't that export was forbidden. It just wasn't specifically *allowed*," McMeekin explains with a laugh. Since then, he says, the proper people have been seen and permits and papers signed. McMeekin now hires local people in the Oriente to cut down the fast-growing tree and strip the bark, which is bundled or bagged and goes to DTM's warehouse in Quito, where it's dried on a chain-link fence suspended above the floor. A month's worth of shipments to Shaman in 1992 amounted to about two thousand pounds of bark. "It's not enough to pose a deforestation problem," McMeekin assures. "It's a common successional species." Besides, he says, he and Neill have hired people to collect seeds and seedlings from the wild to create nurseries like the experimental one that Nixon tends at Jatun Sacha. Still, there is some suspicion in Ecuador about Shaman's intentions, in part because of McMeekin's involvement with oil companies.

The earliest reference to sangre de drago dates its use to the 1600s. A Spanish naturalist and explorer, P. Bernabé Cobo, recorded the use of sangre de drago during his voyage to Mexico, Peru, and Ecuador in the first decade of the century. Cobo said the indigenous peoples of Mexico had a tree called *ezpua huilt*, which meant tree that makes blood. It was a large tree with dark red latex and wide leaves, and the curative powers of the sap were widely known in the New World as well as in Spain.

Ironically, Richard Gill may have "discovered" sangre de drago fifty years before Shaman got to it. The villagers of Gill's Pacayacu region used something they called *languiki*, a Quechua word that Gill translated as bloody water. In the Napo region, Gill wrote, the Quichua called it *yaguarhuiki*, meaning bloody gum or paste. It was used in both Ecuador and Peru as an anti-hemorrhagic, as well as for intestinal fevers and pyorrhea. In Peru, it reputedly was popular for its effectiveness in stopping vaginal hemorrhaging. The medicine came from a tree fifty to sixty feet high with a diameter of eight inches and white flowers. Gill took a specimen of the plant to the New York Botanical Garden, where it was identified as *Croton*.

With its discovery of a compound in the plant that seems to work for respiratory syncytial virus and herpes virus, Shaman has shown not only that the tropical flora are far from exhausted as a source of new compounds, but that even the old dogs of medicinal botany know tricks we've never seen before. Moreover, Shaman has shown that the ethnobotanical approach may be the quickest route to new discoveries, which will no doubt lead others to follow the shaman's trail. That may be good, and it may not be. Brad notes that the growing interest in sangre de drago has pushed its price up severalfold, fine for dealers in Quito, but not so good for poor people who have seen the price skyrocket in their village markets. As for Shaman's promises to cut in indigenous peoples, the Quichua as a group are not partners in Shaman's collecting venture; Doug McMeekin and his hired day-laborers are. Shaman officials say they intend to share profits if and when SP-

303 is approved and starts selling. However Shaman works out the details, expectations among the Ecuadoreans are likely to run higher than what Shaman can or will meet; the worlds of the rainforest Quichua and corporate investors are galaxies apart. That's why Brad keeps North American business at arm's length, and why, as he prepares to make the first botanical expedition into the farthest reaches of Chachi country, he advises his team not to expect, or even hope, that some miracle drug will drop from a tree. "Rainforest drugs are a long shot," he warns. "If we find something, it's a long way to making it as a drug. If it does make it, the Chachi should share the profits, but it's tricky. A big influx of attention, or of money, can tear apart an indigenous community." It's like most of the romantic notions about the rainforest and its people, he says: it doesn't last long in the heat of the tropical sun.

10

The Vainilla Express

Ecuador's three million indigenous people are divided into seven major ethnic groups. Some, like the highland Quichua, have become largely acculturated, while others, like the Waorani and the Achuar in the Oriente, are still living much as they have for centuries. Beginning in the 1960s, a variety of organizations representing indigenous peoples in the Amazon, such as CONFENIAE and CONAIE in Ecuador and COICA in Peru, have sprung up. Federations representing subpopulations of many ethnic groups also have formed, such as FOIN, which represents the Quichua of the Napo region. Some have begun to win a certain amount of political clout, which they are using primarily to gain control over traditional lands. But the federations don't always agree with one another, or within their own organizations, on how to share the spoils. The Quichua, for example, consist not of one nation but hundreds of communities, and getting a majority to agree to anything is, as Charles de Gaulle once remarked ruefully of France, as likely as getting unity in a country where there are 265 different kinds of cheese.

Besides timber, one of the principal spoils at issue in Ecuador is oil. Much of Ecuador's oil lies under land traditionally claimed by indigenous peoples, and oil companies have taken advantage of the lack of solidarity among many indigenous groups to win their cooperation. The Texas-based company Maxus Energy Corporation, for example, has agreements with Waorani people who live on their own land in and around Yasuní Natural Park, a large tract of forest in the Oriente about two hundred miles east of Quito. The oil company CONOCO had spent years negotiating with the Waorani through the umbrella group CONFENIAE, but talks fell into disarray when the federation charged the North American groups Cultural Survival and the Natural Resources Defense Council, who were brokering the deal, of negotiating without Indian participation. CONOCO dropped out and Maxus moved in. A Waorani-only group formed, called ONHAE, but it was never clear who was in charge and whether it represented all the Waorani. Meanwhile, Maxus hired an anthropologist and provided local Waorani communities at Yasuní with goods and services, obviating the need to deal with ONHAE or any other indigenous organization. They now keep local Waorani communities happy with medicine, boat motors, and coloring books for children extolling the virtues of saving the forest, in the meantime driving a ninety-four-mile-long road into the park. Maxus has hired an Ecuadorean environmental group to plant commercially useful trees along the road for the Waorani, while manning checkpoints along the way to keep colonists out, the latter something no one has ever found a way to do once a road is built into an Amazonian forest. The company understands the necessity of keeping good relations with the Waorani; the people have a reputation for fierceness. In 1956 Waorani warriors killed a group of missionaries not far from where Maxus is drilling, and in the 1980s some Waorani got angry with the behavior of oil workers in their forests and killed several of them.

Oil companies also know how to keep the scientific community neutral. Oil exploration crews go places by helicopter that are otherwise unreachable, where they clear forest and set up air-conditioned living quarters for their field workers. Scientists who are invited along get into virgin territory, where they can also get flowers and fruits from the tops of felled trees they otherwise could not reach. They call this "salvage" botany and don't advertise the fact that the oil companies provide the free ride.

Environmental groups are trying to negotiate with indigenous groups and scientists as well, but with a different agenda. The richest groups are still the North Americans and Europeans, and among the more active now is SUBIR, short for Sustainable Use of Biological

Resources. SUBIR is backed by about $13 million from the charitable organization CARE International, the environmental group The Nature Conservancy, and the U.S. Agency for International Development. Its goal is to promote sustainable development of the kind of products that can be harvested renewably. Paul Dulin is SUBIR's director in Quito.

"Some groups, like the Shuar, know how to stand nose to nose with ministers or companies and tell them to eat shit," says Dulin. "Others, like the Chachi, are nothing but bait for loggers, coca producers, and so on. They're easy prey." SUBIR has been trying to help the Chachi federation learn the intricacies of landholding laws. "But they want guns, dynamite to fish with, booze, and batteries. So how do we balance this?" SUBIR is already running behind; a timber company, with help from the World Bank, is paying the Chachi five dollars a tree for their timber. So SUBIR wants to find alternatives to timber, like the fruit of the peach palm, part of the Chachi diet, to put into commerce. Traditional medicines used by the indigenous people have been low on SUBIR's list of potential products, but that has changed. "Now," says Dulin, "there is sangre de drago."

The people of northwestern Ecuador are not known to use the Quichua medicine, but their pharmacopoeia and their forests could very likely contain equally useful compounds. The region harbors some of the least-studied rainforest on the planet and is home to some of its most isolated indigenous people: along with the Chachi, there are the Awá and the Tsachila. But to find new plant products, SUBIR needed a first-class plant-hunter. There were few with credentials as good as Brad Bennett's. And Brad, long interested in the botanical knowledge of the Chachi, needed help to get to where the Chachi live. So, despite misgivings on both sides — Brad regards government-backed bureaucracies with suspicion, while his free-wheeling style strikes some at SUBIR as unpredictable — an informal collaboration was agreed to. SUBIR would help Brad and his team get up the Onzole and Cayapas rivers to the Chachi village of San Miguel, where he could stay with a Peace Corps worker, Patricia Jo Terrack. Terrack had been living with the Chachi for the better part of a year in a house built by missionaries in the 1970s but recently abandoned. Brad would get the lay of the land and help find informants among the local people. After that, some of his students would stay on through the summer, performing the first ethnobotanical survey of the region. At least, those are the plans as we climb a hilly side street in Quito to meet with Dulin at SUBIR's offices.

*   *   *

"Things don't look good," says Dulin, a tall man with dark hair parted down the middle, broad shoulders, and a fashionable European sports jacket worn over a starched Hawaiian shirt. Brad and his team — Jim Burch, a Ph.D. candidate at Florida International, and Lauralyn — sit around a conference-room table. Dulin is pointing to a spot on a wall map of Ecuador.

"There is a roadblock right about here," Dulin says. "And that is the only road into Borbón, where you were supposed to get a canoe for the final leg of the trip." Brad's eyes are fixed not on Dulin but somewhere in the middle distance, a sign that he is not happy. SUBIR has got itself in the middle of a political melee. Although they number only about twenty thousand souls, the Chachi are hardly close-knit. The Chachi federation, a fractious organization that SUBIR has been courting, is in dispute with San Miguel, one of its eight *centros*, or local communities. The federation views San Miguel as separatist. For its part, SUBIR is not terribly happy with the federation, having just given it fourteen thousand dollars that promptly disappeared, along with the federation's president. SUBIR now says handing over cash to indigenous groups is "counterproductive" and is offering "organization and services" instead. In the meantime, though, the Chachi are feuding among themselves. "We have to back off to avoid any exacerbation of this touchy political situation," says Dulin. "So you can't stay with Patricia Terrack, she's linked with San Miguel and you are linked with SUBIR. That would jump protocol and go against the wishes of the federation, although the federation is illegal anyway."

Seeing that the story's twists are losing his audience, Dulin recounts the previous two months' events. The federation recently held an election of its officers in Esmeraldas, the nearest city to Chachi territory. But the necessary quorum of members — 50 percent plus one — failed to attend. They voted anyway, but now those Chachi who were left out, most especially those in San Miguel, are protesting. The reason they could not attend, Dulin explains as he returns to the wall map, is the roadblock. Villagers there created the roadblock to protest against the logging companies. Dulin's second-in-command, Jody Stallings, a fair-haired, bearded biologist, takes over. "You see," he says with jungle-seasoned weariness in his voice, "the logging trucks have ruined the road, and people can't get to the markets. So they blocked the road. They call it a strike." He shrugs. "Things get complicated in Ecuador."

Dulin says if Brad *were* somehow to make it past the roadblock, he would have to camp out near San Miguel at a building owned by the

Ministry of Agriculture. "It hasn't been used in a long time," he says, adding dismissively, "There may be a stove there."

"Are there, like, bathing facilities there?" Lauralyn asks with a hopeful smile.

Dulin laughs. "Bathing facilities? Well, there's the river."

"What about the boat motor you promised us?" Brad asks.

Dulin's gaze remains fixed on the pencil he is rolling between his fingers. "Uh . . . that's another problem," he says. "They're still in boxes, unassembled. Regulations won't allow us to send them out until the technicians have put them together and test-run them."

"You could hire a canoe in Borbón," Stallings offers. "But I wouldn't spend too much time there. It's a hellhole, full of drug dealers. Get in and out fast, and keep your noses clean."

Burch, stroking his beard with quiet anxiety, ventures an observation: "One wonders about one's personal safety with this, uh, 'disarticulation' of the Chachis."

"Oh, no," Dulin assures, "no danger from the people. Just the bushmasters."

"They *are* pretty bad up there," says Stallings with a twisted grin. "Fer-de-lances too. The Chachi lose people fairly often. But there's always 'Thunder Woman.' "

"Thunder woman?" Lauralyn asks.

"It's a personal defense device," says Stallings, "a stun gun, shoots you with fifty thousand volts or so, but low amperage, so it doesn't kill you. You press it just above the snakebite and shock the victim three times, two seconds each time. It denatures the protein in the venom or something. They say it knocks you kind of silly. But Patricia has saved two Chachis and a dog in the last two months. Before they had it, the Chachi were shocking people with jumper cables from boat motors."

"Can we take one with us?" asks Lauralyn.

"Don't have any now," says Stallings. "If you get bitten, you should have enough time to canoe over to where Patricia is."

Dulin stands, explaining that he has some work to finish for an afternoon meeting. "Oh, and I'm sorry but you can't take our van to Borbón, the roads are just too bad," he says. "Actually, you just might want to relax and enjoy Quito for a while."

"And if you do decide to go anyway," Stallings adds with a wave as the botanists file disconsolately out the door, "be *careful* out there."

The hitch in plans is not unexpected: another law of the jungle states that few things happen on schedule. "It's always political," Brad says. "You have to play personal politics, and then practice diplomacy with the Ecuadoreans and the indigenous federation, then the gringos and the Ecuadoreans, then the gringos and the Indians. It's a lot of work." Brad knows it means including Ecuadoreans in his classes and expeditions, getting his scientific papers translated into Spanish and if possible into the language of any indigenous people who are involved, and offering his services and specimens to the herbarium in Quito. "Ecuador is still one of the best places in the world to do this kind of work," Brad explains as we ride in a taxi back to our hotel. "No guerrillas shooting at you like in Peru. There, you'd duck whenever a bus backfired. But even Ecuador is getting difficult. Nowadays there is a growing resentment about 'scientific imperialism' — you know, gringos down here doing it all."

At the hotel, Brad decides to find another way to get to San Miguel and starts calling his network of contacts in Quito. The rest of us read up on the Chachi and the Cotacachi-Cayapas reserve.

Despite almost five hundred years of European colonization in western Ecuador and perhaps thousands of years of indigenous civilization before that, only the Chachi and a few descendants of African slaves have lived in or near Cotacachi-Cayapas. There are no roads, no villages, not even a permanent research station inside the reserve, and no scientist has ever surveyed it thoroughly. Ecuador made it a reserve largely because nobody wanted anything to do with it. It's one of the wettest places on the Earth; eight meters of rain fall a year, the rivers are swift and flood frequently, and the soil, though volcanic, is poor and leached of nutrients — a classic primeval rainforest writ large, too dense, too difficult to negotiate, too forbidding to live in. And therefore safe, for the moment.

The reserve covers about as much area as Utah's Great Salt Lake, and lies on the margin of one of the ten biodiversity hot spots in the world, the Chocó formation, a biological crown jewel extending down from Colombia that is believed to be *the* most biologically diverse ecosystem on the planet. Why is this place so biologically diverse? To start with, the region straddles the equator. Biologists know that as you move toward the equator, the number of species grows, a phenomenon called the latitudinal diversity gradient. Greenland, for example, has 56 species of birds. Moving toward the equator, Newfoundland has 118 bird species, New York State 195, and Colombia, where the Chocó begins, has 1,525 bird species. The same trend applies to flowering plants. Of the roughly 250,000 species that are known now, 170,000, or 68 percent, occur in the tropics and subtropics, mostly in rainforests. In the United States and Canada, you will find only 700 native species of trees. Go south to the three Andean countries of Colombia, Ecuador, and Peru, and you will find tens of thousands in an area that covers only 2 percent of the world's surface. Alwyn Gentry established a world record for tree diversity at a site near Iquitos, Peru: about 300 species in each of two one-hectare plots. The diversity gradient applies to butterflies, ants, reptiles, just about anything that lives. The beetles alone are overwhelming — 18,000 species in a one-hectare site in Panama.

The Chachi legends say "the people," as many indigenous groups translate their names, moved into the Cayapas River area about four hundred years ago. The reason is unclear, although it may be more than coincidence that they left the Andes about the time the Spanish arrived. Their settlements are scattered around Cotacachi-Cayapas, but the Chachi rarely venture into the reserve. It is a forbidden place.

Laws protecting Chachi land are largely ignored, and colonists have slowly been encircling and invading Chachi territory. Colonists number about five thousand now, mostly subsistence farmers or loggers. There are laws protecting the Cotacachi-Cayapas reserve too, but that commitment is about as durable as the paper it's written on. There are supposed to be fourteen park guards, but in fact only two work there full-time. Logging companies have begun to chip away at the boundaries, and poachers occasionally make forays into the reserve, cutting timber and floating it down one of the six large rivers that traverse it. Moreover, Ecuador's Ministry of Public Works is building a road right through Cotacachi-Cayapas, which will doubtless bring in colonists.

Up until now, the world has for the most part ignored the Chachi. There is no complete dictionary of the Chachi language, nor any written history. One westerner who visited the outskirts of Chachi country is Bruce Cabarle, a forester with the environmental think tank World Resources Institute (WRI), in Washington, D.C. He went to the region to study how the local communities manage their land and agriculture. "Africans went there centuries ago to escape slavery," Cabarle says. "The Chachi probably were avoiding the Spanish. The area has been a lost world for the last three hundred years. These people are marooned."

Two days after Dulin put the damper on the expedition, SUBIR's Stallings calls Brad's hotel room to report that the political situation has shifted. The Peace Corps worker, Patricia Terrack, has negotiated passage for the botanists through the roadblock. "You'll have to find your own way to get there, though," he says. Brad hangs up and turns exultantly to his team. "Let's throw in an extra dozen Hershey bars for Patricia. And some cigars."

The next morning we are to fly to Esmeraldas on the Pacific coast. We have been joined by Fred Ogden, a twenty-one-year-old Yale biology student. Fred is a climber, and has brought ropes and pitons to scale trees and snare arboreal flowers, fruits, aroids, and bromeliads. Clean-cut and athletic, he has never been to a rainforest, and he is anxious to get started, although the soiled, ragtag look of Brad and his crew, the signature of weeks already spent in the forest, seems to have given him pause.

The next day, we stand outside the warehouse that serves as the Esmeraldas airport with twenty-five bags of gear around our feet. Brad tries to hire a truck to take us to Borbón. There is a roadblock, the driver says somewhat incredulously, as if it were worldwide news. He agrees instead to take two of us the fifteen miles into Esmeraldas, where we can look for someone more foolish than he.

Our search begins at Esmeraldas's waterfront street, a pot-holed, semi-solid rivulet of mud and trash alongside the Río Esmeraldas docks. This was the grand river that La Condamine traveled, whose hummingbirds, orange-feathered cock-of-the-rocks, and friendly natives had charmed the Frenchman. He wrote to his fellow Europeans that this was no fierce hinterland, no "land" at all, but a green element suspended in the treetops. Now the residents look a stranger up and down as if mentally sizing up his clothes for the time when, after they have been emptied of cash and stripped from his lifeless body, they might be put to better use.

Not all glances are so inclined, however. An employee at the local office of the Ministry of Agriculture introduces himself as Eudoro and tells Brad that although there is little chance of getting to Borbón, he will help the "American friends" look for a driver anyway. He leads us to one of the colorful rancheros parked by the river, inside of which several drivers are drinking their breakfast from a bottle in a brown paper bag.

"To *Borbón?*" one replies to Brad's question. "Forget it."

"They will throw nails beneath our wheels," says another.

"Unless they shoot first," says a third.

"Besides," says the first man, amused by the request, "even if there was no roadblock, the road is ruined from the logging trucks." He smiles, without benefit of several front teeth, and takes a drink of *pisco*. "Stay in our nice town for a while instead."

Several more discussions like this take place up and down the street, and Brad begins to lose hope. Then a truck pulls up across the street and a teenager jumps out. Eudoro hails him. "Sure," he says to Brad, "I'll take you there. Fifty dollars." Brad bargains but the driver knows there's no competition to undercut him, and simply smiles, showing the Esmeraldas insignia of abbreviated dentition. Brad pays and we agree to meet after lunch. As we walk past the back of the truck-bed, the odor of farmyard is unmistakable. "Oh, I'll clean that out," the driver says cheerfully. "It's just from the pigs I was carrying."

Brad repays Eudoro with a late breakfast at a local place called the Cafe Israel — four tables, two items on the menu (beans and rice with meat, beans and rice without meat), dogs underfoot, and a Jesus crucified in plastic over the threshold. Eudoro, who sports a pencil-thin mustache and buffed fingernails, wipes his cutlery clean before using it and tucks his tie into his shirt. He practices his English. "It is very cold here, yes?" he ventures. "You should tell the *New York Times* about Esmeraldas," he advises.

By the time the sun reaches its zenith, the team has been picked up and put in the truck-bed, and the journey to Borbón continues. Segundo, the driver, has brought along a friend whom he calls his "assistant." Soon, the paved road turns to dirt and the ruts begin. These are the Grand Canyons of highway hazards, though Segundo proves deft in negotiating them. He is equally deft when the engine sputters and dies, climbing all the way into the engine compartment and squatting on the engine block to extract the fuel line. Segundo is proud of his truck, his only means of income. Blowing a thimbleful of gunk out of the fuel line like this, he says, demonstrating, is what it takes to maintain such a fine vehicle. His assistant earns his title by crawling under the truck to help put the fuel line back in place. In ten minutes, we're rolling again.

The forest begins to close in around the road, the temperature rises, and we enter that state of suspended animation that travel on tropical roads induces in natives and foreigners alike. The monotony of the dirt track and the shadowy corridor of trees creates the feeling of traveling down a copper-colored river, with no end in sight. So it's with a mirage-like dreaminess that, three hours out of Esmeraldas, the roadblock hoves into view, far in the distance, like an island floating in an ocher stream.

What passes for a roadblock in the backcountry of Ecuador is an orange John Deere earthmover parked sideways on a bridge across a small stream. A couple of rancheros, empty of passengers, are parked on the other side of the bridge. About a dozen shacks constitute the town around it called Vainilla. Segundo stops three hundred meters short of the bridge and leaves his engine running. For the first time during the trip, he is not smiling.

Brad and I get out and walk toward the roadblock. On the bridge, about one hundred people are standing in a rough square, in the middle of which smolder remnants of burned tires, their smell clinging to the still, humid air. The people are a motley group: mostly men, some black, some Chachi, most a mix of the two with a little European blood blended in, and a smattering of women, many holding babies. These are country people, the colors in their shorts and thin cotton shirts faded from too many washings, their skin hatched like the leather of their broken-down shoes. Blue veins bulge from their calves; these are people who walk, and who carry the commerce of their lives on their backs. Yet their eyes are electric, not the impassive wells of the highland Quichua, and they flash as they take in these two gringos walking toward them.

Brad is thinking: "Uh-oh, I'm probably going to have to make a speech in Spanish here. What am I going to say to keep these people happy, that will let us get across but won't offend somebody and won't also make me look like some kind of politician-fool?"

Suddenly, a woman bursts through the crowd and runs toward us. She looks as if she just strolled off the boardwalk at Miami Beach, with thick red hair held high with what looks like a Hermes scarf, and a lurid purple blouse and matching terry-cloth shorts. She reaches Brad and lunges toward him with her arms outstretched. "Brad," she cries, giving him a hug. "You made it." It's Patricia Terrack, the Peace Corps worker from San Miguel. She gestures toward the square of people. "Isn't it wonderful?" she says. "These people are really standing up for their rights. I just *love* these people."

Patricia is known here as a friend, and her welcome puts the truckload of gringos at least in the category of non-foe. People return their attention to the speaker of the moment, a black man in a torn white T-shirt and khaki pants who addresses the crowd through a battery-operated bullhorn. The gist of his presentation is that the logging company in Esmeraldas and its allies in the central government in Quito do not care about the people who live out here. "You have seen the roads," he shouts to the crowd. "You know that we have asked the timber company to fix our roads," he continues, the pitch of his voice rising with each sentence. "And you can see what they have done. They have left us to take matters *into our own hands.*" He raises a hand skyward and the crowd shouts, *"Viva el paro"* — Up with the strike.

The bullhorn is passed around and the discussion continues along similar lines, punctuated now and then with more shouts and applause. Many in the audience stand silently, however, looking glum.

"Well, welcome to Vainilla," Patricia says with a tight laugh. Although invigorated by this Latin American version of 1960s-style street politics, the kind of demonstration she once marched in herself, she's as jumpy as a doe on opening day of deer season. "Things aren't going exactly as planned," she notes with sarcasm. "Don't worry, though, they don't plan to *do* anything to you."

Just what is planned is anybody's guess. It soon becomes apparent that many of the people here are travelers like us who have been stopped and forbidden to leave. Even if they were to sneak away on foot, Borbón lies some forty kilometers away. Some people have been here for days, sleeping on the ground, under the bridge, or in whatever shelter the actual residents of Vainilla, all fifty-odd of them, will offer. Like it or not, everyone here is a participant in the strike.

Hoping to negotiate our way through, we unload the gear and pile it into a canvas and nylon hillock by the road. Segundo, who views the abandoned rancheros by the bridge as an ugly omen, immediately guns his engine and backs down the road for half a mile before risking a slow U-turn in the narrow road. In moments, he is dust. We sit by the road and wait. Soon, young boys wander by, bored by the speechifying at the bridge but interested in what is inside the twenty-five bags. Most carry machetes soldier-style over their shoulders. Armed boys behaving vaguely like soldiers rarely bodes well, so we move ourselves nearer the bridge, hoping that a crowd of adults might exude some sense of civic duty not to rob strangers.

Hours pass, speeches are made, and the sky darkens. "Well, we could do some botanizing while we're here," Jim Burch offers with his signature palms-up, nervous shrug. "I've noticed quite a few interesting Orchidaceae by the road." There are no takers. "Well, I guess it'll be dark soon anyway," he concludes, a disturbing thought. Patricia has been looking for the right moment to press our case with the men who are running the show here, but it doesn't seem to come. She says they had first agreed to let the team through because we were scientists trying to help Ecuadoreans learn about sustainable development. But now they say letting us through would break the strike's momentum.

The sun sets behind the John Deere. For the moment, there is a feeling of safety sitting next to this big, all-American machine, as if somehow it can protect citizens of its own country. The strikers light up the truck tires in the middle of the bridge, and the flames cast the scene in garish hues of yellow and orange while shadows dance under a cloud of oily smoke. Another ranchero arrives and is ensnared. Its passengers, dazed and sulky, walk over and around our twenty-five-bag hillock to find a spot to sit. Bottles of sugar-cane alcohol have materialized, and the speechmaking among the strike leaders devolves into joking and shouting. Someone with a guitar plays two songs over and over: one about revolution, the other a love song. Perhaps because he is a Yanqui and therefore reckoned to be a musician, Fred is offered the guitar, and he plays a serviceable tune or two and passes the guitar around. True to our culture, several of us play, albeit poorly. Cajun tunes are an instant hit, and for the moment, our captors seem a little less intimidating.

The revelry soon begins to get rowdy, however, and Brad suggests that we hoist ourselves and our hillock onto the roof of the most recently arrived ranchero. "We'll have a night under the stars in the tropical paradise of Vainilla," Brad says as we clamber up to the roof. "And free, too." We search our memories for jokes, swat mosquitoes, and sing. Brad croons country songs with a high tenor that won't win any rodeo sweethearts, but he hits the notes well enough on Hank Williams standards and bluegrass ballads. We have decided not to break open any supplies for fear of starting a food riot, but we make an exception for a bottle of Bacardi rum Brad has thoughtfully stowed in his backpack.

The moon rises full and incandescent and the dark shapes on the surrounding hills materialize into palms, banana groves, and clots of somnolent cattle. We run out of songs and talk about ourselves. Jim, markedly less nervous now that the botanical gear is relatively secure, grows uncharacteristically talkative. He was raised in upstate New York, he says, and his earliest memory is of his mother cooking him dandelion greens with milkweed. As a young man he lived in Corpus Christi for a while, working on a tugboat. "They eventually accepted me as much as they could for a Yankee," he says. "But I wasn't a Baptist. So I told 'em I was a Methodist and they seemed to warm up a bit after that." Jim, somewhere past forty (he refuses to say just how old he is), didn't turn to biology until his thirties. Like Brad, he is an outdoorsman at heart. "I always liked going off into the woods," he says. "It never mattered much what I did there. Sometimes I'd go out to bow hunt for snakes. They taste pretty good and they're a lot easier to shoot than rabbits 'cause they don't move as fast." He says he feels more comfortable out in the field than in an academic setting, or for that matter, just about anywhere else. He looks up at the buttery moon and sighs. "I'm a misfit, I guess. Kinda anti-social." Fearing the moment has waxed too sentimental, he suddenly launches into song:

> Cabin boy, oh cabin boy,
> You dirty little ripper,
> You lined your ass with broken glass,
> And circumcised the skipper.

"Pass the rum, wouldja?"

We settle back onto pallets made with the flat cardboard boxes for the plant presses. Some local boys who have climbed aboard have the same idea and, true to the axiom of Ecuadorean buses, even stationary ones, all are soon squeezed together like seals on a sunny rock. Fred and I crawl back to the luggage rack, a jerry-rigged pen of two-by-fours screwed onto the back of the ranchero to carry goods and small live-stock, and collapse among the bags. A pig has settled on the ground underneath the rack, and together we drift off toward sleep.

Soon, however, the ranchero's driver appears and climbs to the edge of the roof to quietly negotiate with Brad. He says he can get us out of here, to Borbón, for seventy-five dollars. "Too much," Brad says. Considering the situation, he seems to be taking his bargaining impulse a bit too far. "Don't worry," Brad whispers. "He'll come down." Sure enough, within five minutes, the driver is back suggesting fifty dollars. Despite the stale essence of alcohol on the driver's breath and the sly history in his voice, the rest of us hold our breaths in anticipation. Brad says no. The driver pauses, spits, and grimaces. Okay, he says, twenty-five. "All right," Brad replies. The driver disappears toward the bridge, promising to return. "Don't get your hopes up," Brad advises.

We awake to gunfire. The ranchero is slowly moving. Loud voices oscillate as people shout on the run. Someone fires a gun again, its flat little pop suggesting a twenty-two. I try to climb up to look over the edge of the luggage compartment but the bags keep rolling underneath my knees. All I can see is a huge plume of smoke that roils above the bridge, glowing a smutty white against the starless sky and peppered with sparks.

When I finally pull myself up, I see several dozen people running up to the ranchero. *"Pare! Pare!"* shouts a woman with a red bandanna wrapped around her head. *"Nadie vaya!"* she yells — Nobody goes. By now people are pounding the side of the bus. Men shake shotguns in the air and wave machetes. Someone fires a rifle again, very close this time, which convinces the driver to turn off the engine. He climbs silently out of the cab and the crowd envelops him like ants around a sliver of cinnamon cake. For a moment, it looks as if some rude justice will be handed out here and now. The driver escapes with a tongue-lashing for his duplicity, however; after all, when the strike is all over, he will still be their neighbor and ranchero driver. We are ignored in our rooftop nest. Brad sighs. "It's just as well," he says. "The only place worse than here is Borbón in the middle of the night. 'Night, y'all."

Sunrise the next morning illuminates a scene like a fresco of the Last Judgment. Sleeping forms lie along the roadside, while those who are awake, or who never went to sleep, sit listlessly waiting for the sun to warm them into movement. The buildings, all of rude wooden plank-ing, look like an abandoned western-movie set: doors hang askew on their hinges, house walls do not quite reach to the eaves, steps tumble out of line like bad teeth. Through the window of a house below us by the road, I can see a bedroom containing a single piece of furniture, a bare mattress on the floor, above which hangs a mosquito net like a cloud of vapor. Above the house, a metal sign on a bamboo pole advertises hope: "Trust in the Evangelical Church, *Apostolica del Nombre de Jesus.*" A chicken pecks in the dirt underneath the front stoop.

"How's everything up there?" a voice asks in English. Below is a head of bright red hair. Patricia. "No progress yet, but this has *gotta* break soon." She had a rough night. "Thirty people on the floor in one room," she says. "You couldn't sleep for all the noise and the mosqui-toes." Her legs and forearms show abundant evidence of the latter. "The men kept pissing through a hole in the floor. Man, *that* stank!" Perhaps the roof of the bus was not such a bad idea.

Another Peace Corps worker, Sondra Klingle, climbs up to the rooftop redoubt. She has lived in the area for several months and has found food, of a sort: a plastic soda cup full of brown gruel. "We call it *quacker,*" she explains — Quaker Oats, some water and powdered milk, a little powdered chocolate, and about half a cup of sugar, the only thing that seems to be in good supply. She also has one boiled plantain.

As the sun rises higher and hotter, it bakes the rooftop and our spirits along with it. We are almost out of water and our jokes are running thin. Lauralyn, sitting with her back to the sun in a wide-brimmed straw hat, looks as if she is heading for a picnic. She says what everybody has been thinking. "At first I joked that we'd been taken hostage. But now I guess it's sorta true." The mood of the others dragooned into the strike is getting ugly too, and the organizers are feeling it. Their leader, an African man who goes simply by the name of William, has been caucusing with his men. William is a large, muscular, and quite beautiful man, with a square face and a glowing, disarming smile. He's flashing that smile now for Patricia, who stands squarely in his face and isn't about to be disarmed. They are out of earshot, but she clearly is giving him every bit of hell she can muster up, pounding him on the chest and stamping her feet. He puts his arm around her and they walk down Vainilla's only street, as if they're lovers engaged in a spat.

An hour later, we're on our way. Patricia convinced William that an honorable man doesn't go back on his word. Besides, William has heard that the army is on its way to wrest control of his bridgehead from him. He doesn't tell the poor souls on the road that, however, saying instead that it's time to suspend the strike to get food and water. Women, children, and scientists are free to go, he announces magnanimously over the bullhorn. Everyone seems to qualify, however, and within five minutes the abandoned rancheros and trucks are packed. As we watch Vainilla recede in a wake of dust, the strikers who remain on the bridge wave their guns good-bye. No one waves back.

11

San Miguel

We arrive in Borbón four hours later, so completely painted in dust that Fred can inscribe his name in the film covering his bare thighs. The ranchero slides to a halt near the river, the Santiago, and we stare down at a place that looks as if it has ruptured up out of the riverbank: a shamble of spattered, tin-roofed dwellings; a few shops of ill-painted concrete block congregated near the waterfront, their goods and customers spilling out into the road; and rutted dirt streets with trash floating in permanent pools of rainwater. Motorbikes rev and slide through the mud while crowds of people of all colors stand, walk, run, lounge, loll, or lie supine in the shade. The place climbs into your nose with fruit hovering near rot, roasting meat, and the river's algal windrow. Merchants buzz at passersby like bees dancing the route to nectar. At first, we're too stunned by it all to move.

Brad and Patricia go in search of last-minute supplies, while the rest of us are eyed with only momentary curiosity, for this is the edge of the wilderness, and eccentrics, adventurers, and fools pass through often enough. Most of the faces in the street are black. While the interior is predominantly indigenous South Americans, in Borbón, the races mix.

Although colonization has long since transformed Esmeraldas, outlying areas like Borbón have not changed too much since La Condamine came through the region. Popular Ecuadorean opinion holds the local people to be just a bunch of lazy banana farmers. Actually, says WRI's Bruce Cabarle, who has visited several times, they have a complex land management system. "These are people from another continent who escaped slavery and built up their own system, adapting some things perhaps from the Indians too," Cabarle says. "But people from outside came in and at various times have tried to rip them off. So they have shunned the outside."

Unlike most Ecuadoreans, the people here divide their land into farms, reserves, and pastures for cattle, with rules about when and how to use each one. People farm about twenty different crops, including cacao, guava, cedar, citrus, chiles, plantain, orange and lime trees, tagua, and chonta palm. It's a diverse mix so that something is always in season. Ecuador does not recognize community land, however, so there has been a lot of land grabbing. Under a set of complicated regulations, government land can be developed by anyone who comes up with a management plan that will "improve" it. Logging companies have capitalized on this incentive and are moving in quickly, and Borbón is fast becoming an enclave economy run by intermediaries.

We haul our gear to the town dock to wait and watch. A farmer wrestles a squealing pig out of one canoe while ten-year-old boys hoist bags of rice half their own weight up the quay. These are a canoeing people, and their upper torsos show it. At noon our ride arrives, a long dugout that takes passengers upriver on its daily run to San Miguel. We load the canoe until the gunwales sink to near-waterline. The captain, Salvador, points the canoe eastward and opens the throttle on the Evinrude outboard, and we resume our journey.

The Rio Santiago links Borbón with the interior and is dotted with villages strung like beads along its length. We pass stilt houses huddled two or three along the muddy riverbanks and rickety fish traps that stand half-submerged in the shallows like duck blinds on the Chesapeake Bay. Soon the houses grow fewer and the forest thicker as the Santiago ends and the Río Onzole begins. The blue cone flowers of water hyacinth drape the shallows, and broad galleries of bamboo march down to the riverside, their parchment-thin leaves so dense and delicate they seem like a lime-green cloud that has descended from the sky. Occasionally we pass a shirtless, glossy black man standing in a canoe, gliding along at the edge of the main current. Lauralyn, more ebullient with each mile we put between us and Vainilla, waves to every paddler. They smile and wave back, their palms flashing pink.

We pass from the Río Onzole onto the Río Cayapas. Finally, five hours and two thunderstorms out of Borbón (during which time Brad extracts yet another surprise from his bottomless backpack — a large, bright yellow umbrella), the rooftops of San Miguel appear just over the high riverbanks, the tallest being a clapboard steeple with a cross. Well before we reach it, however, we pull over at a spot marked with logs laid along the shore as a makeshift pier. Somewhere above, up a steep slope of tall grass and channels of red mud, is the house that its missionary builders called Loma Linda.

Laughing Chachi children materialize as we pull ashore, and they pounce on our bags, hoisting them onto their shoulders and jogging up the hill to the house, while the rest of us shimmy up step by slippery step. By the time we reach the top, we're covered in red slime and sweat. The view, however, is worth the climb. From the curves of the blue Andes, the green pelt of the Cotacachi-Cayapas reserve undulates toward us until, just ahead and below us, it swallows the last curve of the Río Cayapas. A few of San Miguel's wide-hipped, thatched roofs lie at the river's vanishing point. Tree branches show bone white amid the mass of foliage, and clouds hang low in the middle distance, seemingly brushing the tops of the trees. Having so far been mostly inside rainforests looking out, we suddenly grasp the great monarchy of life here, its absolute rule, and are momentarily struck dumb.

Patricia Terrack's house is a large post-and-beam structure with the main floor built ten feet off the ground. Most of each day's activity takes place on an open veranda with benches, a table, and two hammocks. Inside the house are a large main room, a kitchen, and four small bedrooms. Rainwater is captured on the tin roof, then channeled by gutters into aluminum tanks in a loft, and finally directed down bamboo pipes into the house. The furniture is utilitarian, consisting of a round wooden table, folding chairs, a desk, and a small wicker divan. Woven grass carpets cover much of the wood plank floor, and postcards of native peoples, waterfalls, and Swiss mountains adorn the walls, while seashells, glass crystals, and baskets woven by the Chachi hang from the walls. Bookcases, their contents neatly arranged by size, contain the likes of *Rainwater Harvesting, The Jungle Camp Cookbook, In the Rainforest,* and *Where There Is No Doctor.* The kitchen has a porcelain sink and a variety of tightly sealed tins and plastic tubs sitting on a table whose legs stand in old coffee cans half-filled with water — ant moats, Patricia explains. The bedrooms are simple, with wooden frame bunks and nails in the walls to suspend mosquito netting. Screened windows keep the air moving and, for the most part, the insects out. The place is noticeably spotless. Although she loves the forest, Patricia relentlessly keeps it out of her house.

Chachi oral history holds that the people came here from the vicinity of Ibarra in the Andes on the advice of a wise shaman who had asked a jaguar to find the Chachi a new home. The jaguar chose this region, which the Chachi called Pueblo Viejo, but soon after they arrived, they were attacked by a warlike tribe to the west, the Indios Bravos. Indios Bravos wore skirts and, the story goes, ate human flesh. After years of being harassed and eaten, the Chachi finally retaliated and destroyed the Indios Bravos. Some escaped, however, and their descendants are said to practice their old habits in the rivers to the east — in the Cotacachi-Cayapas reserve.

The land the jaguar chose was certainly diverse. The alluvial, volcanic soils of the western Ecuadorean peneplains support twelve life zones. According to SUBIR, the Chachi territory "contains the country's most pristine conditions in any of Ecuador's protected areas." Its isolation has kept it from being explored much, and little is known about its flora and fauna. As for the Chachi culture, the most comprehensive study was compiled by one S. A. Barrett, an anthropologist who lived with the Chachi for nine months between 1908 and 1909. In his account, daily life for this riverine people revolved around the canoe and the garden. The men tended their fish traps and nets and hunted with lances and blowguns made from chonta palm and darts tipped with an unknown plant poison. Chachi women tended the gardens, cooked, and cared for children and the households. Families lived separately, each with a two-room house, one room for cooking and the other for living and sleeping. The houses had no walls — to keep babies from crawling over the edge of the floor, mothers would wrap them tightly. The pillars of their houses, like the ones supporting Patricia's house, were cut from the *guayacan* tree and joined with a vine called *piquihua*, both of which were chosen because they resist insects. The Chachi made no metal, having little need for it, and spoke a language, full of glottal stops, called Cha'apalachi that few strangers mastered.

For the most part, the Chachi still live as Barrett described. Machetes, guns, boat motors, an occasional radio, and some modern medicines have had their influence, however, and the pace of change is accelerating. To get cash for manufactured goods, the Chachi are hunting more and selling the meat, which is killing off the mammals. Cattle ranching and cash crops like cocoa and coffee are replacing subsistence farming and the various native cultivars the Chachi once grew, and some Chachi have moved to the coast to work for foreign mining companies. Those who stay are moving into larger settlements to reach larger markets for their goods, to get better health care, and to send their children to school.

It's hard to imagine oneself as a member of a culture reduced to twenty thousand people scattered across an area about the size of Connecticut. A road or two, a few more Ecuadorean schools, a half-dozen logging camps, and the children of the Chachi will become the children of Ecuador, the children of Latin America, the children of the Americas, and finally Everychild. "If that's what they want, that's their decision," Patricia says firmly, as she says most everything. Yet she regrets the absorption of one more unique people into the multitude. Moreover, without the Chachi and places like San Miguel, Patricia and Brad wouldn't be the people they are.

Patricia came here after her first Peace Corps assignment in the Philippines. There, she had lived with an indigenous group, the Aetas, in the mountains of Luzon near the volcano Mount Pinatubo. She was evacuated a few days before Pinatubo erupted in early 1992. Most of the people she lived with took refuge in a cave and were buried alive. Looking for a new place as far from civilization as possible, Patricia picked San Miguel as her next assignment, not so much because of the Chachi, since no one knew anything about them, but because it was one of the most biodiverse places in the world. "It needed saving," she says. When she arrived, the missionaries' house on the hill was falling in on itself. The Chachi wouldn't live there, for they believed the place was haunted. When Patricia stood atop the hill and looked out over the river to the Andes, she knew that she would put Loma Linda together again and make it her home. "It needed saving too," she says.

The next morning, Chachi children congregate on Patricia's veranda to find out who the new people are. Patricia chats with them in Cha'apalachi, and the children vie for various chores that Patricia might need done that day, knowing that she rewards work with candy. Meanwhile, Brad heads off for the village to meet its prominent families: like many Ecuadorean cultures, the Chachi don't traditionally have an official leader. He returns in the afternoon with Miguel Chapiro and River Nazareno, two young men whom Patricia has recruited as informants. Miguel is a sturdy young Chachi of twenty-four, a family man who despite his youth is of high standing in the village. His father is one of the two practicing brujos here. Though Miguel has decided not to follow in his father's career, he knows more about the traditional use of plants than most Chachi. River is African, barely twenty, and tall and soft-spoken, the son of one of the two park guards who patrol Cotacachi-Cayapas.

Miguel and River want to learn more about the outside world, and Miguel wants his children to go to school, to speak Spanish and perhaps some English, and to learn skills valuable in the world that is closing in around his forest. Yet he knows also that his children are losing touch with the traditions he learned from his parents, and that these traditions could die with his generation. Brad explains that he wants to study those traditions, and that by doing so he hopes to preserve them. He points out that he doesn't pay for knowledge, only for a person's time, and as a scientist he will publish his findings for all to see. Miguel and River agree to help for a wage of five dollars a day, the same pay they get for cutting timber for the loggers. They shake hands and agree to start that afternoon.

The team gathers around Patricia's dining table for a session on plant collecting. It's much like being back at Jatun Sacha: cups of instant coffee with clumps of powdered milk floating on the surface, swarms of gnats chewing on the ankles, and the day's first sweat starting to soak our shirts.

"I believe in more data on fewer plants," Brad says. "You want fertile plants in fruit or flower, and at least three or four samples of each individual. Describe the plant. Here's an example." He reads from his field notebook. " 'Carludovica palmata, Ruiz and Pavon, shrub to four meters tall, leaves to three meters, petiole one point five meters, blade one point five meters. Infructescence to one point five meters, fruits fleshy, dehiscent seeds with red aril.' That's the tree they make Panama hats from.

"Now with informants, it's best if they're in the field with you, rather than you just bringing stuff back in for them to look at. They'll notice things in the field they might not back here. And keep in mind the categories of use. There's construction, food and food processing, forage for animals, fishing, fiber, hunting, medicinal, veterinary, ritual and mythical, and dyes, fuel, and tools. Remember to ask lots of questions. If it's used for, say, baskets, ask who makes the baskets. How much do they get for a basket at the market?

"The medicinals are the most complicated. You can ask, for example, What part of the plant do they use? For what kind of illness? Do you mix it with hot water, cold water? And how long is it cooked? How often is it taken? Ask for the Cha'apalachi word for it and say it back to them. They'll laugh and correct you without being asked, and that's good. The more you talk about it, the more you'll remember it when you get back and do the chemistry. And be careful with names. They may have different names for different parts of the plant, and then another name when that part is actually used for something. You'll want to go into gardens too, of course. Get permission first. Even the bananas are worth collecting. Extra credit for anyone who can put a raceme of bananas through a plant press. Climb when you need to — those palms with the two-inch spines on the trunk are especially fun.''

"Yeah, I'm looking forward to climbing those," Fred volunteers.

"Just climb the tree next to it and reach over if you can," says Brad. He counts more items off the tips of his fingers. "If you don't recognize the plant's family, take better notes. What's the position of the ovary of the flower? for example. Then start a one-hundred-meter-square plot. Lay it out with a compass, mark it off with flags at the corners and also every twenty meters. Number every tree in the whole damn place that's greater than ten centimeters diameter at breast height. Then after that you can start . . ."

"Whoa," says Jim. His normal expression of undirected anxiety creases into near-panic as he tries to take all this down. "Uh, maybe we should start with the top three priorities?" he suggests.

Brad stares at Jim for a moment. "Okay," he says with a sudden smile. "World peace, baton twirling, and, uh, juggling with burning bowling pins."

"And how to paddle a canoe," Lauralyn adds.

"Don't worry," Brad says, "you'll get the hang of it. Anyway, let's quit talking and get going." The team heads for their rubber boots and insect repellent. "Just remember," Brad calls after us, "be careful. It's a jungle out there."

Now, finally, into the forest — out the door a stone's throw and we're in it. Patricia leads the way, swinging her machete through the undergrowth with a fluid nonchalance that comes of much practice, until we reach a shallow stream we can follow to keep from getting lost. The forest here is punctuated with glades, the result of a hurricane that swept through about two years before. These spots are good candidates for useful plants, since secondary forest species tend to be the most commonly used by indigenous peoples. In fact, Miguel soon spots a shrub that he knows. "This is *bu'chui tape*," he says, giving the Cha'a-palachi name. It's an herb, about knee high, and in flower with small orange blossoms. "We treat snakebite with it," he explains. He says his father also cuts lengths of it to strike the body of a patient at the end of a curing ceremony. "Okay," Brad says happily, snipping some flowers and leaves, "one species from the family Gesneriaceae." He wades on, stumbling over rocks as he scans the banks for plants in flower. Miguel spots something on a tree limb. "*Nantape*," he calls out. "We put the sap on the bites of conga ants," he explains, referring to the coal-black, inch-long ant whose bite can lay its victim up in bed for two days. Brad, using all of his six feet two inches of height, brings down some leaves. "An epiphyte, Araceae, the genus I think is *Syngonium*." It goes into the potato sack he has slung over his shoulder.

As Brad's bag gets fuller his spirits rise. "Oh, to be young, a botanist, and in the rainforest," he sings. His head swivels side to side, his botanist's antennae tuned to some vegetable wavelength. "I don't much like being in Quito," he volunteers. "Or any city. This is what I like." He sits down on a fallen tree trunk astride the stream and stares up into the canopy while Patricia and the others forge on. "Sometimes you just have to sit and look for a while to see things. You go into a sort of trance. Darwin wrote about it. Some botanists just go for the numbers, they get as many specimens as they can. But I don't get the sense that they enjoy themselves that much. There is really something to be said for focusing on the forest and losing a bit of everything else for a while." He pulls out his pouch of Red Man and digs in. "I lived in a tent in Big Cypress swamp when I was a graduate student in Florida. I'd go in on my motorcycle with a shotgun and a fishing pole and live mostly off what I could hunt. Alligators, sometimes. I was out with some students one time and I stepped over a log without tapping it, like you should always do there. I had one leg over when I looked down. There was a water moccasin coiled right below me, eyeball to testicle. I had a shotgun but I was too scared to move a hair. The students were off in the bush yelling for me, but I couldn't make a sound. I stood there, it seemed like forever. Finally, I started to slide away, as slowly as I could. I got about ten yards away and turned and shot at it with my shotgun. My hands were shaking so bad I missed him. I *missed* him, from *ten yards!* He moved off fast and I didn't get him 'til the third shot. I figured he deserved to die for scaring me so bad. I mean, I hadn't had kids yet." He rouses himself and smiles. "This is paradise," he says, "compared to that."

Miguel leads the group to a chacra belonging to some of his relatives. It's more like managed wildness than the kind of garden a North American would recognize. Brad reaches up and pulls down a vine that has wrapped itself around a low-hanging branch and shows it to

Miguel. *"Upi chi,"* Miguel says automatically. "Cook five leaves in one or two liters of water, and drink once a day for fevers. Also, it is for snakebite." The number of treatments here for poisonous bites, be they from snakes, ants, or scorpions, is in itself alarming. "You ever been bitten?" Fred asks Miguel. The Chachi chortles and holds up his right hand, which bears a white cicatrix like a small smile between the thumb and forefinger. *"Equis,"* he says, the common word here for the fer-de-lance. "I was lucky. It was a dry bite."

Brad identifies the upi chi as a member of the family Melastomataceae, drawing out each syllable in a musical chant. He marks it down in his orange logbook — pity the botanist who lays down a dark-colored logbook in the densely shadowed forest and tries to find it again. Over the next two hours, we find several more useful plants: a vine whose stem has a delightful lemony taste, which is taken for colds; a tree whose latex is painted on canoes; a six-foot-tall shrub with bright yellow petals used to make a thatch that will last two years; a tall grass, from whose stem a juice is squeezed and put in the eyes for conjunctivitis, an inflammation of the membrane of the eyelids; and more snakebite remedies — apparently, besides generic treatments, there is a preferred plant for every kind of snake.

Back at the house, exhausted, cut, insect-bitten, and happy, the team sorts through the booty. Each plant goes through another identification and description. River, who has now joined the group, compares African uses with Chachi. There are some differences. Only the Chachi, for example, use *pujcui tape,* a small tree from the genus *Solanum,* to make a decoction in which they bathe babies with colic in the light of the full moon. Several species of *Solanum* are in fact used as folk medicines around the world, for eye disease, fever, rabies, gout, whooping cough, bronchitis, and cancer. We learn also that medicine is practiced differently by the Africans. Among the Chachi, the male shamans do much of the healing as well as casting spells, but among the Africans, the women prescribe herbal remedies. "The Chachi shamans also do ayahuasca," Patricia adds. "There was one guy across the river who was chanting for three weeks straight, he was high the whole time. He was doing it before Easter to make sure everything was pure and ready for the Easter fiesta."

Next comes plant pressing. A leaf is placed between sheets of white blotter paper, which then is placed on a sheet of numbered newspaper. That is followed by a sheet of cardboard, then another sheet of the newspaper. The process is repeated with the thick, fleshy parts of the specimen, like fruits, flowers, or large spikes, which can be sliced in half lengthwise and scooped out to speed drying and ease pressing. That stack is followed with a sheet of corrugated aluminum to give some stiffness while allowing air to get in, then another sheet of numbered newspaper and a new specimen, and so on, like a big green-salad sandwich. When the stack is about two feet thick, wooden sheets go at the top and bottom and the whole thing is squeezed tight with straps. "You have to be careful you don't perform 'instant evolution' by putting the wrong flower or fruit with the wrong leaves," Brad says. "That does not amuse the folks at the herbaria back home who do the final identification on these." Finally, the sandwich must be dried. Jim has foraged up the collapsed remains of a chicken coop under the house and built a cage out of it, into which the presses go, and the whole thing is propped up on rocks over a smoldering fire.

By dusk, Brad and his two informants have identified about two dozen plants and their uses. Miguel and River, apparently happy to be paid a good wage for what for them is easy work, politely shake hands all around and stroll down the hill to their canoe. While it's too early to say whether the botanists have been accepted by the community, at least these two are happy to help. For the first time, the expedition is going smoothly — proof, Brad notes, that things are always better in the field.

Patricia has volunteered to cook dinner, a performance by candlelight from start to finish. As she works, she describes what she has learned about the Chachi.

"They have no clue of how valuable their traditional knowledge might be," she says as she spoons canned tomatoes into a pot. "Miguel's father, the brujo, is considered a quack by the educated Chachi and the federation leaders, who've been educated in Esmeraldas or Quito and have spent their whole lives there. But the traditional leaders certainly respect the old knowledge. If anybody falls ill in Franco's family — he's one of the canoe operators — they will go to a brujo." She deftly slices an onion in the semi-darkness and throws the rounds in the pot.

Brad wonders whether the Chachi are aware of the interest in indigenous botanical medicine that has reemerged in the States. "They're so disorganized they can't capitalize on anything right now," Patricia replies with exasperation. She says SUBIR brought some advisers from the Shuar peoples federation to talk to the Chachi. "They said, 'Geez, you gotta get your shit together or you're going to get walked all over.' But no way, they're not ready for it." She slits open a package of noodles and pours the contents into a pot of boiling water.

"The Chachi have a very complicated spirit world," she continues.

"They didn't come up here after the missionaries left. This was 'brujo hill,' where they used to hold shamanistic ceremonies. They would ask me, 'How can you stand to be alone here? Aren't you afraid of the spirits?' The Chachi are never alone, always in a group, because they have so many malevolent spirits. I wish they had a few more nice ones. They also believe that you travel when you sleep. They ask me, 'Do you go to Nueva York?' I tell them I go to the beach. I actually *have* left my body a couple of times, as I was nodding off to sleep. It wasn't planned though." She whacks the side of the pot with a metal spoon. "Okay, everybody, time to eat."

Over dinner, Patricia is persuaded to tell some of her own history. She left home in Florida at the age of fourteen on the back of a boyfriend's motorcycle, ending up a year later in California with a different boyfriend and no country left to explore. The two of them volunteered to make an overland trip from California to Tierra del Fuego, at the tip of Argentina, that was being sponsored by several businesses as a publicity stunt. They traveled in an M36 military transport specially fitted out with communications equipment and were resupplied along the way by helicopter. The toughest part of the trip was getting through the Darien in Panama, a trackless jungle as dense as any in the world. "My main memory," Patricia says, "is swatting huge mosquitoes and watching the blood splatter." She was well-prepared, however. Before the trip, she had taken a jungle survival course in Panama. The culminating "exam" consisted of being dropped into the Darien and given three days to get out alone. She was the second one in her class to reach home, she says.

At the end of the trip to Patagonia, Patricia discovered she was pregnant. She married her boyfriend and they settled in Colombia, making a living as expedition outfitters. When the marriage broke up seven years later, she and her daughter moved to California, where she taught school. "The money was terrible, so I bluffed my way through a heavy-equipment test. Hell, I'd driven that M36 for seven months and I'd learned how to repair diesel engines. I got first place on the written exam." She made heavy equipment her career, even competing in a contest in Las Vegas where she won ten thousand dollars by picking up a dime with a backhoe blade. When her daughter left home to join the Army, Patricia decided it was time to travel again, and joined the Peace Corps. "My daughter's an MP in Germany now," Patricia says. "She tells me she can't find a man who's tough enough." She laughs sardonically. We suspect she has run into the same problem.

*   *   *

The Chachi project was looking to be, by ethnobotanical standards, relatively easy. In the tropics, the first contact with a new culture can be a test of one's constitution. Brad's first in Ecuador was with the Shuar people in the Oriente. He was just out of his twenties, spoke little Spanish, and knew almost nothing about rainforest cultures. As for the Shuar, they were best known as recently reformed headhunters.

The Shuar are one of five indigenous groups who once were lumped under the name Jívaro, a fierce people who have always rejected assimilation. In the 1520s, the Inca emperor Huayna Cápac tried to subjugate them and was sent packing, never to return. In 1549, Spaniards tried to establish a town near Jívaro territory in the province of Macas, but found the Jívaro more than happy to kill or be killed to keep them out. Eventually, Spanish gold miners won an uneasy coexistence with the Jívaro that nonetheless gave the habitually warring Jívaro communities a reason to stop fighting one another and confront a common enemy. They did just that in 1599.

The Spanish governor of the province of Macas imposed a tax to be paid in gold on Spaniard and Indian alike, against which all parties rebelled. The governor rescinded the tax for his Spanish subjects but said nothing to the native people, most of whom submitted to the order. Not the Jívaro, however. They retreated to their traditional lands, elected a leader named Quirruba (Big Frog), and enlisted other indigenous groups to help them wipe out the Spanish.

According to nineteenth-century Spanish historians, when the governor paid a long-awaited visit to the town of Logroño, some twenty thousand Indians attacked the town. Quirruba seized the house where the governor was staying and put everyone to the spear but him. The Jívaro, apparently not without a sense of symbolism, stripped the governor naked and tied him hand and foot, then set up a forge in the courtyard and melted gold they had brought with them. With an animal bone, they propped open the governor's mouth and slowly poured the molten metal that the governor had so coveted down his throat.

Logroño lost twelve thousand souls, almost the entire population save those women the Jívaro chose to carry off, and the nearby town of Sevilla del Oro was sacked as well. Understandably, Spaniards put down few roots in Jívaro country afterward, except for one small town, Macas, in 1870. When anthropologist Michael Harner lived with the Jívaro during the 1950s and 1960s, he noted that they had no oral history of the uprising of 1599 except for a vague tale of white men whose arms were all bone to the elbows and who carried machetes at the hip and rode mules.

Steel, especially in the form of machetes, finally seduced the Jívaro to trade with the citizens of Macas, the Macabeos, who by the nine-teenth century were themselves a polyglot of indigenous and Spanish blood. Among the items the Macabeos asked for in return were the shrunken heads, or *tsantsa*, that the Jívaro collected. When the Jívaro obliged them, their reputation flourished anew; few things focus the mind quite like a shrunken human head.

These tsantsa of the Jívaro served an important utilitarian purpose. The Jívaro had always raided villages of other Amazonians or, within their own culture, settled serious disputes by killing one another. In-deed, a saying common among Jívaro men is "I was born to die fight-ing." Killing, however, is not as clear-cut as it is, say, in Washington, D.C., or Los Angeles. Each person possesses a *muisak*, an avenging soul that will pursue the killer and return the favor either directly or to members of the killer's family. To avoid this spiritual tit for tat, the Jívaro soldier must decapitate his victim and shrink the head in order to capture the victim's muisak before it can do any mischief.

The task of shrinking begins as a war party retreats. The warriors stop by a river or stream and peel the skins from the heads, throwing the skulls into a river as a gift for *panji*, the anaconda spirit. The skin is boiled in water for about half an hour, then dried and turned inside out so that the flesh can be scraped out. Turned right-side out again, the skin is filled with a handful of heated egg-sized stones that are rolled around to facilitate drying and shrinking, accompanied by some knead-ing to keep the skin flexible. The process continues with smaller and smaller stones, and finally with heated sand. A red-hot machete is used to dry the lips, which are then lashed together with string made from tree bark. To prevent the muisak from seeing out of the head, the skin is also rubbed with balsa wood charcoal. The whole process takes about six days and produces a tsantsa, including hair, about the size of a small cantaloupe.

Lest one get the idea that headshrinking is all work and no play, it should be pointed out that the process is not complete until the cul-mination of two or three feasts back in the home village. During these feasts, a man holds his tsantsa aloft while two female relatives hold on to him. In this way, all gain power from the muisak, the men for hunting and fighting, the women for working in the gardens and rais-ing livestock. There is much drinking and celebrating, although the feast is conducted with careful attention to proper decorum. At the end of the final feast, the spirit in the head is released and sent back to the village from whence it came. Subsequently, the owner is free to sell it. As one might expect, there is a high price on such heads.

The Ecuadorean government frowns on the practice of headshrinking, and it's believed to have disappeared about the same time lynchings stopped in the United States. When Harner visited the Jívaro in the mid-1950s, they had also decided to rehabilitate their name. The word *Jívaro* had earned a common pejorative meaning something like *savage*, so the Jívaro began calling themselves *šuära*, pronounced Shuar. The largest group became the *Untsuri* Shuar, meaning "numerous Indians." The Shuar's new, more pacific lifestyle paid dividends. In 1957, the Shuar population was estimated at 7,830. By the late 1980s, that number had swelled to forty thousand, making them Ecuador's second largest indigenous culture next to the Quichua.

It was the lot of a young Brad Bennett, newly hired in 1988 by Mike Balick at the New York Botanical Garden, to go live with the Shuar. Brad had defended his Ph.D. dissertation at the University of North Carolina on a Monday and was scheduled to leave for Ecuador the following Friday. "Balick told me, 'Here's some money. Go to Ecuador. Good luck,' " Brad recalls.

Brad went to the Shuar federation headquarters in Sucúa, but the federation leaders were unimpressed and told him to go away. Brad luckily had hired a young Ecuadorean botanist, Patricia Gomez, who convinced the federation that a scientific study of their plants would be of historical importance. By April, the scientists were accepted into a *centro* called Yukutais, a village of about thirty Shuar families situated on a bluff overlooking the Upano River. "We explained what we were doing and they seemed interested in it, surprisingly so," Brad recalls. "We made it clear that we were trying to preserve a part of their history, and that our idea of ethnobotany wasn't just medicine or drugs, but all the plants they use, and that we would get a record that would be available to them and their children." They also brought books for the schools. "And we bought a soccer ball. In fact, we had to play with them several times in the tropical sun. I could play up to about a four- or five-year-old, but once they hit six, forget it, I was no match for them."

Brad got tipsy the first day he arrived. The Shuar custom for getting acquainted — indeed, for almost any occasion, even getting up in the morning — is to drink chicha. Brad tried to meet each family, and managed eleven houses. For lodgings for himself, Gomez, and another Ecuadorean botanist, Efrain Freire, he rented a shack from the family of

Domingo Antich, one of the two prominent families in the centro. The scientists diplomatically took their meals with the family of Pedro Kumkumas, the other prominent household in the village. They had with them essentially what they could carry in — rubber boots, machetes, and plant presses.

Over the next two years, Brad visited the Shuar seven times, staying for a week to a month each time. Each time he would collect a few hundred vouchers and haul them back to Quito. Each voucher consisted of a twelve-by-sixteen-inch sheet of acid-free paper on which leaves, stems, and flowers had been pressed. Written information with the voucher included the plant's family name, genus, and if known, the species; the collector's name; the nearest community; and a physical and geographical description of the place where the specimen was collected (soil type, type of tree canopy, proximity to rivers or ridges, and so on). Such information can be crucial. For example, plants now being investigated by the National Cancer Institute are being collected by scientists who have never seen the real thing, only vouchers. For interviewing the Shuar, he followed guidelines suggested by the New York Botanical Garden's Brian Boom. In Boom's "artefact interview," the botanist visits a home and asks about the plants used to make common household items like baskets, food, utensils, benches, pots, or thatch. That done, the botanist collects plants in the field and brings them back to ask villagers what uses they might have, in what is called the "inventory" technique.

Eventually, Brad and his colleagues became accepted as village fixtures, more than guests if not quite residents. For his part, Brad found the Shuar far healthier and happier than the image he had come with of poor South American peasants huddled in shanties. Soon he was invited to participate in *minga,* a communal work period common in western Amazonian and Andean indigenous cultures. The gesture of comradeship, however, had an unforeseen drawback. "We were clearing around the schoolhouse, cutting down trees. I worked like a son of a gun, but I enjoy working hard, swinging my machete, whack, whack, whack. Pedro Kumkumas saw me pause for a break and he started berating the women. 'Look at him, he's working so hard, go over and give him some chicha, he needs some.' They'd been digging in the fields all morning, and they come out with the chicha, with a couple of gourds of water from the river, not boiled, and they mix it together, stirring it with their hands. I *had* to drink it, of course. So I decided not to take a break again. I'm just going to work like a madman. So Pedro looks and says, 'Look at him, he works like a madman, give him some more chicha.' Then the third time, I said 'I'm just going to go sit down and rest.' So Pedro yells at the women, 'Look at him, he's tired, he hasn't had enough chicha.' I must have had about five or six bowls of the stuff."

The dropout rate among young ethnobotanists on their first expedition is high. Besides the discomfort — in Yukutais, the cocks crowed at three A.M. and chickens roosted in Brad's bamboo-slat bed — there's the tedium, the strangeness of an alien culture, the language barrier, and of course the cuisine. "You've got to be flexible," Brad says. "You have to adapt very quickly to different cultures. I can find the good and ignore the bad in a new culture or food. Every time I go somewhere new I feel like I'm living anew. What I *don't* adapt well to is being away from my family."

Brad and his partners collected over 9,000 vouchers representing 985 taxa, of which 673 have some use among the Shuar. The Shuar use a phenomenal 245 different plants as medicines, and another 196 for food. They build with 88 different plants, making logs, flooring, rooftops, and lashing from them. Necklaces are made from seeds; bags from the fibers of the plant *Astrocaryum chambira;* and red dyes for fabrics, pottery, and face paint from the seed pulp of the shrub *Bixa orellana,* known as *ipiak.* They make meals called *ayampakus* from broad-leafed plants filled with meat and yuca (manioc), and a special chicha from sweet potatoes that women drink.

Of their medicines, the Shuar employ 104 plant species just for gastrointestinal ailments, not surprising given the catholic Shuar diet, the means of preparing food, and drinking habits that would humble a sailor on shore leave. Other frequent complaints are bruises and tumors, with 23 specific plants for their treatment. For headaches there are 15 plants, while fever can be treated with any of 19 different plants. Skin ailments such as fungus are rampant, for which the Shuar have 98 species of medicinal plant.

This eclectic use of plants isn't unique to the Shuar. Boom studied the Chácabo of eastern Colombia and found that they employ 82 percent of the species and 95 percent of the individual trees found in a twelve-thousand-square-yard plot of forest. The Quichua living around Jatun Sacha were found to use over 90 percent of the trees in a sample plot. Different cultures in the Amazon may call these plants by different names, but most of the medicinals are used for the same ailments in each culture, lending credibility to the argument that they do indeed contain compounds that work. Indeed, forest peoples often are remarkably healthy before colonists bring in disease. Former Schultes student

Wade Davis and anthropologist James A. Yost were among the first westerners to live among the Waorani, over a period of nine years in the 1970s and 1980s. They found a robust population with few signs of epidemic disease, internal parasites, or bacterial infections. The Waorani treated themselves with only thirty-five medicinal plants, and thirty of them were used to treat just six conditions: fungal infections, snakebite (eight types of venomous snake live in Waorani territory), dental problems, fevers, tropical warble-fly larvae, and various stings. Among their medicines is the resin extracted from the inner bark of *Virola calophylla,* known there as *tegidewe,* which they use for fungal infections, scabies, and infestations of mites.

The Waorani are in fact among the world's most efficient forest foragers. They eat forty-four different kinds of plant, twenty-five of which are gathered wild from the forest, including a gelatinous fungus that grows on fallen logs and the stems of a begonia, which Davis says tastes like rhubarb. Davis marveled at the depth of their understanding of forest ecology. They know a great deal about such complex phenomena as pollination and seed dispersal, and about the interdependence of animal and plant cycles, which enable them to predict animal behavior. They anticipate the flowering and fruiting cycles of edible forest plants and know not only what species most forest animals prefer to feed on, but also what part of the plant they prefer and in what stage of development the plant is eaten.

The belief that almost every plant can be used sustainably runs consistently through all these forest cultures. Brad was once chastised by the Shuar for discarding fruit seeds that could be saved for planting. The Kayapó of Brazil and Venezuela carry seeds with them while they are walking on their trails to plant wherever they stop to defecate. The Kayapó even use insects to their advantage, placing nests of what they call "smelly ants" near gardens and fruit trees because their pheromones repel leaf-cutter ants. These findings cast the notion of "virgin rainforest" into doubt, according to the anthropologist Darrell Posey. He found sections of forest once thought to be natural that were actually islands of useful vegetation created by the Kayapó.

Notions of illness and the ceremonies surrounding plant use are remarkably consistent among Amazonian cultures. The Shuar and the Chachi, for example, believe that the vast majority of illnesses and nonviolent deaths are caused by spirits, either at the behest of a shaman or, especially among the Chachi, through a person's own mistakes. Remedies are usually divided into the practical herbal and the supernatural. The supernatural cure requires a shaman, who often takes an hallucinogen to give him the power to enter the supernatural world and perform his work. For the Shuar, shamanistic power is incorporated in magical darts, called *tsentsak,* which are actually supernatural forces believed to cause illness and death and which a shaman can accumulate and control.

In Yukutais, the local shaman was one of Brad's hosts, Pedro Kumkumus, a robust forty-five-year-old whose profits from practicing medicine permitted him the luxury of two wives. He invited Brad to a healing ceremony, and Brad accepted, expecting it to be the highlight of his expedition. But sometimes a glimpse into the heart of darkness is more comic than awe-inspiring. Brad's account of the ceremony follows.

Pedro places a *tumank* on the table where we sit in his house. This traditional Shuar instrument is a hollow bow about two feet long. I've not seen one in Yukutais before. Pedro takes a bottle of trago (sugar cane alcohol), pours some over a wad of tobacco in a small cup, then puts a quartz stone on the tobacco. The quartz, called *namor,* is passed over a patient's body to draw out evil.

Mariata, Pedro's daughter, brings us roasted meat (we learn later that it's duck), ají (hot sauce), and boiled bananas. The bananas are bland but the duck and ají are excellent. They remind me of Sonny's Real Pit Barbecue. After we eat, Mariata brings us a finger bowl to wash our hands.

Pedro begins preparing for the ayahuasca ceremony at 8:45 P.M. Ayahuasca is used throughout northwest Amazonia. While under the influence of the plant's narcotic alkaloids, a shaman diagnoses physical and psychological illnesses of his patient. Natem is ayahuasca's Shuar name but Pedro uses the Quichua term which means death or soul vine. Pedro's fourteen-year-old brother-in-law has stomach ulcers and is unable to gain weight. A doctor in Quito diagnosed the problem as a "tired stomach" and charged thirty thousand sucres for his assessment — more than forty dollars or two months' salary for the average Ecuadorean. Since modern medicine failed, Pedro returns to his people's traditions.

Pedro places three small cups on the table. They look like those from a toy dinner set that my daughters use. He fills two cups with trago. He drinks one, passes the other to me, then refills them for Patricia and Efrain. . . .

As we wait, Pedro describes his preparation for becoming a

shaman. For several months he ate no meat and had no sexual relations. Eventually he was permitted to eat some kind of fish. He did not bathe for one month nor did he eat any processed food . . .

The tin roof amplifies the sound of light rain, making it difficult to hear. Someone hands Pedro an eight-ounce medicine bottle containing a few ounces of ayahuasca. Pedro prepared the hallucinogen earlier from the stem of the ayahuasca vine (*Banisteriopsis caapi*) and leaves of *yaji* (*Diplopterys cabrerana*), *kuishinkiap* (*Herrania*), *wais* (*Ilex guayusa*), *winchu* (*Heliconia stricta*), and *mukayashu*, an unknown species.

The sooty yellow light of a kerosene lamp barely illuminates the room. I can see nothing beyond the table. After offering us each a cigarette, Pedro describes visions he sees while under ayahuasca's influence. Boas, frogs, tigers, dogs, and trees are frequent. Many of these can transform into other forms. Tobacco is an important element of the healing ceremony. Like the evil spirits that cause illness, smoke rises and is amorphous. It cleanses and protects the room. Pedro frequently turns to spit. . . .

Pedro pours one and one half ounces of ayahuasca into the third small cup. Taking a match stick he stirs it, patiently removing small particles from the mixture. Pedro takes the cup of ayahuasca, blows smoke into it, then sucks air from the cup and spits. He begins to whistle. He repeats these actions, then pours more trago, placing it to the left of the ayahuasca. Removing his shirt, Pedro lights another cigarette and blows more smoke into the cups of trago. He makes the sign of the cross and then meditates. After meditating he begins to rub his upper body and head.

At 9:20 P.M., Pedro drinks the ayahuasca, chasing it down with trago. He grimaces as he swallows the bitter alkaloid. He then drinks the tobacco-soaked trago, covers his mouth, grunts, and stretches. Pedro pours the remaining tobacco juice into one hand, then cups his hands and drinks. After spitting again he washes his upper body and hands with another cup of trago. Sweating noticeably he wipes his face with a handkerchief and shouts "ay yow." In a few minutes he begins to spit more frequently. He burps loudly. The rain increases. My butt hurts. We've been sitting for ninety minutes.

For another ten minutes, Pedro continues to drink glasses of trago and smoke cigarettes, encouraging the others to join him. Suddenly, the table begins to shake. Brad realizes that they're experiencing an earthquake. It's a chilling thought — not because of physical danger from the quake, but from what it might mean to the Shuar. Had they been among the Achuar or the Waorani, such an omen would surely have meant immediate expulsion from the village, or much worse. Among the Shuar, they apparently are safe, for Pedro says nothing and continues to smoke and drink trago, tobacco juice, and more ayahuasca, as tremors rattle the furniture for another half an hour. When he's not consuming something, he sings or plays a simple four-note melody on the tumank, which sounds like a Jew's-harp. Finally, he makes his sick brother-in-law, also named Pedro, drink ayahuasca.

At 10:22 p.m., Pedro (the shaman) throws up. The moon's reflection off the clouds abruptly illuminates the room as the rain stops. Pedro drinks more tobacco juice. He lights another cigarette . . . Pedro sings . . . we smoke another round of cigarettes . . . Pedro says he feels drunk but can hear voices from other places. He prays to heal young Pedro "in the power of the Son of God." He imitates an evil shaman. He pours more trago. By now the trago and cigarettes have numbed my mouth . . . Young Pedro rests his head on the table.

The ceremony ends when Brad cannot drink any more trago or smoke any more cigarettes and collapses into his sleeping bag in the corner of the room. "Pedro didn't make any attempt to cleanse his patient," Brad recalls. A Shuar cleansing involves blowing tobacco smoke on the patient, followed by a mimed act of sucking the evil spirits out of the body. "I'm not sure if it was because we were present or because Pedro received no clear vision of the ailment," Brad says. "The kid probably had an ulcer that didn't appreciate a dose of alkaloidal ayahuasca. By then I'd seen shamans do all sorts of things. One added a Valium to his herbs for a snakebite victim, and another one put in an aspirin.

"At any rate, at six in the morning after that ceremony I walked down to the stream to wash my face and hands. I was exhausted. And there was Pedro, returning from a predawn hunting trip, none the worse for wear. I think the guy who gets to be shaman is the guy who can out-drink and out-smoke everybody else."

A week after arriving in San Miguel, Jim gets his own chance to experience some Chachi shamanistic medicine. The occasion arises in a roundabout way. The Chachi have invited the team to attend a fiesta, and Jim and Fred accept. That evening, they hire a Chachi to paddle them up the river — in the hands of an amateur, the narrow dugouts soon submerge. When they arrive at the village, the party has begun under a large thatched roof on poles. The scene is lit up by copal torches, and syncopated rhythms of Latin dance music from a battery-powered tape player throttle the air. The village men stand at one side of the clearing like quills on a nervous porcupine, while the women stand expectantly at the other side. The first couples out onto the hard-packed dirt are Africans, who slide into what looks like a samba. The Chachi hang back for a while, and when they finally do dance, they stand stiffly and avoid one another's gaze.

Fred dances with a young Chachi woman, being careful to select someone who apparently is not attached, and her friends titter and smile. Aguardiente, a cane alcohol, flows freely and the dancers soon loosen up. Jim, not one to dance under any circumstances, watches from outside the circle of light, occasionally perusing the contents of the closest houses, there being no walls to hinder his view. Hammocks and gourds hang from ceiling posts, clothes are draped over baskets woven of palm-leaves, and shotguns and machetes lean against the door frames. Lost in observation, he at first does not notice a wiry old man who approaches him. When he does, the old man smiles, his cheeks breaking into a sheaf of deep lines. Jim uses most of his Spanish. *"Hola,"* he says. *"Cómo está?"* The man responds by offering a cup of cloudy liquid from a milk jug, and Jim diplomatically downs it. It seems to be some sort of homemade whiskey. They drink another cup and the old man, who seems to be in charge of the communal bottle, waves good-bye and moves on. That's the last Jim sees of him that night.

The next morning, Jim sits on the veranda with Fred drinking instant coffee and talking about San Miguel. "I'm getting to like this place," he muses. "It's like where I grew up in upstate New York. It's got that small-town feel. People are sincere and honest, and everybody knows all the gossip." As he talks, a figure appears over the crest of the hill and approaches the house. It's the old man who was passing out the hooch at the fiesta. "Well," says Patricia through the screen door. "This is a surprise. I never thought *he* would come up here."

"Who is he?" Jim asks.

"He's a brujo. A medicine man."

The brujo introduces himself as Horátio Lopez and makes small talk about the fiesta and recent happenings along the river community. Eventually, he gets to the point. He's heard that the son of the other brujo in the community is advising the scientists on Chachi medicine.

They should know, he says, that he's an expert too. It appears he wants in on the action. Jim decides that a second opinion on Chachi medicine might be enlightening, and he hires Horátio to help.

A competition of sorts soon develops between Miguel and the old brujo. Miguel usually contradicts whatever advice Horátio has on plant medicines, and Horátio offers little resistance, whether in deference to Miguel or because he's confident in his own knowledge, no one can determine. But one thing Horátio does know for sure is how to perform a Chachi healing ceremony. Jim decides this is an opportunity that cannot be passed up. One day he asks if Horátio can cure his bad back. At first, the brujo declines, without saying why, but when pressed he reluctantly agrees. He sets the price at four thousand sucres, or about one dollar and fifty cents. Miguel, shaking his head, complains that they're being overcharged, but makes no objection.

That evening Jim goes to visit Horátio in his house, taking Fred along for support. From the copy of Barrett's 1909 ethnography in Patricia's house, they know that the Chachi attribute illness to evil spirits that live in small, black, water-worn stones, in ancient pottery, in mammals, snakes, insects and the like, and enter the body unawares, perhaps when the soul is traveling out of the body. To draw out the spirits, the shaman rubs the affected part of the body with a decoction of rum and herbs and may massage the affected part. There is much blowing of tobacco and the shaman occasionally takes a slug of the rum decoction and sprays it with his mouth over his patient. Jim wonders if this will be his fate.

Horátio meets them at his house across the river and they settle in a dimly lit room furnished with mats, a hammock, and a small table. A wooden carving of a forest spirit looks down from its place over the doorway. Jim takes off his shirt and lies prone while the brujo lights a candle and then a cigarette from a pack labeled "Full Speed" and transfers trago from a bottle he asked Jim to bring into another bottle containing branches and herbs. He hands Jim a cup of this mixture to drink, then instructs another Chachi man, an assistant brujo, to scrape Jim's bare back with an unlit candlestick. Meanwhile, Horátio chants solemnly, blows smoke over Jim, and spits trago over a collection of smooth stones, pigs' teeth, and a carved figurine representing a spirit that assists Chachi brujos. Next, the brujo takes the candle that has been rubbed on Jim, presumably now containing the evil spirit, or *Bu'chulla,* and lights it. As it burns, Horátio takes another mouthful of trago and noisily sprays it over Jim's back, then chokes on it and retches. When he recovers, he gives Fred and Jim some more trago to drink for good measure. That done, he strikes Jim's back with bundled herbs (one bunch, Jim notes diligently from the floor, is from the family Fabaceae, another is oregano), then presses the smooth rocks onto Jim's back and slaps them with his hand. They all drink more trago, Horátio applies his not-so-fine mist a few more times, and the ceremony ends.

Jim and Fred teeter home, glowing.

"So, how do you feel?" Lauralyn asks.

"Great," Jim says with a crooked grin, and collapses into a chair. After dinner, he gets up and stumbles to his bed. "Well," he says, "it felt okay till the trago wore off."

It's an hour before dawn on the day before Brad and I return to Quito. We're packing for a day-trip into the Cotacachi-Cayapas reserve, a three-hour journey upriver by motorized dugout. The destination is a waterfall and rapids where the Río Bravo, rushing clear and strong down the west slope of the Andes, spills into the Cayapas River.

The collecting has gone well. The Chachi seem enthusiastic about the collaboration, and Miguel has even learned how to handle a pinch of Red Man. Lauralyn has set up a small lab and begun analyzing plant samples for sentinel chemicals, while Patricia has put out the word in the African community that the women healers are invited to visit and share their healing methods over lunch. The team will stay for six more weeks, establishing, Brad hopes, a relationship with the Chachi that will last indefinitely.

By sunrise we're aboard two canoes and headed upriver. We stop at San Miguel to pick up Miguel, some of his friends, and one of the two park guards, Cristóbal Medina. He's a Chachi in his late thirties, with a square, set face under the only part of his clothing that qualifies as a park uniform — a short-billed hat with the word *Guardia* stitched across the front in bold green thread. Miguel whispers to us that Cristóbal never, ever takes his hat off. Having married an African woman, Cristóbal is considered something of an eccentric in San Miguel. The other park guard, Nelson Nazareno, is African and thought to be more mainstream, having two African wives and twenty-four children, among them our other informant, River.

Rapids become more frequent and larger the farther we travel upriver. The boatmen approach each torrent at a crawl, standing in the stern as the dugouts hang in the current below a jumble of rocks, foam, and marooned tree limbs. When our boatman finds a clear route, he commits us with a turn of the throttle and powers up through a sluice that only he could have seen. On several occasions we jump out and push, knee deep in the roar and splash. Ground is hard won, and we're grateful for the dugouts' narrow bottoms, which slide over the water like reeds. Eventually, we hear the rapids where the Cayapas officially begins. In fact, we can feel them on our skin, as the air fills with mist from water shattered into droplets against volcanic rock and transformed into a cloud that flickers with rainbows. The trees here extend their branches well out across the water, and the banks are studded with rocks burnished by the rub of the river to the smooth glossiness of a young palm stem.

We pull over to the bank beside two empty canoes that are tied to trees on the river's edge. Cristóbal looks them over and confers with Miguel in Cha'apalachi but says nothing to the rest of us. We clamber out, swing our day-packs onto our shoulders, and follow a path alongside the falls. Mosses are abundant and thick here, clinging to branches and tree roots that twist acrobatically over and around rock like the tentacles of octopuses. Rotting logs are everywhere, festooned with rows of creamy white or pale orange mushrooms, which on closer inspection are the homes of tiny flies. Miniature ferns poke up through the flaking bark. Below us, the river falls some sixty feet over three huge ledges, like the mythical cyclops Polyphemus's rocky footpath down his Sicilian mountainside. At the top of the falls, a house-sized rock sits at the edge of a wide pool that swirls and curves before sliding down into the falls. Atop the rock, we can see above the falls to a river, the Río Bravo, as clear as any Caribbean lagoon. The place could well be the gate to Elysium.

A few years before, two Chachi went into the reserve from here and never returned. Patricia says the Chachi believe they were done away with by the Indios Bravos. "Miguel believes it too," she says. "He believes there's a monster that lives under this very rock, and there are others in the waterfall. And most of them believe that Indios Bravos eat Chachi."

"They think that Indios Bravos are white, don't they?" Lauralyn asks.

"Yeah," Patricia replies, "and we most certainly are demons." She tears open an orange and stuffs the peel into her backpack. "They're all convinced that there is danger lurking everywhere."

After lunch we walk upriver to where the water is calm, strip to our shorts, and dive in. The water is cool and so clear that we cannot imagine anything unsavory lurking within it. Even Miguel and the Chachi boys dive in, shouting and laughing with uncharacteristic abandon. Cristóbal, however, sits on a rock looking dignified. When we come ashore, he tells Brad that there are poachers somewhere nearby. The canoes left below the falls belong to them, he says, and he suspects they have gone upriver to fell trees and float them through the falls to where they can be lashed together and floated at night past San Miguel and on to Borbón. He wants Brad to go with him to investigate.

Brad, Miguel, and I swim across the river to find a small dugout that Miguel has hidden in the woods for his occasional trips upriver, while Cristóbal forges ahead on foot through the shallows. Aboard the dugout, Miguel tries gamely to pole us into the current, but our top-heavy North American bodies capsize the boat. We try to push it up through the shallows, but our bare feet find little purchase on the mossy rocks. Brad grunts and grimaces as his injured toe — somewhat the better from the sangre de drago but still painful — is mauled. We decide to ditch the boat. "Let's just swim," Brad suggests.

We stick to the river's edges, where the current is slower. King-fishers swoop overhead, and we hear the call of a bellbird in the riverine gallery. Below the surface the riverbed is scoured with hummocks of smooth, black rock that look like the backs of sleeping manatees. Clumps of long-stemmed, rust-colored weed billow up toward the surface, swaying with the current. I can see how someone on the bank could mistake these shapes for dormant beasts. We grab hanging lianas and the branches of fallen trees to pull ourselves along, and soon establish a regular pace behind Cristóbal, who's plowing ahead upstream.

We don't know how far we have to go, nor what, or who, we'll meet when we get there. But what ill could befall us when above we're escorted by such a dazzling pair of morpho butterflies? Their wingspan is a good ten centimeters across, and the upper sides of their wings are an intense blue like nothing else in the forest. They're ungainly fliers, inscribing a series of U's in the air as they rise and dip. On the upswing, the blue surface shows like a beacon, and when they gather their wings behind them for another thrust, the brown undersides of their wings blend with the backdrop of trees. The result is a flickering, strobe-like effect, a clever camouflage against predation by birds like the jacamar, which can swoop down and pluck a butterfly out of the air.

As we swim, I remember that von Humboldt once wrote of a Río Guancabamba, another river that falls from the Andes. The river people there had a very singular manner for the conveyance of correspondence, called the *correo que nada*, or the swimming courier. A young man would swim for days at a time from one village to another, carrying letters in a large cotton handkerchief wound around his head like a turban. Sometimes the swimmer would throw his arm around a piece of wood (which the ever-observant von Humboldt noted was of the family Bombacaceae) when he got tired. Good citizens living along the way would provide food and drink.

There are no signs of food or drink on this river, however, and after an hour of swimming and walking along gravel bars, we're beginning to question our sanity. Around a turn, finally, we come upon Cristóbal. He stands ankle deep in red mud, peering around a boulder. Ahead, the riverbank looks like a boil that has burst. The lateritic soil, full of aluminum and ferric oxide, runs red and sticky down to the water, where the vegetation has been cut and cleared, and the ground is rutted where logs have been rolled into the river. In the forest, shafts of yellow sunlight penetrate where cedar once stood. We walk quietly up behind Cristóbal, unsure of what to do next. Brad looks at me, then down at himself, and laughs. "Look at us," he whispers. "These poachers carry machetes, they have chain saws, and they have shotguns to hunt with. What are we gonna do if we *do* find them? Wave our swimming trunks at 'em?" This disparity in firepower doesn't faze Cristóbal, who now strides up the slippery bank. Perhaps he's reassured by some perceived aura of scientific authority that a half-naked North American botanist radiates. More probably, the bravado comes from his hat, soggy but still square on his head and emblazoned with that authoritative green stitching — *Guardia!*

No gunshots ring out, nor challenges from grizzled frontiersmen or Indios Bravos. The place has been abandoned. Cristóbal finds a few plastic bags half-submerged in the muck, some cigarette butts, and a tin cup. Brad walks into the woods with Cristóbal to identify some of the felled trees and do a little on-the-spot botanizing. I turn to walk down to the bank into the sun to dry, but before I can put my foot down, Miguel grabs my arm and pulls me back. He points to the ground. Where I was about to step, the oddest creature slithers across the rocks, the biggest caterpillar I've ever seen, fully a foot long. On closer inspection, I realize that the creature is actually seven caterpillars, lime green, hairy, and attached front to back like a line of freight cars. Miguel smiles. He takes a stick and writes a word in the sand. *"Wacha,"* he says. "Patricia taught me this English word," he says in Spanish.

"Oh, you mean *watch out*," I reply.

"Si, *wacha*," he nods, pointing to the caterpillars. "They sting." I agree that *wacha* is indeed a useful word of English to learn if one lives in the rainforest.

Brad and Cristóbal return and we dive into the river for a free-float back downstream. This is a belly-up float trip, with a three-knot current and deep water to carry us back to the falls. Cristóbal loosens up and joins us as we swing on hanging lianas and float with our feet up in the air, while Brad sings. "Take it easy, take it easy, don't let the sound of your own wheels drive you crazy," he warbles, then switches into a sing-song botanical chant as he identifies the passing trees: "*Me*-la-*sto*-ma-*ta*-ce-ay, *Ma*-ran-*ta*-ce-ay and *Palm*-ay, *Cy*-clan-*tha*-ce-ay, A-*can*-tha-ce-ay." We come to a rapid and Brad yells to Miguel, "Let's do it." They swim to the middle of the channel, point their legs downstream, and rush into a standing, foamy wave. For a few long seconds they disappear, then bob to the surface, whirling like corks, too breathless and scared to laugh but grinning like kids on a Ferris wheel.

As we float back down to the falls, I reflect on the nature of this craft and science, ethnobotany. The ethnobotanist spends half his time amid the sacred, trying to separate mumbo jumbo from ancient if primitive genius, and the other half amid the profane, looking down the barrel of a microscope and deciphering the code of taxa, alkaloids, symbiotes, and the ephemera of ecology. More than most other sciences, ethnobotany has continued to run on the radiant energy of great but long-dead men. Ask an ethnobotanist to name the lights of the discipline, and most of the names will be of people born in the last century. Even the totemic personality of twentieth-century ethnobotany, Richard Schultes, was born during World War I. He still writes in Latin and acknowledges that he has patterned his career after a man who died a century ago.

But now the discipline is changing. Scientists are embracing the new realities of Third World politics as well as the demands of drug-makers and conservationists back home. In the meantime, they watch helplessly as the traditions they study slip from their grasp like puddles of mercury. That is one reason why, probably more than any other type of scientist, tropical botanists are willing to put limb and even life on the line for their work. The risks can be dramatic: a capsized canoe on a flooded river, a poisonous snakebite two days' travel from medical help, liana bridges of questionable engineering. Usually what gets them is something more mundane, however — muggers in Lima, a plane crash, an overturned ranchero, or, probably most feared, some insidious parasitic disease. The common topic of conversation in the halls of herbaria is who got malaria or what the latest drugs are to treat giardia. We get to have all this, they laugh, and an assistant professor's salary too.

Few dwell on the dangers, however. They would rather talk about what you have to be to become an ethnobotanist. The night before our trip to the Río Bravo, Brad described the qualifications. "People who like adventure, who like the outdoors," he said. "And while you have to be a people person, you also have to remain objective. There are some who worship native peoples, the 'noble savages.' There has never been a noble savage. They're just like everybody else. They're as selfish as we are, as cruel, greedy, kind, generous, loving." And you have to be patient, he said, because if you push at the wrong time, things won't happen. You also must be able to handle disappointment. "And, most of all, you have to expect the unexpected."

These ruminations are too heavy to carry along the Bravo for long, however. It's enough simply to watch the trees that have risen from the earth, merged, and overtaken the horizon. For a moment, I can forget *wacha*, plants, loggers, and undiscovered alkaloids, and simply surrender to the river, to be pulled gently through this green fuse, back to the beginning.

12

The End of the Pipeline

Spread out a map of the world and stick a green-headed pin into
northern Ecuador. Put another pin into the center of Belize for the Ix
Chel farm, another in the forests of Cameroon in West Africa, another
on the Caribbean island of Dominica, and yet another on the Southeast
Asian island of Sarawak. Each represents a source point, a well from
which new compounds from plants are being drawn. That map, peppered with scores of pins, hangs on the wall of an office at the heart of
a military base in the green hills of northern Maryland.

At Fort Dietrick, on the edge of the Catoctin Mountain ridge, two
groups of scientists toy with the chemistry of death and life. One group
studies how microorganisms and chemicals can kill people. The other
scans the planet for substances to rescue us from cancer and AIDS. Fort
Dietrick is an irony of convenience, pairing the U.S. Army's chemical
and biological warfare program with the drug discovery group of the
National Cancer Institute (NCI). Were Americans more given to symbolism, we might fashion a logo for Fort Dietrick, depicting the forces
of good and evil locked in conflict, perhaps a pair of notched cog-
wheels, enmeshed but turning in opposite directions.

As it is, most people do not know much about what goes on at Fort Dietrick. The town of Frederick has grown around the military base like ivy around an old potting shed, and people here are accustomed to shuttered buildings and cryptic cargoes rolling through the streets. So the windowless, squat brick building near the railroad tracks, where trucks with "US government" license plates pull up and unload lumpy linen bags and unmarked cartons, is so much backdrop. Yet there is no other place like this in the world. Inside this building, in rows of two-story-high freezers, lies hope for millions of people dying of cancer or AIDS.

If you walk inside one of these twenty-eight custom-made freezers, you can look up through the swirling mist and the perforated aluminum floors and see racks and racks of boxes and fiber bags. The bags are tagged with dates, identifying numbers, and brief descriptions, such as "New York Botanical Garden: H. Beck. Dominica," and "Cameroon, D. Thomas, Missouri Botanical Garden." Inside the bags are the raw materials, leaves and branches and bark, frozen to a brittle −20 C. In the boxes are scores of vials filled with gooey residues squeezed from the tissue of plants and marine organisms.

This place is NCI's Natural Products Repository. Hundreds of collectors began filling it with plants, fungi, protozoa, and microorganisms from all parts of the world in 1986, when NCI's plant discovery program was restarted after several years of neglect. By early 1992, over twenty thousand terrestrial plant specimens had arrived at the repository, as well as seventy-five hundred marine animal specimens, and over two thousand marine plants. Fungi have recently been added to the list and are coming in at a rate of about twenty a week. All the lines drawn from all the green pins converge here.

Beginnings are difficult, and this repository was no exception, though not so much because of nature's obstinacy but science's. The man who convinced the skeptics it was worth creating is Michael R. Boyd, a restless man of forty-six, compact and quick and possessed with a nervous energy that, like an object charged with static electricity, constantly seeks an outlet. He holds a medical degree as well as a doctorate in pharmacology, drives a big pickup truck, and flies planes for fun. He is of a scientific species called the lab jockey, whose forte is detail and technique. In the quest for new drugs, he designs the equipment, marks off the false trails, and ensures that the path taken is the shortest and truest. Boyd may not be the kind of blue-sky theorist who wins the Nobel Prize, but he is the kind of person who is likely to make it possible for someone else to.

In 1982, the cancer research community and its Mecca, NCI, had literally dumped its phytochemistry program. Over a period of twenty-five years, NCI had screened over one hundred thousand plants and close to two hundred thousand microorganisms against cancer, yet none had led to development of a successful treatment. NCI decided to pack it in, and gave away most of its extracts to academics. Synthetic chemicals became almost the sole reservoir for experimenters to draw from.

Boyd, a senior scientist with the drug development program at NCI at the time, believed the institute was throwing out the baby with the bathwater. Boyd's faith in natural products had been inspired by a medical mystery he helped solve as a young chemist twenty years before in his native Tennessee. Cattle had been dying of a mysterious ailment after eating moldy sweet potatoes. The mold, the young scientist discovered, created a toxic chemical that destroyed the cows' lungs. Boyd helped show that this compound, ipomeanol, also killed lung cancer cells. That discovery put Boyd's name on an article in the prestigious journal *Nature* and started his career in parsing the chemistry of nature. (Ipomeanol, meanwhile, is currently an experimental drug for lung cancer.)

The failure to find many new drugs for cancer lay not with nature, Boyd reasoned, but with the methods humans had devised. By the early 1980s, close to half a million chemical compounds had been tested against cancer — on mice. Only those that worked against either one of two forms of mouse leukemia, a cancer of the blood, proceeded to trials against human cancer. The philosophy was, cancer is cancer is cancer; what works against one should work against others. Indeed, many of the "winners" did work against human leukemia, but very few affected cancers of the brain, liver, lung, kidney, and other organs.

After decades following this line of reasoning, drug-screeners had produced about sixty cancer drugs, mostly from synthetic chemicals. The majority of them worked pretty much the same way, by interfering with the way cells make DNA when they are dividing and reproducing. Few worked very well, however. Scientists were frustrated. "We just had damn few good drugs," Boyd recalls. "I had just lost another uncle to lung cancer. I mean, hell, people would call me because I worked at the cancer institute. Well, what could I do? There was nothing you can really treat that disease with. . . . I had told my uncle, basically, 'Forget it, enjoy your days because the drugs are worse than the disease in many ways.'"

Boyd argued for a radical change in drug screening. The mice should get a rest. What the war on cancer really needed was a defense of infinite variety to match cancer's seemingly infinite powers of disguise and infiltration. That meant better reconnaissance and a wider variety of weapons to choose from, weapons that the human mind had never imagined.

In 1984, Boyd took over the job of associate director of NCI for the Developmental Therapeutics Program, the arm of the institute that searches for new drugs. He was young for the job, just thirty-seven, and brash: in short, a thorn in the side of the graybeards who ran the nation's biggest cancer research operation. NCI had been spending much of its time squeezing tiny improvements out of existing drugs by mixing them into unusual cocktails or by putting them into patients in new, more efficient ways: laudable efforts, but not likely to produce remarkable advances. Cancer researchers meanwhile were being harried by critics in Congress who had tired of spending billions for the war on cancer with so few victories. It was not a good time for a newcomer to barge into the war room and accuse the generals of blowing the campaign.

NCI had kept a small budget for natural products, which it handed out to a coterie of researchers who made a comfortable living testing them against cancer. Boyd wanted to set up his own plant-testing operation, an idea that set the existing plant-testers into a lather. Boyd lobbied hard, knocking on doors up and down the gray hallways at NCI's headquarters on the sprawling campus of its parent organization, the National Institutes of Health (NIH), in the suburbs of Washington, D.C. He was a paradoxical character, with his buttery, Smoky Mountains drawl yet relentless, rapid-fire delivery. Many among the white-coated, Ivy-league scientocracy at NIH viewed him as a dreamer, and he set the needles quivering in the normally tectonic cancer community. "I was getting shot at at every turn," Boyd recalls, "and everybody at NIH was under the table." So Boyd went outside the cancer club for support. He assembled an informal advisory group of scientists, mostly from abroad, with good reputations and no stake in the status quo at NCI. They met regularly with Boyd to whip his plans into shape. "We would yell back and forth and argue all day," Boyd recalls. After two years in this intellectual forge, Boyd's plan for a new natural products program was wrought and, he believed, close to ironclad. The core of his argument was the undeniable contribution that natural products had made to medicine. The most spectacular were the vinca alkaloids, vincristine and vinblastine, from the common ornamental the rosy periwinkle. But there were other experimental compounds with promise, too, like homoharringtonine, from the Chinese plant *Cephalotaxus*. There was podophyllotoxin from roots of the mayapple, *Podophyllum peltatum*, whose roots had been used by Native Americans for worms, fevers, jaundice, and constipation. It had been tested in the 1950s by NCI (although it killed tumor cells, it was too toxic for humans), but a new version of it had been made into the experimental cancer drugs etoposide and teniposide. Etoposide was approved in 1983 for use against forms of leukemia, lung cancer, testicular cancer, and lymphoma.

And what about the oceans? Boyd argued. Marine organisms had barely been looked at. Two that had — the sea squirt (species of the genus *Didemnidae*) and the sea hare, *Dolabella auricularia*, had produced experimental compounds that were quite potent cancer inhibitors. There were also bacteria from the Bahamian sea floor that made chemicals called macrolactins that worked in the test tube against skin and colon cancer cells. Even traditionally conservative drug companies were hiring divers and marine biologists to start searching the ocean floor for new compounds.

Natural substances also were producing other drugs besides cancer treatments. Scientists at Johns Hopkins University and government laboratories were testing a new compound called artemisinin, from the plant *Artemisia annua*. The fragrant herb grew wild in China and, called "qing hao," had been used for centuries there against fever, and now artemisinin was believed to work against forms of malaria that were quinine-resistant. And bacteria from jellyfish in Florida had been found to contain compounds called salinamides, found to be effective against inflammation and potentially a new treatment for arthritis and asthma.

Skeptics pointed out that most of the natural product drugs had been discovered long before. The fabulously successful vinca alkaloids for childhood lymphocytic leukemia and Hodgkin's disease were products of the 1950s, and, moreover, had been found by accident. If there were more hot compounds out there, they would have been uncovered already. Besides, natural products required too much luck and carried too much risk, while drug companies would be reluctant to develop them because their patentability was often in doubt. What was left unsaid was that natural product chemistry lacked prestige. Synthetic drug designers considered themselves to be the pharmaceutical world's fly-fishermen, stalking their prey with knowledge and calculation, the "rational" way. Natural products people were viewed as simple empiricists, like worm fishermen who sat with their bait bouncing on the bottom, hoping that something big would come along and take it. That was the most generous view. Many simply lumped phytochemists in with fringe herbalists and their ilk. Laetrile was an example of such pseudo-science. Rejected as ineffective by cancer researchers, the peach-pit extract was embraced by unconventional healers and legalized in twenty-one states. Laetrile eventually failed and sank from sight, and the gulf between mainstream and unconventional medicine widened. In the late 1980s, the government's Office of Technology Assessment tried and failed to find common ground between the two groups. "The sides are closely drawn," the OTA reported, "and the rhetoric is often bitter and confrontational. Little or no constructive dialogue has yet taken place."

Boyd, however, believed natural products research could be made rational. For cancer, it amounted to viewing the illness more as a series of related diseases than as some monolithic monster. What might stop cancer in a woman's ovaries could not be expected to stop skin cancer any more than an antibiotic for an infected wound could be expected to cure a fungal infection. Being smart — rational — involved creating better screens.

"I spent years trying to convince people of this," Boyd recalls. In 1984 he got his first break: NCI gave him permission to develop a pilot program for testing plants and marine organisms for anti-cancer potential. It was, in essence, an invitation to stick his neck out. He started small, at a laboratory at the Frederick Cancer Research Center at Fort Dietrick's chemical and biological warfare operation in Frederick. It seemed an odd place to put scientists who were working on new ways to cure the sick, recalls chemist John Beutler, one of Boyd's collaborators in what was dubbed the "grind 'em and find 'em" operation. Then again, cancer, AIDS, and chemical weapons revolve around similar biochemical processes, whether they be life-giving or life-ending.

Prospecting for drugs from plants was all a matter of how you looked, Boyd told his colleagues at Frederick. A compound that fails against one kind of cancer might do better against another — a philosophy not so different from what the Quichua shamans and Belize bush doctors espoused: that somewhere on the planet there is a plant for every disease of man. Unlike the brujos, however, Boyd did not have to rely on generations of trial and error to prove it; he had millions of dollars and some of the world's finest laboratory technology at his disposal. Instead of patients in thatched huts, he had cancer cells from patients with seven major types of cancer: lung, melanoma (skin), kidney, ovarian, brain, blood, and colon. The plan was to grow sixty variations on these cancer cells in dozens of tiny wells punched into plastic sheets, each the size of a school notebook. Into each well would go extracts from nature, up to three hundred a week, in a continuous production line. Anything that slowed or killed the cancer cells would move on to tests with tumors grown in mice. If it passed that test, the long process of analyzing the chemical's structure, its toxicity, and its potential for human use would begin.

To feed all these screens, Boyd wanted to take a huge slice of the planet — almost all of its tropical biota. That meant half the species of organisms on the Earth. Who could satisfy such a huge appetite? Boyd convinced NCI to give him $1.2 million to pay for a legion of new plant-hunters to vacuum the world's tropical ecosystems. On September 1, 1986, his laboratory signed contracts with three organizations to do the job: the New York Botanical Garden, the Missouri Botanical Garden, and the University of Illinois in Chicago. Keeping this botanical foreign legion going became the full-time job of Gordon M. Cragg, a soft-spoken, wiry South African expatriate who left his position at Arizona State University to join Boyd's operation in 1984. For five years, the three contractors would sniff out unusual plants, marine organisms, fungi, cyanobacteria (blue-green algae), and protozoa. Their territory would encompass twenty-five tropical countries, with New York exploring Central and South America, Missouri searching Africa, and Illinois traversing the forests of Asia. Each institution was to collect at least fifteen hundred specimens per year. It was the biggest search for medicinal plants in history, with scores of plant-hunters whose peregrinations were marked by the pins in Cragg's wall map.

For botanists, this amounted to an ocean of plants. Yet for chemists, the project would at first be fishing in a rather small pond. Drug experts say a good hit rate is one worthwhile compound in every one thousand plants (not to be confused with the rate of one in ten thousand chemical compounds that drug companies cite). And NCI was just looking for activity against cancer. So the odds of quick success were long. Boyd, however, convinced NCI that his new screens could do better than one in a thousand. They had to. "A lot of people thought it was a boondoggle," Boyd recalls. "All the experts in the field said this was not possible to do and not worth trying."

In 1986, Boyd's group decided they should cast their net a little wider. If natural products could produce cancer drugs, why not also medicines for humanity's newest and most puzzling pathogen, the human immunodeficiency virus (HIV), the cause of AIDS? Nobody, said Boyd, had ever looked systematically. Within a year, Boyd had a set of HIV screens up and running at Frederick.

Boyd's grind 'em and find 'em bunch began to win some influential allies. David Korn, dean of Stanford University's School of Medicine and a member of NCI's advisory board, backed Boyd's approach. Drug companies were quietly supportive, too; after all, they would have access to this new larder of compounds stocked by the government. But Boyd needed a hit soon to keep the skeptics at bay, and the news from the cancer screens was bad. They were proving very difficult to manage. Growing human cancer cells in a lab is not like kneading yeast into warm water and flour and watching it rise. Each type of cancer cell is different and endlessly quirky. Most were very sensitive to things like the nutrients they grew in or temperature, and when a plant extract was added and altered the cells, lab technicians had be sure it was indeed the extract that did it and not some environmental effect or accidental contamination.

Then the researchers had to learn how to read the screens. Extracts that killed all types of cancer cells, for example, were generally use- less — these might stop cancer, but they would probably kill the patient too. They wanted compounds that were more selective, that might kill some kinds of cancer but have little or no effect on others. The scientists found that each compound created a kind of fingerprint that could be quickly read as success or failure. On paper, these prints took the form of a bar graph that looked like a comb missing some of its teeth. Each tooth of the comb represented the effect of a compound on one type of cancer. Where the teeth remained, the extract had killed lots of cancer cells. Where they were short or broken off, the extract had had little or no effect.

The fingerprints led Boyd to the suspects. For example, compounds that turned out to be false positives, that is, that seemed to work against cancer at first but eventually failed, often had distinctively similar fin- gerprints. Other fingerprints might resemble those of drugs known to work against cancer, like Adriamycin or Mithramycin; Boyd's lab had 176 prints of known anti-cancer compounds like these for comparison. Some new fingerprints were bizarre, and thus especially interesting. Whenever extracts looked intriguing, they would be fractioned into their chemical subparts — there could be scores in one extract — and recycled back through the screens in what Boyd called bioassay-guided isolation, until the individual compound that actually worked was found. Learning to do all this took time, however, and it generated amounts of information that only computers could handle. "A lot of people in the beginning said this would be impossible to do," Boyd recalls. "It wasn't. It was just a nightmare."

One year passed with nothing of interest to report from the AIDS screens, then another, and then a third. The cancer screens finally got working properly in 1990. Still nothing materialized. With the end of the first natural products collecting contract just over a year away, the Frederick team still had no drug candidate to show for the effort. Unless someone found a wonder plant soon, Boyd suspected that the program would be killed.

In 1990, that wonder plant materialized. It did not come from Boyd's shop, however. In fact, it was not even from the tropics but from North America. Yet it worked against cancer like nothing ever seen before, and if it lived up to its promise, it would give Boyd and his plant-hunters a new bargaining chip because the source of the excitement was a tree, a trash tree, unprepossessing and considered worthless. It was the Pacific yew, from the remnants of the Pacific Northwest's great temperate rainforests. From its inner bark came the extraordinary substance, taxol.

13

The Yew

Taxol begins as tree bark on the steep slopes of the Cascade Range that runs from Washington State down to northern California. A typical bark-peeling day in August 1992 starts at first light along a gravel logging road on the range's western slope. A pickup truck with heavy-duty shocks and a permanent coat of dust pulls to a stop at a lonely spot along the road and a crew of young men climb out. The bark-peelers pull on their caulks, the clunky, spike-soled boots that loggers wear to keep their feet attached to the thirty-five-degree slopes, hoist thirty-pound chain saws and stacks of burlap bags, and start up the slope. The sun is just rising above the hills to the east, the direction in which the bark from the yew trees they seek will eventually go.

Most of the mountainside has been clear-cut, the fate of the great majority of Oregon's privately owned, old-growth forest. The Douglas fir and cedar that grew on this unit of some two thousand acres is now plywood, studs, or furniture in homes from New York to Tokyo. In its place is waist-high scrub of Oregon grape, sword fern, red cedar saplings, and tangles of blackberries, whose thorns rip at the palms and ankles at every step. The peelers climb for twenty minutes to where the clear-cut ends and the forest begins again. There, the ground turns spongy and treacherous with rotting branches and knee-deep piles of evergreen needles. The sun does not penetrate here, and at this hour the late-summer air still holds traces of night coolness and the dampness of rain that fell weeks ago.

Martin Thiele finds the tree he is looking for and drops his gear. Thiele is an ex-logger in his early thirties, slat thin and slow-talking, with a springy, nut-colored beard, who has learned to peel bark for a living. His felled yew tree lies precariously across a small ravine, perpendicular to the slope. Fellow members of his crew fan out to look for other yews to cut and strip. Stripping the bark kills the tree, so the workers generally cut them down first to get at all the available bark. This is the last chance to get the yew out of this unit; loggers will be here soon to clear-cut the rest of the hill.

The peelers number a half-dozen and have the logger look: straight-legged denims and checked cotton shirts, one man with a ponytail, several with faces almost hidden behind rangy beards, all thick through the chest and shoulders with blunt fingers and hands engraved with small wounds that come with working with sharp instruments in the woods. At one time or another, they have felled or set choker cables on Douglas fir, or driven the skidders and Cats that haul or "yard" out big Oregon trees. But the timber industry in the Northwest slumped in the mid-1980s, victim of overcutting if you listen to the environmentalists, or of government overregulation if you listen to the logging industry. Now loggers find work wherever they can get it.

The yew trees in these forests used to be considered trash. They grew in among the taller firs, and clear-cutters felled and dozed the yew into slash piles where they were left to rot and then burn in the fires set after logging to clear undergrowth so that new fir seedlings could be planted. Then in 1988, a company called Hauser Chemical Northwest arrived in Cottage Grove in western Oregon, set up an office on a large lot on the edge of town, and put out the word that they would pay for bark from the Pacific yew. The news spread quickly through this community of hard-nosed lumberjacks, men who had left the woods to drive trucks, work farms, learn new trades, or collect unemployment in towns like Roseburg, Drain, Umpqua, Mohawk, Springfield, and Riddle. The work would be steady and safer than handling eighty-foot logs that could crush a man's leg or snap a cable that would arc through the air and cut off an arm, logs that could release a bent sapling like a catapult and knock a big man down like a matchstick. And the "tree-huggers," the kindest term here for the environmentalists who fought to save the old growth forests and the spotted owl that lived within them, could not get in the way. This bark cured cancer.

Thiele kneels next to his yew and works the bark off with a metal tool like a paint scraper. This time of year, late summer, the bark tends to seize up on the trunk. Many foresters here say just leaving a tree cut and down for a day or two will do that. On the other hand, the drought the region has been suffering from may be doing it. "Sometimes I'll get a tree where the bark is stickin' real bad, and I'll curse the day I ever started this job," says Thiele. He peels as he talks, making a longitudinal cut with the corner of his scraper, then working the edge of it under the bark and jimmying up a piece. Moist, it feels like stiff boot-leather, an eighth of an inch thick, with pink-white cambium on the inside. "My worst day was thirty-seven pounds," Thiele says. "My best day was one hundred ninety-one."

Thiele was hired by one of about fifty-five contractors who collect for Hauser. The U.S. Forest Service and Bureau of Land Management (BLM) set rules for collecting on federal land. They require collectors and timber companies to leave some yews standing on every unit to preserve the genetic pool. When a tree is cut, a stump twelve inches high must be left so that it can regrow vegetatively. Bark must be stripped down to the point where branches are no more than one inch thick. These rules came after Hauser and the government took a thrashing in the press. A former schoolteacher named Wendell Wood of the Oregon Natural Resources Council (ONRC) snuck into logged sites and found felled trees where bark had only been partly stripped. There was too much waste, Wood argued, in part because bark strippers were being paid by the pound and would pick over the easy parts of the tree and leave the rest. There were too few yew trees to waste anything, said Wood. They grew in isolated clumps and only in old growth forests, averaging perhaps one per acre or fewer. And no one knew the total yew population — estimates ranged from four million to over one hundred million, so broad a range as to render the estimate useless. Besides its western range, the right kind of yew tree grew only in parts of Idaho and Montana, and environmentalists worried that a few years of unrestricted cutting could wipe out the yew before taxol even got beyond the experimental stage.

So in 1992 the Forest Service and BLM required collectors to haul trees out of the woods if they could not strip them clean right away, and finish the job at the Hauser yard. They also encouraged Hauser to pay peelers by the hour or day, not by the pound. Hauser now has inspectors, like Jeff Schutte, a broad-shouldered, twenty-one-year-old woodsman and college student who started working in logging at the age of fourteen. Schutte had planned to learn forestry engineering, to run the machines that cut and haul the massive trees, but demand for those skills has all but evaporated, and Schutte studies forestry management instead. In the meantime, he drives hundreds of miles a week from unit to unit to check on Hauser's peelers. Today, he is visiting Thiele's crew.

Thiele says he was "just doin' whatever fell into place" before this job came along. "I like working in the woods," he says, stripping and bagging as he talks. "This seems like a level-headed compromise, a wise use of the woods. There is rhetoric about yew wood being wiped out, usually from people who ask questions like, 'Do the yew trees live after you take the bark off?' You kinda have to keep from smiling too big and explain to them what's going on. It's a slow process. Human beings are prone to making lots of mistakes before they do what's right. But people are waking up to the fact that they ought to leave a little bit of everything to grow."

By day's end Thiele and his fellow peelers have three or four bags of bark each. Sweaty and stiff in the joints from climbing and squatting all day, they toss the bags down the embankment and follow them, legs bent at the knee against the pull of gravity, to the road below. Their boss weighs the bags and attaches "trip-tickets" to each indicating where, when, and by whom it was collected. Sometimes poachers come in and strip whatever they can reach, killing the trees and wasting most of the bark. Two men were tried, convicted, and fined for poaching yew bark in 1992. The tags are meant to discourage poaching, although the practice continues. Schutte says when Hauser hears about poached trees, it sends peelers in to salvage what is left.

The peeling today has been slow, and Thiele's boss hammers his crew with a workingman's frank profanity for cutting down a large, old yew and failing to strip it right away. Its bark is now as tight on the trunk as white on rice. "Who needs this?" mutters one tired-looking young man. Still, it could be worse: in some units, cutters have to fell the trees with hand saws — they call them "misery whips" — rather than risk setting the drought-dried brush afire with a spark from a chain saw. And one hundred dollars a day is hard to pass up when jobs are scarce. Moreover, these woodsmen can go home and tell their families that instead of leveling forests they are helping to fight cancer.

When taxol got its first trial in humans, in 1983, it made them very sick. Their blood pressure dropped, their muscles ached, they vomited. Trials were suspended and many cancer researchers wanted to drop it altogether. Ten years later, it would become the hottest new cancer drug in the world. Its story is a lesson on how circuitous a drug's journey is from the forest to the patient.

The Pacific yew, *Taxus brevifolia*, is an evergreen tree with a fleshy aril, or berry, instead of a cone. In the moist temperate forests of Oregon and Washington, its spindly branches collect moss, giving the trees a soft, almost hairy appearance, like the legs of a tarantula. There are six other species of yew besides the Pacific yew, though each is closely related and hybrids are common. The yew is a slow grower, a mature tree adding an inch in trunk diameter every ten to fifteen years, and a tree fifty feet tall is considered big. There are living European yews (*Taxus baccata*) that were seedlings before the Goths sacked Rome.

Throughout history, the yew has been associated with death, and the tree was often planted in graveyards. In the second century b.c., the Greek poet Nicander warned about people being poisoned with an oil of crushed yew leaves, bark, or seeds. In *Macbeth*, the three witches spice their bubbling cauldron of brew with "slips of yew sliver'd in the moon's eclipse." Greek mythology held the yew sacred to Hecate, the goddess who represented the waning moon and had dominion over the land of the dead. But the yew also had its defenders. Chinese healers used it to treat arthritis, while Native Americans prescribed bark extracts for kidney disease, digestive distress, scurvy, and tuberculosis. The wood is extremely hard and dense, and the oldest-known wooden implement is a spear made of yew found in Great Britain, said to be fifty thousand years old, according to Hal Hartzell, a forester and author of the book *The Yew Tree: A Thousand Whispers*. The yew was especially favored for bows; the reputedly five-thousand-year-old man whose corpse was recently found frozen in the Italian Alps was carrying a yew bow.

In 1962, a bag of yew bark was just one of many samples collected by foresters in Washington State to send back east to NCI. Little was known about the tree's chemistry except that it contained alkaloids. It would take three decades to find out what magical properties the bark actually possessed.

When yew extract was put through the standard test against cancer cells in a laboratory, it appeared to slow down the cancer's growth. So NCI got more tree parts, made extracts, and sent them to one of its best consulting chemists, Monroe Wall at Research Triangle Institute in North Carolina. Wall found that crude extracts worked against mouse leukemia, and he set about ferreting out the chemical compound in the plant that was responsible. It took several years of painstakingly eliminating one compound after another in the extract until, in 1967, Wall and colleague Mansukh C. Wani found the right one. They called it taxol, after the tree's genus, and Wall told NCI it deserved special attention. By then, the U.S. Department of Agriculture had indeed been looking for more abundant species of the yew to see if they would yield taxol. Wild trees were peeled and cut in the United States, Italy, Mexico, Florida, and in a nursery in Maryland, but none matched the Pacific yew for taxol content. And the Pacific yew was proving difficult to find.

At the time, there were thousands of compounds with some sort of activity against cancer floating through the NCI system, and none so far had panned out. Taxol was put on hold and might have joined the effluvia of rejected plants but for the continuing efforts of Wall and others intrigued with this odd material. In 1971, Wall published taxol's molecular structure. It was a dauntingly complex molecule, a diterpene, a compound common to plants but with an unusual, clunky structure: a core with twenty carbon atoms arranged in three linked rings, with a side chain of atoms extending from one ring and a fourth ring hanging off another. It was a conundrum, and not something that was going to be synthesized from scratch anytime soon.

Taxol's novelty, however, was still not sufficient to push it into the research mainstream. True, it did seem to work in some tests against a form of skin cancer in mice, done in 1974. But it was not until 1977 that NCI made a serious effort to find out how taxol worked. Chosen for the job was Susan B. Horwitz, a professor of molecular pharmacology at the Albert Einstein College of Medicine in the Bronx. Horwitz noted that it certainly was odd-looking stuff, something that only nature could have dreamed up. With ten milligrams of taxol, not enough even to coat a fingernail, Horwitz and graduate student Peter Schiff tested it against several cultures of human tumor cells. What they observed under the microscope was like nothing ever seen before.

The cancer cells were not dividing, the very thing that cancer cells normally do best. Inside each cell were parallel bundles of microtubules, spindle-like structures of a substance called tubulin that form a framework when a cell is about to divide. Microtubules are needed at this critical point, when the cell's two sets of chromosomes are rearranged just prior to separating into what will soon become two daughter cells. A cell must dismantle its microtubules, like scaffolding in a building under construction, before this final division takes place. But these microtubules had gone rigid. "Taxol had gummed them up," says

Horwitz, who, like Wall and other taxol pioneers, continues to study the substance to this day. Even when she tried, Horwitz could not cause the cancer cells to pull apart the taxol-treated microtubules, and the cells soon died. It was indeed a rare and bizarre material, one that Horwitz guessed might well be a completely new class of anti-cancer drug.

That uniqueness was exactly what cancer researchers like to see. So NCI finally started putting money into tests of taxol against human cancers transplanted into mice, a technique that had just been developed. Taxol worked well. That was no guarantee, however — plenty of compounds could slow cancer in mice but did nothing for humans with cancer. But it was looking better all the time. If taxol proved not to be toxic to other, *non*cancerous cells, cancer patients would get a chance to try it.

The glitch was the supply line. Yew bark was scarce. Most Pacific yews were less than ten inches in diameter, and many were only shrubs. Peeling bark was not a skill loggers knew much about. And with some forty thousand new compounds being tried out every year at NCI, scientific attention spans were short; a reputation for being hard to get could ruin a drug like taxol. Worse, taxol was not soluble in water, which meant it was very difficult to get into patients. Scientists thought they could solve that problem by combining taxol with cremophore, a mixture of alcohol and castor oil, and a saline solution.

In 1982, exactly twenty years after yew bark was first gathered, the first patients were chosen, all advanced cases for whom conventional therapies had failed. Preliminary trials were not expected to cure anyone, but simply to ensure that the drug was not dangerous and to determine what dose levels would get effects, if any.

The first experiments were disastrous. Patients got very sick and at least two died from allergic reactions. It was soon determined that the probable cause was the cremophore, however, not taxol, but some trials were stopped anyway and a few physicians argued it was too dangerous to continue. Instead, patients were given steroids or anti-histamines to combat allergic reactions, the drug was given slowly over a twenty-four-hour period, and there were no more deaths. Other side effects cropped up, such as suppression of blood-cell production by bone marrow, aching muscles, nausea, loss of feeling or tingling in the extremities, and fever, and it took several years for physicians to learn how best to control them. And while the Phase I trials eventually showed that taxol, if used properly, at least did no serious harm, there were no stunning improvements either. Interest in taxol waned, and it was not until 1985, in Baltimore, that taxol's true potential was revealed.

It was William P. McGuire III's first year at Johns Hopkins University's medical center. He had been a young mover and shaker at NCI, where he had served on the drug decision network that determines which drugs deserve human trials and which are worthless. Like many oncologists, he had chosen cancer as his specialty because it was the most challenging human disease to fight. When he arrived at Hopkins, he was eager to try this latest weapon, but the university was on the verge of ending its taxol trials. It was a single patient who walked into McGuire's new office that altered that decision. She was a Baltimore native whose ovarian cancer had resisted almost every treatment. She knew that there were no more medicines on the shelf for her, but she had heard of this experimental drug taxol, and she wanted to try it. McGuire examined her and realized that she had nothing to lose. He recalls the day he gave her the drug: "I told her two sons to come back and see me, but I said I did not think she would live beyond three weeks. Well, a week to ten days after she got the drug, one of the sons called and said, 'You know, my mom's really a lot better.' So I brought her back early and looked at her and clearly her tumor had responded dramatically in that ten-day period. Now, I had spent fifteen years of my life taking care of patients with ovarian cancer, and that was so unusual that I petitioned the NCI to do an in-depth study of the compound for ovarian cancer."

McGuire and others who got similar results urged the government to stay with taxol. NCI did, taking taxol into Phase II studies, where a potential drug's effectiveness is more closely examined in a large group of patients. McGuire found several more women with ovarian cancer and gave them taxol, and again, the results were remarkable. With most drugs, treating ovarian cancer that has spread through a person's body — metastasized, in the medical jargon — is like trying to hold back a flood with sandbags. Taxol, however, was more like a seawall. It might not be a miracle cure, but it could stop tumors from growing and even shrink them. Word spread that ovarian cancer seemed to be taxol's forte.

In August 1989, McGuire, Eric K. Rowinsky, and their colleagues at Hopkins published their first results. They reported improvement in 30 percent of patients. That was six times better than standard drugs like cisplatin. Others who had tried taxol on ovarian cancer patients reported unofficially that they too had good results. Taxol was no longer just a curiosity. Within a year, NCI decided to try it on other cancers as well: head and neck, breast, cervix, colon, stomach, lung, and prostate.

It was now dawning on NCI that scientists would need a lot more yew bark. And if taxol went beyond experimental use, the demand could be astronomical. It then took about thirty pounds of *Taxus brevifolia* bark to make a gram of taxol. A patient needed an average of two grams for a course of treatment, so each patient needed sixty pounds of bark. While NCI estimated a mature tree could produce about twenty pounds of bark, Oregon peelers often got a lot less, sometimes only five pounds per tree. So that worked out to at least three trees and as many as a dozen per patient. With twelve thousand women dying of ovarian cancer yearly, that was as much as 144,000 trees a year. Then there was breast cancer. Close on McGuire's heels was Frankie Ann Holmes, a cancer researcher at the M. D. Anderson Cancer Center in Houston. Using taxol, she got partial or complete remissions in advanced breast cancer patients in almost half of twenty-five women she treated. Forty thousand women die of breast cancer yearly in the United States alone. That market could consume another half million trees.

In January 1991, as data from trials continued to roll in, NCI agreed to give the drug company Bristol-Myers Squibb exclusive rights to make taxol. The company would have access through Hauser to yew trees on federal lands, and taxol would get orphan drug status, giving Bristol-Myers seven years as sole maker. In return, NCI would get free supplies to distribute to doctors while it was still experimental. NCI does not develop cancer drugs, instead encouraging drug companies to finish what its own researchers have begun. The deal saved the government a lot of money, since taxol was costing some six hundred dollars a gram to make, according to NCI officials.

But the arrangement looked very cozy. Congressman Ron Wyden, Democrat of Oregon, challenged NCI for turning over not only its taxpayer-supported research but "an entire species" to a single company without opening taxol up to wider competitive bidding that could have cut costs and economized on the bark supply. NCI scientists saw it differently. Several who worked on taxol at the Frederick cancer center say that in the early 1980s Bristol-Myers had shown the most interest in taxol. When bids were taken for someone to develop the drug, Bristol-Myers chemists knew more about it than anyone else.

More troubling was the future of the species. Some biologists and environmental groups urged the government to get off the bark habit and find new sources of taxol. McGuire recalls that as early as 1988, he told his former colleagues at the institute, "To put it mildly, 'Get your ass in gear and start looking at alternative sources.' We would not be as far behind as we are now if some people had listened back in the mid-1980s. They didn't, so by the time it was clear that this was an active drug, they were sort of behind the eight ball."

NCI had in fact looked at yew needles as a source of taxol in the 1970s, recalls NCI's Matthew Suffness, now the institute's program director for natural products. But the needles had about one-third the taxol content of bark, and lost much of it if it was not extracted quickly. Meanwhile, attempts to synthesize taxol from scratch had failed utterly. And the government's arrangement with Bristol-Myers asked specifically for taxol from bark, not from needles. As a result, complained groups like the Environmental Defense Fund and the Audubon Society, Bristol-Myers had little incentive to develop other, renewable sources. Soon, these groups warned, the yew could be extinct.

On a summer evening in 1992, pickup trucks laden with Oregon yew bark pull into Hauser Chemical's gravel lot in Cottage Grove, empty their goods, and head home. It is past six o'clock, the wood chippers are quiet now, and the lumberyard is darkening under the lengthening shadows cast by the young fir surrounding the lot. Inside a double-wide trailer, however, men in rolled-up shirtsleeves and cowboy boots are still working the phones at their cheap metal desks and swigging from cups of coffee that have that late-afternoon, overcooked aroma. They are making yew deals with landowners and logging companies, scheduling times when they can send in collectors before a stand of forest is logged. Pinned to their cubicle walls are Polaroid snapshots showing the men posed proudly next to dead deer. They look more at home in the photos than they do at the desks in this cramped office.

Behind the trailer is a building the size of a barn where chippers break up the bark and conveyers shunt the pieces into steel canisters, dryers originally designed for filbert nut harvesting. When the bark is cut and dried its weight is down by half and it looks like Grape-Nuts cereal. The plant works at about 60 percent capacity; it would be higher, say Hauser officials, if the government would open up more old growth forest to logging. "It's the spotted owl thing, you know," says Hauser's Jim Sharr, puffing on a cigarette as he shows a visitor around. The owl gets the blame for most everything in Oregon. "Next time you run out of toilet paper," suggests one Oregon bumper sticker, "wipe your ass on a spotted owl." The owl is like God or Lucifer; if it did not exist, people would have to invent it.

Mike Trumbull runs the Hauser operation in Cottage Grove. When yew collecting first started in a big way in 1988, no one knew much about the tree and how best to get bark from it. They made mistakes, he acknowledges, though a bit defensively. Loggers would clear-cut a unit and leave the yews behind to be yarded — dragged out by tractor and chain — and much of the bark would get scraped off and lost in the undergrowth. "That's all in the past," Trumbull assures. Now, Hauser goes into units before they are logged to hand-peel the bark, and, if necessary, collectors will bring back the whole tree to be stripped by Hauser's big Swedish debarking machine. Trumbull is proud that Hauser is putting close to one thousand people to work. "They're usually 'bullbucks,' " he says, logging contractors who know their way around trees. "We've got whole families that were out of work that are now peeling," he says, "even the grandfathers." Hauser has hired peelers to strip yew in Montana as well, where the yew tends to grow as low-lying brush. There, they work in a tight circle, never more than ten feet apart, he says, because of grizzly attacks.

All the bark goes to Hauser headquarters in Boulder, Colorado, where it is put through a bath of methylene chloride and water to get a crude, red, honey-like extract of raw taxol that is purified in several more steps. The taxol content of the bark is tiny: about three hundredths of one percent of dry bark, says Trumbull, like three drops in a cup of water. The raw taxol is dried to powder and sent to Bristol-Myers to be formulated into a drug.

Before Hauser got involved, NCI got bark on an irregular basis from almost anybody who could find it. Much of it came from what one NCI official describes as "hippies living in a commune," who would dry it on their driveways. After 1987, however, demand skyrocketed, and soon there was not enough for all the patients who wanted it. The Forest Service and BLM were taken by surprise; they normally serve the needs of the logging companies and knew very little about yew trees. To find out, they are now sending foresters like Kent Tressider, an Oregon native, out in a helicopter to track down yew and monitor the harvest.

"It's an unprecedented effort," Tressider shouts over the noise of the rotor as the Bell 206 Ranger hovers over a clear-cut hump of Oregon's Coast Range. The low mountains, five hundred feet below, extend west some twenty miles before plunging into the waves of the Pacific to give the state its famous shoreline postcards. "Some of our districts moved quickly to get yew out," he says. "They even went in with helicopters and hauled out the yew trees." Elsewhere, however, where yew was not properly peeled, hundreds of trees now sit in stacks, called "cold decks" in logging parlance, on government land, their taxol probably gone. Tressider, a six-footer as lean as a sapling and sincere the way farm-raised men tend to be, grew up along this coast, where the yew are fewer than inland and grow mostly on steep slopes. From above, one can easily spot these steep slopes because they still have trees, while the flatland has mostly been stripped and looks like the back of a dog with a bad case of mange.

The helicopter lands on a sixty-two-acre unit on BLM land that was clear-cut the year before. BLM had originally calculated that there were 236 pounds of yew bark to be peeled on the unit. Hauser did not get to it for several months after clear-cutting and peeled only fifty-one pounds; the rest, they said, had seized up. "Perhaps they were going to the most productive areas first, to get the most pounds in the shortest period of time," Tressider speculates. The undergrowth of huckleberry and rhododendron can grow twice the height of a man after clear-cutting. "Under those conditions," says Tressider, "it can be almost impossible to see the small yews. They might only be six inches diameter at breast height and twenty feet tall." Whatever the reason, the inefficiency seems to contradict the claim by Hauser that the spotted owl is to blame for having to run at less than full capacity.

Claims such as that are what got environmentalists involved in yew politics. They suspected that logging companies would try to get the government to reopen protected old growth forests for clear-cutting in exchange for collecting yew and then accuse the environmentalists of choosing owls over women dying of cancer if they objected. Indeed, environmental groups have decided to downplay their early opposition to harvesting yew. "We are not saying the yew should not be cut," says ONRC's Wood, who works out of a rambling bungalow on a leafy residential street in Eugene. "But for every tree that is killed for a person now, it means there will be none for five people in the future." Wood and other yew-defenders say taxol-makers should have tried harder to conserve the yew and get the extract from renewable yew needles.

In fact, even up until 1992, doctors and patients were told there was not enough taxol to go around. The government told Bristol-Myers in 1991 that the peeling season's haul of 60,000 pounds of bark was far short of need, and asked for 750,000 pounds, a twelvefold increase, the next year. It was anybody's guess whether that much yew even existed.

*   *   *

By the end of the summer of 1992, Hauser had collected over one and a half million pounds of bark, twice what NCI had requested, churned out 280 pounds of raw taxol, and predicted that they could double that the next year. While the kinks in the supply of taxol seemed to have been straightened, the hose was still too small. And although BLM and the Forest Service had finally begun an inventory, they still had no idea how much yew existed. If taxol proved to work for other cancers, shortages would recur.

Some one hundred laboratories, many of them with money from Bristol-Myers, now were trying all manner of tricks to find a substitute, or at least get more out of the bark. A company in Ithaca, New York, was trying yew tissue culture; that is, starting a plant from a few cells grown in a petri dish, while others were growing yew cells in a nutrient "soup" much the way bacteria are grown in fermentation tanks to make penicillin. At Stanford University and Ohio State, chemists were attempting total synthesis of taxol, starting from common substances like pinene, found in pine trees. At the University of Mississippi, chemists were trying to get raw taxol out of the needles of common forms of yew. The biggest operation was a string of huge nurseries of various ornamental yew species planted by the timber company Weyerhaeuser in Washington and Oregon. The company had fifteen million cuttings planted in 1993, with the goal of finding varieties that grew fast and had lots of taxol, especially in the needles.

The man who first broke ahead of the pack was a chemist named Robert Holton. In 1991, Holton, a faculty member at Florida State University in Tallahassee, had discovered a way to synthetically create taxol's large side chain. He locked up the method with a patent and then got over $1 million from Bristol-Myers to find a way to make taxol using something other than the Pacific yew bark core molecule. In early 1992, Holton succeeded with a core molecule called 10-deacetyl-baccatin III, found in the needles and other renewable parts of common species of the tree like the English yew. Bristol-Myers found a natural products company in Milan, Italy, called Indena, that was able to provide 10-deacetylbaccatin III from needles and twigs of European and Asian yews.

Finally, in January 1993, the thirty-year taxol marathon crossed the finish line. The U.S. Food and Drug Administration approved taxol for general use in women with advanced ovarian cancer, making it an official cancer drug. Cancer specialists predicted that it would soon be approved for other types of cancer as well. That same month, Bristol-

Myers announced that, with the help of chemists like Holton, it could get all the taxol it needed from semi-synthetic processes using common forms of yew. It no longer needed the wild-growing Pacific yew.

Taxol will doubtless make headlines again. While Bristol-Myers may no longer require the Pacific yew, others who want to make cancer drugs may need it. Congressmen Wyden and Robert E. Andress, Democrat of New Jersey, still worry that the lack of competing manufacturers could lead to unfairly high prices, although a European company, Rhone-Poulenc Rorer, now makes an almost identical drug called Taxotere. And a plant pathologist from Montana State University, Gary Strobel, and two colleagues found a fungus growing on yew bark that also produces taxol. Although it makes taxol only in minute quantities, biotechnologists predict that these fungi might be grown in huge vats and secrete taxol in a factory-like operation.

For physicians like McGuire, however, it does not matter where the drug comes from, so long as his patients get it at a reasonable price. "Taxol has extraordinary activity in ovarian cancer," he wrote in 1989. In 1992, as he prepared to start treating hundreds rather than just a handful of patients with taxol, McGuire was even more enthusiastic. "Taxol," he said, "is the drug of the nineties."

14

Disappearing Cures

Taxol's final success and its attendant publicity gave the new plant-hunters a trophy to show off to the skeptics. Never mind that it took thirty years to develop, or that some one hundred thousand *other* natural extracts the government tried produced nothing. Taxol was the hot topic at scientific meetings all over the world, while environmental groups that once fretted about overcutting the yew cited taxol as evidence of the foolhardiness of cutting down rainforests.

More drug manufacturers began to invest in plant-hunting. Smith, Kline, for example, which had abandoned its natural products efforts a decade before, opted for exploring the oceans, hiring a young marine biologist and diver and collaborating with academics at Scripps Institute of Oceanography in California to collect unusual creatures from the deep. Soon other companies, like Monsanto, Ciba, Pfizer, and the British company Glaxo got into collecting. The new demand even spawned a globe-trotting plant "broker," called Biotics, that collected exotic plants for drug companies for a fee.

Ahead of all of them was Shaman Pharmaceuticals. The little California upstart already had its two plant drugs in clinical trials, one for respiratory syncytial virus, common among young children, and one for herpes, plus several other potential drugs in their pipeline. In January 1992, the company's risk-taking paid off: the pharmaceutical giant Eli Lilly & Company gave Shaman $4 million for the right to develop at least two of the company's antifungal plant drugs over the following four years. No longer seen as a curiosity shop for politically correct investors, Shaman went public a few months later at fifteen dollars a share. By then, the source of Shaman's two drugs in trials, the tropical tree genus *Croton*, had begun to leak out into the botanical community, but patents on the two experimental medicines, Provir and Virend, had been applied for. Securing supplies of the raw materials, however, continued to be "a delicate political situation," especially among indigenous groups, according to Shaman's botanist. Steven King had tried to arrange a deal with the federation that represents the Quichua in the western Amazon to supply bark, but they wanted more than ten times the amount Shaman felt it could pay, and were suspicious of *Croton* supplier Douglas McMeekin's ties to oil companies. Shaman had a collecting arrangement with a Peruvian company for collecting bark there, however, and King stated that both countries' governments were aware of the arrangements and had issued the necessary permits and licenses. As for the royalties that Shaman had promised to return to tropical forest peoples, they remained for future negotiation.

At the Frederick phytochemical factory, meanwhile, word of taxol's first clinical successes came as the contracts with the collecting groups at New York, St. Louis, and the University of Illinois were up for renewal. During that first five years, Michael Boyd's team had tested thousands of new extracts, but Boyd had not announced any discoveries, and the skeptics were looking wise again. What very few people knew was that the grind 'em and find 'em team actually had hits, in fact, several of them. These were nowhere near becoming drugs, but they were exciting enough to keep NCI interested, and Boyd's operation got more money to keep the plant-hunters in the rainforests for another five years.

What the Frederick groups had discovered were several unique new compounds that worked in unusual ways against the AIDS virus in test-tube experiments. Boyd had kept quiet about them because premature promises of new AIDS drugs were even worse than rumors of cancer cures: hope would surge unrealistically, then plummet when the drugs failed to live up to the expectations of desperate people. AIDS research was littered with such wrecked remedies, like the Chinese cucumber and alpha interferon, and Boyd did not want to send more to a similar fate. Besides, NCI had a more serious problem, one that was not discussed outside the small community of medicinal plant-hunters. The botanists who found these anti-AIDS plants were not sure they could find them again.

In September 1987 John Burley arrived in the tropical forests of Sarawak, a state of Malaysia in the northwestern portion of the island once called Borneo. Burley, as unassuming and reserved as one might imagine a British botanist to be, had been teaching at Harvard University when the collecting team at the University of Illinois hired him to gather some plants from Sarawak for NCI. An expert on Southeast Asian flora, Burley roamed Sarawak's tropical forests for almost four weeks, gathering 136 plant species. He had no idea when he shipped off his samples that any would be of medicinal interest.

In those first years, the backlog of plants in the testing pipeline at Frederick was huge, and it was not until 1991 that Burley's plants got to the head of the line. It was to be a lucky day. An extract from a tree sample rang the bells and whistles on the AIDS screen. It came from a single tree identified as *Calophyllum lanigerum*. Burley and his colleague Bernard Lee of the Sarawak Forest Department had found it in a lowland forest, about twenty feet above sea level, near a river called Batang Kayan in southern Sarawak. The tree was not spectacular by tropical standards, standing about fifty feet tall and less than two feet thick at breast height. It was one of about eight hundred species from Southeast Asia sent to NCI during its first five-year collecting effort.

Extracts from the tree had dramatic effects, protecting human cells almost completely from HIV. Moreover, the extract was not swallowed up by the "black hole," what AIDS researchers call the collection of viral strains that quickly develop resistance to the known drugs used to kill them. The compound that did this, one of eight isolated from the tree sample, was unique. NCI called it calanolide A.

Boyd's team was elated. They needed more of *Calophyllum* right away, and the Illinois team arranged for collectors to get more samples. When they returned to the spot where Burley had collected, however, all that was left of his tree was a stump. The tree had been cut down, a fate that did not come as a great surprise: Malaysia and Sarawak are cutting down their forests faster than just about anyplace in the tropics. The botanists eventually found other trees that looked to be of the same species and, with their fingers crossed, sent samples back. The chemists at Frederick added the extracts to their rows of cell cultures infected with HIV. After six days, they looked to see if luck was with them. It was not — the virus had killed the cells. NCI had the wrong plant.

The collecting director for the Illinois team, Indonesian-born botanist Djaja Soejarto, is a small, voluble man with a big name in botanical circles. He was not happy about the turn of events. He had studied with Schultes and had become as insistent a defender of plant-based medicines as anyone in the business. With a scientific reputation to defend, he packed off to Sarawak in the spring of 1992 to find more of this mysterious tree. Wandering in the same swamp Burley had visited, he located the now-famous tree stump. If the world ever needed an example of why forests should be conserved, he thought at the time, that tree stump said it all.

Soejarto recognized other species of *Calophyllum* nearby, however, and took samples from them. This time the plant-hunters were lucky. After several months of tests, they found one sample, later identified as a variant of *Calophyllum* called *teysmannii* var. *inophylloide*, that contained a compound that was almost identical to calanolide. They called it costatolide, and while it is not as powerful as the original, it serves as a chemical sibling for researchers while NCI's plant-hunters continue to this day to look for more trees like Burley's.

The experience with *Calophyllum* made three things abundantly clear. First, there are indeed undiscovered plant-based compounds that can fight diseases, even diseases the likes of which the world has never seen before. Furthermore, these compounds can turn up anywhere and come from plants that, unlike Shaman's sangre de drago in South America, apparently have never been used by humans before, even forest peoples. That lent support to the mass screening approach. Sure, it might look to be as brainless as sifting dirt through a screen to find a diamond, but it got results. At the same time, Boyd's chemists realized that with thousands of compounds zipping through their screens every month now, a momentary lapse of concentration could lose them another calanolide A.

And third, the forlorn tree-stump sitting in the Sarawak swamp stood as a bitter reminder that if they found another calanolide, the plant might well be rare and perhaps even on the verge of extinction. The conservationists might be right; cures might indeed be burning up before our eyes.

There is nothing, Machiavelli wrote, more uncertain in its success than to take the lead in introducing a new order of things. So it seemed at NCI. The plant-hunters were finding more hits, but each one was freighted with unforeseen problems. A botanist with the Smithsonian Institution, for example, collected a type of seaweed near a beach in the Philippines that showed unusual potency in killing cancer cells. When it was recollected, the second sample might as well have been iced tea. The collector found more of it in another location, but a typhoon wiped out most of that population of it. Meanwhile, NCI's attempts to grow the seaweed in tanks continue to fail. Then NCI found another anti-AIDS plant, this one from Cameroon, but again, it could not be found again despite the efforts of teams of botanists from the Missouri Botanical Garden. Also, there were problems with plant chemistry. One plant that killed the AIDS virus was found among the pharmacopoeia of native Samoans by a crusading ethnobotanist from Brigham Young University, Paul Alan Cox. Cox had mortgaged his home in Utah to buy and save a tract of forest destined for clear-cutting that contained the plant. Unfortunately, the anti-AIDS compound in it was a phorbal ester, a chemical that is known to cause cancer.

Perhaps the most persistent problem Boyd's team faced was political. As much as scientists would like people to believe it so, science does not operate free of politics, medicinal botany included. The most contentious issue for the plant-hunting renaissance has become the question of "intellectual property rights." Intellectual property — techniques, methods, know-how — is protected through patents, copyrights, trademarks, and laws governing trade secrets. These have helped protect and encourage industrial development. Now that wild things — plants, insects, algae, microorganisms — appear to be both endangered and commercially valuable, those who control them want similar protection. The question is, can such objects of nature be "owned" in the sense that one owns a factory, an auto design, a computer program, or even a specially bred kind of wheat?

It is a difficult case to make. Only intellectual effort can be protected as intellectual property. No human, for example, may be responsible for the fact that a wild, rare Peruvian potato is resistant to cold weather. Yet if riches are made from the cold-resistant genes and chemicals in that potato, should the people who tend the land where it comes from reap some of the profits? What about the Peruvian government? Then there is the contribution of the researchers who find it and bring it back to a laboratory where its cold-resistance can be "discovered." And of course the company that breeds a new hybrid potato with the Peruvian gene will demand credit as well.

Third World countries have traditionally fought the industrialized world's insistence on protecting ownership of technologies ranging from computer software to hybrid seed. Many do not even allow patents to be taken out on pharmaceuticals. Now they want some of that protection for their biodiversity. It will be an extremely difficult argument to make, for it is not simply new potatoes at stake but ownership of whole ecosystems, a shaman's entire plant pharmacopoeia, or databases containing inventories of organisms.

Take the Amazonian tree *Virola*, for example. Schultes and some of his students advocated it as a potential source of medicines for years, so Shaman Pharmaceuticals went looking for it. They found several western Amazonian peoples using it for fungal infections. Now Shaman is investigating its chemical properties for the lucrative market in antifungals. AIDS patients in particular are susceptible to serious fungal infections. But which ethnic group gets credit if a drug is produced? Conservation International's ethnobotanist, Mark Plotkin, says at least four cultures he knows of that use *Virola* as an antifungal might be cut in, as well as governments of countries that supply it. "Sure, that's a lot of red tape," he concedes, "but what's the market for a cure for skin fungus that affects millions of people around the world? You're not talking about dividing up one hundred thousand dollars a year, but millions or hundreds of millions a year." Helping the local people as you explore their culture, he says, is the "Schultesian tradition." But is the compound or the use of *Virola* as medicine really newly discovered? Scientists over the past several decades have described the tree, its indigenous uses, even many of the chemicals it contains. And is it unique? It is not unlikely that the active compound in the bark is found in other organisms. The neurotoxin homobatrachotoxin, for example, is found both in the feathers of a New Guinea bird, the hooded pitohui, and in the secretions of the Amazonian poison-dart frog.

The debate over intellectual property and biodiversity is taking place in a world that is markedly different from the days when drug and chemical companies could collect exotic plants at will. Third World governments are in principle dead set against turning over what they regard as their genetic treasury. Their mood got particularly testy during 1991 when the United States refused to agree to a draft worldwide treaty for conserving biodiversity. The final treaty was signed by most of the world's governments at the watershed United Nations environment conference in Rio de Janeiro in 1992. Then-president Bush declined to sign, saying it gave away too much Western technology for free and threatened the international patent system (a position many American drug companies say they did not share with Bush at the time). Some developing countries vowed to lock up their natural resources as a result. Indigenous peoples also have grown politically stronger, and while their first order of business has been to win title to traditional lands, they are increasingly aware that valuable biochemical secrets may reside in their forests and in their medical traditions.

Principle is one thing, practice quite another. There is no international rule book on intellectual property rights, and most Third World governments continue to allow plant-hunters into their rainforests. Private companies like Merck have settled the issue with a contract between themselves and their hired collectors — in Merck's case INBio, which has a non-exclusive concession from Costa Rica to prospect. As a private enterprise, Merck is not required to reveal all the details of the agreement. NCI, however, being a government agency, must air its linen in public, and for some critics, that linen is dirty.

To the countries where its plant-hunters roam, NCI has offered a "letter of intent" whose purpose is to assure there will be no rip-and-run exploitation. What NCI promises is that if a plant becomes a drug, the source country, or an institution in that country, will get first crack at supplying bulk material. NCI will also help train scientists from the source country and will share details of its scientific findings. But the patent on any chemical compound, or on the means of making it, will belong to NCI. Moreover, should NCI allow a drug company to develop the compound into a drug or use it as a starting point to synthesize one, NCI promises to make its "best effort" to assure that the source country gets a piece of the company's profits. NCI insists, however, that it cannot promise that private companies will in fact share anything.

At first, the letter of intent did not draw much attention abroad. Soejarto's experience in Sarawak, he says, is typical. In July 1992, when it was clear to him that *Calophyllum* species were a potential hit, Soejarto showed a copy of the NCI letter to the Sarawak forestry department, along with his own proposal to manage and collect the tree. "I said, 'This is important,' " he recalls. " 'AIDS is killing millions. We may be able to produce a drug for it, and income could be returned to Sarawak.' But no one really cared. They did not foresee the importance of this. At first, no one did." The forestry department subsequently lost the letter and Soejarto's proposal, he says, and only when reports about NCI's success with the tree reached Malaysia did their interest pick up. Since then, Soejarto has developed mixed feelings about NCI's letter. "I do not start out by showing the letter," he says. "It can do damage, slow things down." Instead, he either waits until someone asks, or offers it after it is clear that a country has a plant worth investigating.

Back in the United States, however, the letter has been likened to the "dollar diplomacy" with which nineteenth-century North America pried open Latin American markets for the delectation of its own entrepreneurs. One of the critics, himself a rainforest entrepreneur, is Jason Clay, who opened the pipeline of renewable forest products from the Amazon to North American businesses. Clay does not believe that NCI or drug companies have the will to compensate indigenous peoples for their knowledge of medicinal plants. Nor is there much good in shifting First World wealth to Third World governments. "Governments do just fine," Clay is fond of saying. "Indigenous cultures do not." Even if indigenous peoples have no knowledge about a rainforest plant, says Clay, they deserve compensation for rainforest products because they have preserved them by maintaining the forests instead of cutting them down.

Many of NCI's hired plant-hunters are embarrassed by the letter of intent. At a contentious meeting with NCI and several drug companies at the New York Botanical Garden in May 1992, several botanists said they could not in good conscience offer the letter to host governments. What would happen, they asked, if a drug company decided not to play by the rules? Botanists feared that countries where they had collected for years would cut them off. Objections also arose over a "materials transfer agreement" that drug companies would sign to get into NCI's repository. The document implied that extracts that do not initially score a hit at Frederick, along with the botanical information about where the samples come from, would be handed around to any and all drug companies to do with what they pleased. To the botanists, this seemed like a way to scratch them and the source countries out of the picture. One botanist at the meeting describes the drug companies as "staring at NCI like a gold mine, rubbing their hands and drooling over plants we had collected. . . . They considered the plant contractors as just a bunch of technicians, as if we were just stuffing plants in bags."

NCI eventually agreed to tighten up the materials transfer agreement to ensure that all who had access to the repository were obliged to follow the letter of intent. But the institute kept the offending "best efforts" clause intact. Gordon Cragg, NCI's chief plant collector, acknowledges that countries want a firmer guarantee of profit sharing. "But we have discovered through our legal people that the government cannot do that sort of thing" — that is, force a company to make a royalty deal. Cragg points out that NCI, as patent-holder, can still wield a hefty stick — the power to choose and license the companies that bid to develop a drug from NCI's green gold mine.

Several countries — Tanzania, Ghana, Madagascar, and Cameroon — accepted the letter of intent when proffered by the Missouri Botanical Garden. Then NCI ran headlong into serious trouble — a government that refused to play along after a plant-hunter stumbled on what may be NCI's best lead yet for an AIDS drug.

Somewhere in the sprawl of the Western Australian outback, there grows a wildflower that contains one of the most powerful HIV-killers the plant-hunters have found to date. Its potential was first discovered, by accident, in 1989. About all that has been revealed since then is that it is a species of the shrub *Conospermum*. Its full name and description are a secret, says James Armstrong, the Australian botanist who is representing his country's interests in its development. "I am concerned about the madness that will happen when the story comes out that there may be an anti-AIDS plant," says Armstrong. "People are desperate. We have to see if it works first."

The plant was first collected in 1981 for NCI in a sweep of Western Australia by an American botanist on contract with the U.S. government. At the time, NCI's plant-testing project was moribund and about to shut down. NCI shipped the Australian sample to a university lab anyway, where extracts were tested on cancer cells. They had no effect, and the extracts were stored away and forgotten. In 1989, however, Boyd's team in Frederick needed plant material to test a new AIDS assay. One of the samples they took off the shelf was the Australian extract. "When I looked at the results," Boyd recalls, "I said, 'My God, this stuff is hot for a crude extract.'" The Frederick chemists double-checked their results. There was no mistake; this stuff killed the AIDS virus. Moreover, it had a phenomenally good therapeutic index, meaning that the amount needed to kill the AIDS virus was far less than what killed human cells — twenty-five hundred times less.

The team called their discovery conocurvone, and asked for more.

NCI's collector returned to Western Australia in 1990 to get more plants. The Australians inquired about how credit for the discovery and profits from any drug from it would be shared and were handed NCI's letter of intent. "We viewed it as a piece of toilet paper," recalls an Australian scientist who saw it. Australia had its own sophisticated chemists and pharmacologists, they said, and were entitled to a partnership, not a promise. In fact, an Australian chemist, Jack Cannon, had already isolated several compounds from the wildflower in the mid-1980s (though not the one that killed HIV), and scientists at NCI had relied on Cannon's published work to help them trace and then synthesize the vital compound. Synthesis was too complicated to manufacture much conocurvone, however, so the plant remained the only source.

The Western Australian government refused to give NCI's collector a permit to recollect. He left, empty-handed, but reappeared in 1992, according to Armstrong, when he was found photographing information from a voucher specimen of the plant in the state's herbarium. There was nothing illegal in that, but Australians say there was in the bags he checked at the airport on the way back to the United States — 390 specimens of the plant. More plants were found at a house the collector had used while in Australia. "I have many friends in the botanical community," says Armstrong, who is head of Western Australia's Department of Conservation and Land Management, and one of them had tipped him off about the shipment.

The collector was allowed to return to the United States, but there would be no more *Conospermum* hunts. It was not until May 25, 1993, that Armstrong and other Australian officials quietly met with U.S. government officials near Washington, D.C., to negotiate a compromise. The atmosphere in the closed-door meeting, NCI's Boyd recalls, was "very tense." The Australians proposed a deal that would make them partners in collecting and studying the plant and chemical compound, and that would give them a stake in any profits from it. NCI countered that any Australian enterprise would have to bid against other drug-makers when it came time to develop conocurvone into a drug, if indeed the compound actually worked. Negotiations continued through the end of 1993, when the Australians won the right to extract the compound and prepare it for NCI experiments. It remains to be decided who will have the right to turn it into a drug. "We are hoping for the best," Cragg says of the negotiations. In the meantime, NCI has just enough of the substance to continue preliminary experiments.

15

The Flowers of
Ancistrocladus

Linnaeus, prime mover of botany, observed that nature does not proceed in leaps. His advice applies as well to those human enterprises that are built on nature, which does not unveil itself at the viewer's demand but at its own pace, one geared more to creation than to human acts of deconstruction. So the medicinal plant-hunters of the 1990s have discovered. While they have retooled the ancient craft of medicinal botany and have tracked down tantalizing leads for new drugs, each step of the way has been marked by false starts and unexpected setbacks. Now, finally, almost a decade into the effort, comes the kind of lucky strike that could reward their efforts and prove the medical worth of the rainforest.

The story of *Ancistrocladus* begins with a family of unconventional adventurers. Duncan and Jane Thomas set out for Africa in 1983 with their daughter Rhiannon and most of their worldly goods packed into the back of a Land Rover. They headed east from Great Britain, crossed the Channel, the low countries, France, North Africa, the Sahara Desert, and the forests and savannah of west central Africa before reaching their destination: the rainforests of Cameroon, a country pinned like a green barrette at the nape of Africa's neck just beneath its northwestern bun.

Duncan Thomas loved Africa. He had first studied botany in North Wales, a land of delicate lines, shale mines, and hills scoured of trees by Atlantic winds and the saws of British fleet-builders. Africa was Eden. He and Jane had first gone in 1977, and Duncan spent two years in Cameroon studying its plants, its French and Pidgin dialect, and its people, the Ekoi, Ibibio, Bantu, and Mbo. A loose-limbed beanpole of a man with a shaggy head of mottled hair like a pinto pony's and the preoccupied dreaminess that seems to be the professional seal of field botanists, Duncan was a taciturn Tarzan next to the bubbling, enthusiastic Jane. If he was unpolished obsidian, solid but barely reflecting light, Jane sparkled like quartz, an ebullient woodswoman and ornithologist who clucked over the exotic birds and other animals, who climbed the trees in harness to photograph the shyest canopy creatures, and who recorded the family's adventures on film, videotape, and in notes and stories.

In the 1970s, the rainforest was not yet trendy, which was fine with the Thomases; they called themselves "the lost causes people" — experts on what nobody has heard of. With their toddlers in tow — Emily was born in 1984 — they returned several times, living in Land Rovers, in tents, in thatched huts, or, if they were lucky, in rented bungalows. They sold their expertise to a variety of sponsors: Great Britain's Royal Society, the United Nations, the U.S. National Science Foundation, conservation groups, and, luckily for NCI's plant-hunters, the Missouri Botanical Garden.

When NCI asked the Missouri Garden to collect plants in Africa, Thomas, who now lives in a suburb of Corvallis, Oregon, was the Garden's man in Cameroon. He was a "straight" taxonomic botanist, he recalls as he sits one July evening in 1992 in his Corvallis garden beneath several towering Douglas firs; that is, he collected and classified plants for their own sake. In Gabon, he had discovered what he believes was the largest leaf in the world, from a raphia palm — sixty-five feet from the base of the stem to the tip of the last frond. He sent the measurements off to the Guinness people, who have yet to respond. "It may not have been the biggest leaf *in the world*," corrects twelve-year-old Rhiannon as she toys with her dinner of ham and pineapple pizza. "But it was the biggest anybody has ever *found*." Thomas, weighing this subtle point of definition with the same dubiousness as he does his slice of pineapple-covered pizza, notes that there was one thing he discovered in Africa about which there is no question: a new begonia.

It now bears, somewhat awkwardly, he concedes, his full name: *Begonia duncan-thomasii*. It is not a particularly remarkable plant, he concedes, "But I suppose it's better than having a stinging nettle named after you."

Thomas got into ethnobotany in Cameroon, provoked by the big tree farms and plantations that were replacing natural forests that he believed were quite capable of supporting people just as they were. He recorded local plant uses to prove that rainforests could be sustainable sources of income, and found Cameroon's economic botany extraordinarily rich. Outside the city, every village had its own herbalists who treated minor ailments, as well as a flourishing class of professional healers, like Professor Jerome Ngwa in the town of Buea, whose spiritual-healing home advertised folk treatments for "madness, gastric pain, heart pain, stomach ache, pile, sterility, witchcraft, poison, yellow fever, epilepsy, rheumatism, etc."

Thomas then believed that medicinal plants were fine for primary care but had little promise of generating much income. "They could earn more money from the hooch they make than from pharmaceuticals," says Thomas, who as a home brewer is not unfamiliar with the subject of hooch. One obstacle to getting outsiders interested in their medicinals, he notes, is the fact that a good half of them are administered as enemas. Nonetheless, some of them have become commercial products locally, like the bark of the tree *Prunus africanus*, which is said to shrink the prostate gland, and the alkaloid-rich seeds of the plant *Strophanthus*, which is traded as heart medicine. Some plants have a small international reputation, like *Pausinystalia johimbe*, a source of the aphrodisiac yohimbine. "It's primarily sold to the French," Thomas notes dryly, "but if it catches on in Japan, it'll be the end of the species."

The Thomases had been working mostly in a national park called Korup, a reserve several hours by car northwest of the capital city of Yaoundé that is maintained by the government and the World Wide Fund for Nature. It is not an especially large park, about one-fourth the size of the Grand Canyon, but it is relatively undisturbed, with few inhabitants and a wealth of plants and animals. Outside of the handful of local residents, only the Thomases knew much about what grew inside.

In March 1987, Duncan Thomas was wandering through an area of Korup he had occasionally surveyed before, a remote section in the south and accessible only by several days' trek by riverboat and footpath, including a stomach-churning river-crossing over a swinging liana bridge. It was mostly dense, closed-canopy forest, evergreen and undisturbed except for a few hunters, and laden with many endemic species. Thomas had been stuffing bags with plants for the Missouri Garden about a quarter mile from the Mana River and its liana bridge when he spied an unusual plant tangled in the branches of a fallen tree. Thomas knew right away it was extraordinary. "I thought it was *Ancistrocladus*," he recalls, "but I had never seen one like that before." The name *Ancistrocladus* means, roughly, "hooked branch." The plant is a slender, sinewy vine with ovate leaves and curly tendrils extending from its stem with which it grasps and climbs. Spectacular it was not, but rare it most certainly was. Thomas cut it free from the tree. Its leaves were distinct from other *Ancistrocladus*, curling slightly under at the base in a way that botanists call revolute. The undersides of the older leaves had an unusual yellowish cast, while the young leaves were chimney-brick red. Thomas thought it might even be a new species, but he would need fruits or flowers to be sure and neither was in sight. He bagged a few kilos of the vine and made note of where he had found it before moving on, adding it to his mental list of plants to watch for in the future.

Four years would pass before he saw it again. By then, Thomas had parted ways with the Missouri Garden and he and Jane had started their own environmental consulting business in Corvallis. Out of the blue on a spring day in 1991, the Thomases got a phone call from NCI's Cragg. Cragg had good news and bad news. First, Cragg explained, they had found something quite amazing in this vine from Korup, something that stopped HIV from killing human cells in the test tube. And the bad news? Well, Cragg said rather forlornly, it seemed that the Missouri Garden had sent some other plant-hunters into West Africa for more, but they couldn't find the bloody plant again. Might he, Cragg asked Thomas politely, get some more for them?

For the Frederick team, the elusiveness of *Ancistrocladus* was frustrating. This was the best stuff they had seen so far. When the crude plant extract was added to cultures of human cells infected with HIV, it kept the cells alive well after the virus should have killed them. When chemists managed after much effort to find the one compound that was responsible, they came up with a previously unknown alkaloid, with the formula $C_{46}H_{48}N_2O_8$. Like all alkaloids, it was toxic, yet it had what looked to be a favorable therapeutic index. Even more unusual, the alkaloid stymied the other major strain of HIV, called HIV-2, something very few other AIDS drugs could do. And as a bonus, it worked against viral strains that resisted other new drugs.

It was an extraordinary find. The extraction laboratories at NCI (operated by a private company, PRI/DYNCORP), had been churning out extracts like so much cement, twelve hours a day. Plants alone now amounted to at least twenty thousand specimens, each chopped up with band saws and mechanized hamburger grinders, bathed with methanol and methylene chloride and aqueous solutions, spun in banks of centrifuges, evaporated, freeze-dried, and finally bottled. Pure, labeled extracts then faced the screens. Hundreds of extracts had scored well enough on these to go on to the next step, the painstaking dissection of the extract into its constituents to find the one effective compound. The process was like trying to find a mischievous orchestra musician playing slightly out of tune. The searchers would first divide the orchestra — the extract — into like groups: violins in one group, cellos in another, horns in yet another, and so on, the groups being equivalent to distinct classes of chemicals. Each group would play a note, and the one with the false note would be subdivided into rows and each row made to play the note again, then half the row, then each musician until finally the culprit was found. At Frederick, this process of elimination took place in rows of glass columns, where solvents do the separating work of chromatography. Each solvent divides the extract into two types of molecules, big and small. Each of these two groups is then screened again with HIV and cancer cells. The sample that still works is subdivided again by a more sophisticated chromatograph, perhaps one that separates compounds by their preference for dissolving in one liquid but not another, or by their ability to form hydrogen bonds with different solid surfaces. Each step eliminates the useless parts until, finally, the one true actor is isolated.

Of these finalists, only a handful stop disease without killing the cells they are supposed to save. These few achieve a sort of chemical stardom, like some new substance arrived on a meteorite. With mass spectrometry, the molecular components of these compounds are divined by turning them into gas, bombarding them with a beam of electrons, and watching how the atoms of each element sort themselves out under the influence of a magnet. Each element reveals itself as a characteristic vertical spike or peak on a graph — some nitrogen here, some carbon there, a spike of hydrogen and one of oxygen — as if each were a handwritten letter in a signature. To find how the atoms are packed together — that is, to determine their molecular structure — a compound undergoes nuclear magnetic resonance, in which radiation at the radio frequency plus a magnetic field are applied to it. When and how a nuclear particle, such as a proton, begins to absorb the radiation reveals its chemical environment, or the way in which other nuclear particles are arranged around it.

In 1989, after chasing hundreds of matchhead-sized smears of gummy residue from God-knew-where up dead ends and blind alleys, something from the rainforest finally rewarded all this effort — Thomas's *Ancistrocladus*. Of the chemists who pried the extract apart, it fell to NCI chemist Kirk P. Manfredi to name the new compound. He called it Michellamine, after his wife, Michelle.

As if to mock the teams of scientists and their million-dollar machines, the odd little creeper from Korup was to tease the drug-hunters and then disappear back into the forest, trailing a frustrated crew of botanists behind it. When the extract first proved itself in the AIDS screen, NCI asked the Missouri Garden for more. The Garden no longer employed Thomas and did not consult him, instead sending its own specialists to several parts of West Africa in search of *Ancistrocladus*. They eventually found what they recognized as the species *A. abbreviata*. They sent samples back to NCI, only to find that it did nothing in the HIV lab tests. Months passed and several more collections were made, but nothing worked quite like the first batch. It became clear that only one kind of *Ancistrocladus* would do — the kind Thomas had found in Korup. But no one, not even the Cameroonians with whom Thomas had worked, could identify the right one. That came as no surprise to Thomas. As far as he knew it grew only in untouched, moist, old growth forest along the sandy lowlands of Cameroon's Atlantic coast. Yes, he agreed that day on the phone with Cragg, "it *is* bloody hard to find."

In April 1991 Thomas went back to Cameroon, courtesy of NCI. There he met his old colleagues, Johnson Jato of the University of Yaoundé and Jato's nephew, Emmanuel Jato. Both had worked with Thomas for years in the forest, but neither could find the original *Ancistrocladus*. They returned to the Mana River, over the same liana bridge, and into the same forest. Thomas could not find the original plant, but he found another just like it. He returned to Cameroon again in February 1992 and found more plants. In all, he and his Cameroonian colleagues collected about 220 pounds of leaves and bark and shipped them back to NCI. No fruits, flowers, or seeds from the plant showed up, but at least NCI now had enough of the vine to keep Michellamine clearing the experimental hurdles that every potential new drug must negotiate.

Two months after Thomas's rediscovery, Michellamine B (the compound's most effective variant) became the first of Boyd's hits to go up for consideration as a new drug candidate. Sitting in judgment was the NCI drug decision network committee, the sentries who decide which new compounds are promising enough to merit the ultimate test: use on the human patient. On June 1, the panel sat solemnly around a polished oak table in a conference room at the National Institutes of Health listening to a fast-talking Boyd rattle off the virtues of Michellamine B. Boyd knew that skeptics on the panel still viewed plant-based compounds as good romance and bad risks, and he had prepared as hard for this day as for anything he had ever undertaken. This African plant was his best shot. Michellamine B was not dangerously toxic, he assured. Moreover, it would dissolve in water, making it suitable for a medicine. It was found in fairly high concentrations in the plant, and getting pure compound out was not troublesome. Only one serious drawback could hold it back. "There is precious little of this plant," Boyd warned, only about two hundred pounds in hand, enough to make about two ounces of the compound. Nor was Michellamine B something that clever chemists could synthesize anytime soon. If there were questions, Boyd said, "they need to be discussed now, *right* now." The rainforest from which the plant came could fall to the chain saw at any time.

There were few questions; the data were solid and comprehensive. The chairman of the panel, Bruce Chabner, called the vote. "This sounds like that movie that was just out," he joked, referring to the jungle adventure *Medicine Man*, in which Sean Connery plays a botanist who finds, then loses, the cure for cancer in a South American rain-forest. On that note, the panel voted overwhelmingly to give Michellamine B the nod. That meant the compound would get some $4 million worth of attention. In effect, the panel had said, Let's push this stuff down the path toward human trials.

Boyd beamed as brightly as his fire-engine-red tie. He had his first serious hit. The meeting adjourned and a crowd of well-wishers gathered around him to offer congratulations. On the fringe, a gaunt man looking about as comfortable as a roped calf in his charcoal suit and tight brown shoes stood clutching a leather briefcase to his side. "It seems we've been abandoned," Duncan Thomas said plaintively to his companion, a balding African in a somewhat snappier European business suit. Indeed, the celebrants seemed to have forgotten that the discoverer was among them. They would not forget for long, however. Like a cat proudly showing his kill at the doorstep, Thomas flipped open his briefcase. Inside were the first flowers of *Ancistrocladus*, brought just days before from Cameroon by his well-dressed colleague, Johnson

Jato. These tiny pressed florets, each no bigger than a clove, were no mere souvenirs. They proved that this was indeed a new species of *Ancistrocladus*, and gave Thomas what he needed to name it. Moreover, the flowers would allow botanists from the Missouri Garden (which had laid claim to *Ancistrocladus*'s discovery the week before without crediting Thomas) to identify the right plant every time.

Eight months later, Thomas was back in Cameroon, helping Jato with two nurseries that had been established for seedlings of *Ancistrocladus* that had been transplanted from the forest (cuttings had failed to grow). One nursery, with only about a dozen plants, lies incongruously amid vegetable gardens near Yaoundé, the other just outside the Korup reserve. Their exact locations are being kept secret to discourage theft; if Michellamine B really works, the plants in those nurseries could become the most valuable in the world. As for a name for the plant, the typically unhurried Thomas had yet to come up with one. "Duncan-thomasii is taken," he mused with some relief. "I don't know," he said. "Perhaps I'll name it after my daughters."

The discovery of Michellamine B has given the medicine-hunting enterprise new momentum. Cameroon's University of Yaoundé signed NCI's letter of intent and supplies of *Ancistrocladus* are for the moment secure. Botanists have discovered that the leaves are still potent even after being shed by the plant, meaning that plants do not have to be killed to be harvested. Meanwhile, NCI and the New York Botanical Garden signed a collecting arrangement with the Awá people of northwestern Ecuador, with whom the Garden's Hans Beck had been living for several months. It was the first arrangement between NCI and an indigenous group, and a coup for ethnobotany, especially since the Awá have traditionally been reluctant to allow outsiders into their land. The Garden will pay the Awá federation several thousand dollars for the right to study medicinal botany with their shamans, who will also be paid for collaborating. Shortly after the deal with the Awá was sealed, Mike Balick's Institute of Economic Botany signed an agreement with the drug company Pfizer, which will support the Garden's plant-hunters with $2 million to explore for medicinal plants in North American forests.

Shaman Pharmaceuticals continues to look for collaborations with South American indigenous groups. King speculates that as many as eighty groups worldwide over a five-year period might be involved in the company's *Croton*-based drug project. Shaman has for the moment decided not to set royalties for any particular group. "We will return finances to all the groups we work with when we succeed with a product," King says. This compensation will be in proportion to each group's contributions and how much money a drug makes. Like Merck, Shaman does not reveal how much that might amount to, exactly when those payments would start, or to whom they would go. But in late 1993, Shaman did get votes of confidence from one of South America's largest indigenous federations, COICA, in Peru, and from the council of Peru's Aguaruna and Huambisa peoples, which agreed to help Shaman collect plants for pharmaceutical investigation. In the meantime, the company's charitable foundation, the Healing Forest Conservancy, has hired its first full-time director, Katy Moran. Moran's operation only gets its operating costs from Shaman, however; it must raise money from contributors to donate to indigenous groups. In the spring of 1993, the Conservancy made its first cash donation, two thousand dollars, to the Belizean Healers' Association that Rosita Arvigo presides over (and which has no connection with sangre de drago) to establish a reserve for medicinal plants. The Conservancy also has supported a Peruvian art school that specializes in rainforest paintings, and donated medicine to the Yanomamo people in the Venezuelan Amazon.

In Costa Rica, INBio has built on its success with Merck. It has concluded an agreement with Bristol-Myers-Squibb, the makers of taxol, the cancer drug from yew bark. INBio will supply Bristol-Myers with a set of biological samples different from those it collects for Merck, in return for somewhat less of an advance payment but a higher rate for future royalties, according to an INBio staff member. Also, the British Technology Group has contracted with INBio to investigate a plant discovered the eco-rational way — rodents refuse to eat it. The plant contains a compound that kills parasitic nematode worms that infest crops, animals, and humans. INBio has also been negotiating with agrichemical companies to do "gene prospecting," that is, hunting not for whole organisms but just for genes that might be useful in pesticides.

Perhaps the surest sign that plant-hunting for medicines has reestablished itself in our time comes from the U.S. government. In late 1993, the government began a multimillion-dollar project to create what it called International Cooperative Biodiversity Groups. Loosely patterned after the Merck/INBio deal, the project supports five consortia that will prospect for new medicines in Third World rainforests.

Each consortium includes a developing country with a large stock of unusual biota, both plants and insects; a U.S. drug company; and botanists from American universities and conservation groups.

If any of the experimental ventures into the forest works, what will success look like? That depends a lot on what is discovered and how it is marketed. If the label on a new medicine for, say, athlete's foot says "Made from tree bark from the tropical rainforest," it is doubtful an outpouring of support for conservation will follow. If Michellamine B or some version of it works against AIDS, however, it could inspire a new respect for tropical forests and their inhabitants. Respect may not buy real estate. But victory for biodiversity is not only measured in acres of secured territory, as if this were some kind of jungle war. Another measure is attitude. Victory can be declared when people start to regain their biophilia, their realization that all life is knit together and that its strength, its center, cannot hold if large patches are allowed to fray and fall apart.

16

Time Holds Us Green

In theory, we know that rainforest biodiversity can be a source of wealth. In practice, we know almost nothing.

Rock stars tour the Amazon and motorists affix "Save the Rainforest" stickers to their bumpers, evidence of a nascent biophilia among some parts of the population that makes nice publicity but does little yet to preserve forest. Nor do heartfelt appeals on behalf of biological truth and beauty. So those who would make plowshares into greensward have turned to the allure of the dollar to help them. Some of those who have the dollars are America's drug-makers. Between 1980 and 1993, the industry increased the proportion of its total sales spent on the discovery and testing of new drugs from 11.7 percent to 16.7 percent, and some of that money is now being spent on canvassing the world's last great wild places. More is in the offing, and yet more will follow if — or perhaps it now can be said, when — a prescription for the first new rainforest drug is written.

As biologically rich as tropical forests are, however, they are not drugstores where products sit on the shelf waiting to be swept up. Profit from biodiversity is and will continue to be hard-won. Rainforest species are not clumped together like Canadian pine or Douglas fir but widely dispersed and often hard to find, which makes harvesting difficult. Profit-seeking businesses will prefer plantations or managed plots of valuable plants over collecting from the rainforest. Eventually, they will create semi- or wholly synthetic versions of forest pharmaceuticals, as Bristol-Myers has done with taxol. And conservationists are right to worry that overzealous harvesting could wipe out rare species. As the plant-hunting team from the University of Illinois discovered in Sarawak, one tree can constitute an entire population. Here today and gone tomorrow is no exaggeration in the rainforest.

So the allure of rainforest profits is much like that of an ardent Capulet for a Montague — thrilling, but difficult indeed to consummate. If a plant-drug is found in a tract of Ecuadorean forest, it will probably make money for its North American developers and investors, but one drug may not be enough to convince Ecuador to protect much more of its forests. Nor would it automatically guarantee a better life for people living in those forests. The rubber tappers of the Brazilian Amazon, for example, pioneered sustainable harvesting for a Western market, yet they must supplement their income from rubber with farming and other activities that clear land, and over half of these men and women are in debt and live in poverty. Indeed, no international law clearly states that indigenous people "own" their knowledge or the plants and animals they use or grow on their land. For that matter, personal ownership of such things is often alien to their way of life. To introduce the idea of profit in return for medicinal plants and traditional knowledge might make them wealthier, but it will hasten the westernization of their culture as well.

The advantages of medicine-hunting in the rainforests outweigh these drawbacks, however. The objection that nature should not be reduced to cash value is a romanticism that we can ill afford. Nature is a free good now, and free goods, unfortunately, are too often scorned. And it is naive and paternalistic to argue that profit and materialism will taint "pure" native cultures. There are no such cultures left, and even if there were, it is not the privilege of we moderns to keep them that way.

There is evidence that a more balanced regime for sharing wealth from biodiversity can be forged. Shaman Pharmaceuticals at least has made public promises to share its plant-derived profits with suppliers, even if it has yet to deliver. Merck & Company has established a precedent of paying up front and guaranteeing royalties to a Third World institution for its country's biodiversity, while INBio has initiated the first experiment in charging admission to the greenhouse. Meanwhile, organizations like the New York Botanical Garden are insisting that their business partners agree to share profits with source countries and organizations. True, these are not yet partnerships of equals. Costa Rica's INBio, for example, does not get patent rights to whatever it discovers on Merck's dollar, while Shaman Pharmaceuticals, which also has an arrangement to prospect for Merck, does, so long as Merck has first crack at marketing what Shaman finds. Once valuable compounds are found, however, the balance of power may begin to shift. For example, the prospecting arrangement negotiated between Cameroon's University of Yaoundé and NCI for collecting *Ancistrocladus* is now the subject of debate in Cameroon, and may be renegotiated. And several developing countries are watching to see what kind of deal Western Australia can make for itself in return for its anti-AIDS plant. Indeed, in late 1993 NCI changed the wording of its letter of intent to require U.S. drug companies to address tropical countries' concerns over securing a share of drug profits. As for indigenous groups, there are precedents for trading access to their biodiversity or knowledge for income. In the early 1980s, the Kuna Indians of Panama established strict rules for visitors to their land, such as requiring scientists to get research permits, hire Kuna assistants, and provide the Kuna with copies of published papers. The Awá people of northwestern Ecuador have a similar set of rules and charge for their time and knowledge.

The way for the biologically rich and cash-poor to profit from biodiversity lies in controlling the resource and driving a hard bargain for it, without, however, scaring off those with the scientific knowledge and capital to render biota truly valuable. That means keeping rainforests open but demanding payment not only from drug companies who wish to explore them but also from scientists who plumb them for their dissertations and research projects.

The details of who gets how much should not obscure a more fundamental benefit from biodiversity prospecting. What most prospectors want is to change the way people look at the Earth. Once, our species survived only by understanding and respecting the living things with whom we share the planet. Nowhere was this relationship more vital than in the shamanistic tradition, in which powerful plants and animals were the vessels through which humans reached out to the ultimate arbiters of life. Now we have dissolved our partnership with nature, and treat it like a smashed piggy bank, drawing from it but putting nothing back in. That recent attempts to glue it back together again are imperfect brings to mind the comment by Samuel Johnson about women preaching in church: like a dog's walking on its hind legs, it is not done well, but one is surprised that it is done at all. For people like Michael Balick, Dan Janzen, Thomas Eisner, Steven King, Nelson Zamora, Brad Bennett, or Patricia Terrack, however, it must be done. Like scientific shamans, they have sworn themselves to an *active* engagement with nature. When they go into the rainforest, they risk more than some scientific hypothesis dreamed up at a faculty seminar or university laboratory; they risk their lives, because they know there is too much at stake, and too little time left, to sit in the shade and remark on how beautiful the garden is.

In 1980, *Harvard Magazine* asked prominent faculty members to name what they considered the world's single most pressing problem. Edward O. Wilson responded this way: "The worst thing that can happen — will happen — is not energy depletion, economic collapse, limited nuclear war, or conquest by a totalitarian government. As terrible as these catastrophes would be for us, they can be repaired within a few generations. The one process ongoing in the 1980s that will take millions of years to correct is the loss of genetic and species diversity by the destruction of natural habitats. This is the folly our descendants are least likely to forgive us."

At the time Wilson made that prediction, the species of Earth, as far as anyone knows the only planet to bear life, were disappearing four hundred times faster than at any time in recent geologic past. From their outposts in the rainforests, biologists called in the bulletins of extinctions: half the freshwater fish of the Malay Peninsula, half the forty-one tree snails of Oahu, close to one hundred tree species on the Centinela Ridge in the Ecuadorean Andes. In the United States, about two hundred plant species have disappeared since records have been kept.

What is disappearing is the geography of where we came from. We can draw in uttermost detail the machined universe of the carburetor, recite liturgies on bytes and random access memory, even measure the direction of the rotation of an atom. But how much does any of us remember of what T. S. Eliot once called "the unheard music in the shrubbery" — the value of willow and yew bark, the fermentation of barley malt, or when to tap the rising sap from the sugar maple or the Quichua's red bark tree? We are abandoning fellow living things for a manufactured dreamworld, as if we could grasp immortality by replacing what is born, grows, and dies with that which never ages.

Some middle kingdom where nature and our engineered world can live and let live must be the goal. To achieve this, we must listen to those whose feet are solidly aground in the wilderness, the scientists who have studied biodiversity and the indigenous peoples who still live in and from it. As for those last great wildernesses, they remain as the still points of the turning world. Realizing their economic value may not salve the wounds we have inflicted on life on Earth. But it is a hopeful new direction as we flail about trying to husband the earthly goods that gave us life and then sent us, reeling, on our uncertain course.

References

Introduction

Richard Evans Schultes described myths of the northwestern Amazonian cultures, with coauthor Robert Raffauf, in *The Healing Forest* (Portland, Oreg.: Dioscorides Press, 1990); in his *Where the Gods Reign: Plants and Peoples of the Colombian Amazon* (London: Synergetic Press, 1988); and in personal interviews with the author.

The best history of plant-based medicines is Margaret Krieg's *Green Medicine* (Chicago: Rand McNally & Co., 1964).

Part 1: Return to the Native

Chapter 1 — Paradise Revisited

On life zones, see Gary S. Hartshorn, "Possible Effects of Global Warming on the Biological Diversity in Tropical Forests," in Robert L. Peters and Thomas E.

Lovejoy, eds., *Global Warming and Biological Diversity* (New Haven and London: Yale University Press, 1992), pp. 137–146.

The habits of the strangler fig are described in *Scientific American* 266, no. 4 (April 1992): 25.

Richard Spruce's "I well recollect . . .", along with a record of his entire journey through South America, from Alfred Russel Wallace, ed., *Notes of a Botanist in the Amazon and Andes* (London: Macmillan & Company, Ltd., 1908), pp. 208–209.

The flora, fauna, and ecological mechanisms of tropical forests are outlined for the lay reader in John C. Kricher, *A Neotropical Companion* (Princeton, N.J.: Princeton University Press, 1989). Various phytochemicals useful in medicine are discussed in Chapter 1, pp. 180–210.

A wide-ranging discussion of the variety of useful compounds in plants appears in Olayiwola Akerele, Vernon Heywood, and Hugh Synge, eds, *Conservation of Medicinal Plants* (Cambridge: Cambridge University Press, 1991).

Included in *The Diversity of Life*, by Edward O. Wilson (Cambridge, Mass.: The Belknap Press of Harvard University, 1992), are lengthy discussions of the extent of biodiversity and the speed of the planet's species' depopulation. See also Wilson, "The High Frontier," *National Geographic* 180, no. 6 (December 1991): 78–107; and Wilson's book *Biophilia* (Cambridge, Mass.: Harvard University Press, 1984).

Recent figures on deforestation appear in Richard Monastersky, "The Deforestation Debate," *Science News* 144, no. 2 (July 10, 1993): 26–27.

Habitat diversity in the Amazon is the subject of several papers by Alwyn H. Gentry, including "Patterns of Neotropical Plant Species Diversity," in *Evolutionary Biology* 15 (1982): 1–84; "Phytogeographic Patterns in Northwest South America and Southern Central America as Evidence for a Choco Refugium," in Ghillean Prance, ed., *Biological Diversification in the Tropics* (New York: Columbia University Press, 1982), pp. 112–136; and, with Calaway H. Dodson, "Contribution of Non-trees to Species Richness of Tropical Rain Forest," *Biotropica* 19:149–156.

An entertaining pocket history of eighteenth- and nineteenth-century naturalists appears in Victor Wolfgang von Hagen, *South America Called Them: Explorations of the Great Naturalists — La Condamine, Humboldt, Darwin, Spruce* (New York: Alfred A. Knopf, 1945).

The first and still the most comprehensive review of thinking on biodiversity is found in the proceedings of the Smithsonian Institution's meeting on the subject, September 21–24, 1986, E. O. Wilson and Frances M. Peter, eds., *Biodiversity* (Washington, D.C.: National Academy Press, March 1988).

The loss of plant species and their potential value is discussed by Peter P. Principe, "Valuing the Biodiversity of Medicinal Plants," and Norman R. Farnsworth and Djaja D. Soejarto, "Global Importance of Medicinal Plants," in Akerele, Heywood, and Synge, eds. (see Chapter 4). See also Soejarto and Farnsworth, "Tropical Rainforests: Potential Sources of New Drugs?" *Perspectives in Biology and Medicine* 32, no. 2 (1989): 244–256.

Chapter 2 — Green Medicines

Among the oldest herbals in existence is that of Dioscorides, *The Greek Herbal.* It was compiled in the first century A.D. Almost four hundred illustrations were added by an anonymous Byzantine artist in A.D. 512. It was translated into English by John Goodyer in 1655 but not published until 1933, by Oxford University Press, and edited by Robert T. Gunther.

The prescription for antifungal medicine from the bark of the tree, genus *Virola,* comes from Richard Schultes and Albert Hofmann, *Plants of the Gods* (Maidenhead, England: McGraw-Hill, 1979), pp. 169–170.

The Ebers Papyrus prescription is cited in Krieg's *Green Medicine,* p. 215. The botanical interests of Egypt's Queen Hatshepsut and the Sumerian king Sargon are described in Knowles A. Ryerson, "History and Significance of the Foreign Plant Introduction Work of the United States Department of Agriculture," *Agricultural History* 7, no. 3 (July 1933): 110–128. See also Jack R. Harlan, "The Utility of Plant Exploration," *Twentieth Century Agricultural Science* 8, nos. 1–4 (January-December 1983).

The story of *silphion* from Cyrene is told by John M. Riddle and J. Worth Estes, "Oral Contraceptives in Ancient and Medieval Times," *American Scientist* 80, no. 3 (May-June 1992): 226–233.

The translation and contents of Metrodora's materia medica is described by Marianne Cianciolo, "Deciphering 1,500-Year-Old Greek Text Giving Clues to Medical, Women's History," *Current Research* (University of Cincinnati), March 6, 1992, p. 4.

The leading text on shamanism is considered to be Mircea Eliade's *Shamanism: Archaic Techniques of Ecstacy,* trans. Willard R. Trask (Princeton, N.J.: Princeton University Press, 1964). See also Nevill Drury, *The Elements of Shamanism* (Shaftesbury, Dorset: Element Books, Ltd, 1989); Michael J. Harner, ed., *Hal-*

lucinogens and Shamanism (New York: Oxford University Press, 1973); and Wade Davis, "Sacred Plants of the San Pedro Cult," *Botanical Museum Leaflets* (Harvard University) 29, no. 4 (Fall 1983).

For the Enlightenment's views on natural science, see Ray Spangenburg and Diane K. Moser, *The History of Science in the Eighteenth Century: On the Shoulders of Giants* (New York: Facts on File, 1993).

A history of foxglove, Calabar bean, opium, cinchona, and other early plant-based drugs appears in Norman Taylor, *Plant Drugs That Changed the World* (New York: Dodd, Mead & Company, 1965). See also Krieg's *Green Medicine*.

La Condamine's travels in Ecuador have been described in a translation of the eighteenth-century classic of exploration by Don George Juan and Don Antonio de Ulloa, *A Voyage to South America* (London: L. Davis and C. Reymers, 1758).

In addition to von Hagen's work on Humboldt, see Alexander von Humboldt, *Aspects of Nature* (Philadelphia: Lea and Blanchard, 1849).

For a book-length account of the history of curare, see Philip Smith, *Arrows of Mercy* (New York: Doubleday and Company, 1969).

Cinchona's history has been the subject of many books and articles. Besides sections in the cited books of Krieg, Taylor, and von Hagen, see William Campbell Steere, "The Cinchona Bark Industry of South America," *The Scientific Monthly* 41 (1945): 114–126. See also Anna Koffler, "Quinine," *Natural History* 50, no. 2 (1942). Spruce recalls his hunt for cinchona in *Notes of a Botanist*, Vol. 2, pp. 261–280. Another account of the origin of the cinchona fever bark discovery appears in Alexander von Humboldt, *Aspects of Nature*.

Chapter 3 — The Arrow Poison and the Yam

Richard Gill wrote many books about the Amazon. Some of curare's history, such as Hakluyt's account of Sir Walter Raleigh's encounter with curare, and the story of how Gill got curare in Ecuador, is contained in his book *White Water and Black Magic* (New York: Henry Holt and Company, 1940). Gill quotes from Hakluyt's history of the voyage, *The Principal Navigations, Voyages, Traffiques, and Discoveries of the English Nation* (New York: Dutton, Everyman's Library), Vol. VII, p. 321. Another account by Gill appears in "The Genie in the Ampoule," *Technology Review* (Massachusetts Institute of Technology) 43, no. 7 (May 1941).

For Gill's early days at Río Negro, see Richard Gill, "Curari — The Flying Death," *Natural History* 36 (November 1935): 278–292. Also, "Herbs and Simples — Jungle Style," *Natural History* 41 (January 1938): 29–33.

Ruth Gill also penned stories about Ecuador and Río Negro. See her story (by Mrs. Richard C. Gill) in *National Geographic* 45, no. 2 (February 1934): 133–172.

Medical research on curare is described by Abram E. Bennett, M.D., in "The History of the Introduction of Curare into Medicine," *Anesthesia and Analgesia . . . Current Researches* 47, no. 5 (September-October 1968).

A guide to plants with medicinal as well as poisonous properties is published by Steven Foster and James Duke, *Medicinal Plants (Eastern/Central)* (Boston: Houghton Mifflin Company, 1990).

Medical as well as historical detail of the curare story appears in the magazine *MD* (February 1965): 251–255.

Alexander von Humboldt makes mention of curare and the genus *Strychnos* in his memoir, *Aspects of Nature,* p. 165. His account of the making of the poison is quoted by Smith, *Arrows of Mercy,* pp. 69–70.

Giles G. Healey's contribution to curare's history is described in "Explorer Secures Arrow Tip Poison," *Boston Post,* July 2, 1927.

Gill recorded much of his final curare expedition in field notes now located at the Arthur E. Guedel Memorial Anesthesia Center in San Francisco. He also made an 8-millimeter film of the expedition, also kept at the Guedel Center. Logs from his 1938 expedition and correspondence concerning his subsequent efforts to commercialize curare are contained there, as well as reports, financial statements, and scientific documents Gill either wrote or collected, including identifications of the plants he brought back.

The botanical identifications of the ingredients of curare appear in B. A. Krukoff and A. C. Smith, "Notes on the Botanical Components of Curare — II," *Bulletin of the Torrey Botanical Club* 66 (May 1939): 305–314.

Squibb's curare research and commercialization of the drug are described in *Squibb Memoranda* 22, no. 3 (September 1943); and *Squibb Memoranda* 23, no. 3 (September 1944).

Ranyard West, M.D., "The Pharmacology and Therapeutics of Curare and Its Constituents," *Proceedings of the Royal Society of Medicine* (London) 28 (January 8, 1935): 565.

For a summary of Gill's contribution to curare's history, see Roy M. Humble, "The Gill-Merrill Expedition, Penultimate Chapter in the Curare Story," *Anesthesiology* 57, no. 6 (December 1982): 519–526.

A. E. Bennett wrote several monographs about his work with curare. See A. E. Bennett, "The Introduction of Curare into Clinical Medicine," *American Scientist* 34, no. 3 (Summer 1946).

The Badianus Manuscript: An Aztec Herbal of 1552, translated by Emily Walcott Emmart (Baltimore: Johns Hopkins Press, 1940). A short history of the discovery of the manuscript appears in the magazine *HerbalGram*, no. 27 (1992): 13–17.

Carl Djerassi, credited with the development of the oral contraceptive and a pioneer in steroid chemistry, recounts the story of diosgenin in his autobiography, *The Pill, Pygmy Chimps, and Degas' Horse* (New York: Basic Books, 1992). See also a letter to the editor by Djerassi in *Science* 258 (October 9, 1992): 203–204. Krieg's *Green Medicine* and Taylor's *Plant Drugs That Changed the World* also describe diosgenin's history.

An extensive history of Syntex and the hunt for cortisone and the Mexican yam can be found in Milton Silverman, "The Wonderful Medicine Plant," *Saturday Evening Post*, February 21, 1953. See also (Anon.) "Cortisone Made from Mexican Yams," *New York Times*, August 28, 1949; and Howard W. Blakeslee, "Yam to End Cortisone Scarcity," *Boston Herald*, July 7, 1951.

A Latin American viewpoint on the *Dioscorea* story is offered by Arturo Gomez-Pompa, "La Botanica Economica: Un Punto De Vista," a paper delivered at the Latin American Congress of Botany, Medellín, Colombia, June 1986.

For more on *Rauwolfia* and the discovery of reserpine, see Krieg's *Green Medicine*, pp. 317–339.

The cyclical nature of plant-hunting for pharmaceuticals is discussed by Norman R. Farnsworth and Ralph W. Morris, "Higher Plants: The Sleeping Giants of Drug Development," *American Journal of Pharmacy* 147, no. 2 (March-April 1976): 46–52. An account of one drug-hunting adventure in South America appears in Nicole Maxwell's book *Witch Doctor's Apprentice* (New York: Citadel Press, 1961).

Figures on drug company interest in phytochemicals and reasons for the decline in the science are listed by Farnsworth in "The Present and Future of

Pharmacognosy," *American Journal of Pharmaceutical Education* 43 (1979): 239–243. See also Ara H. Der Marderosian, "The Need for Cooperation Between Modern and Traditional Medicine," *HerbalGram*, no. 24 (Winter 1991): 30–36.

Chapter 4 — Ethnobotany

A discussion of ethnobotany in the New World appears in Richard I. Ford's "Ethnobotany: Historical Diversity and Synthesis," in Richard Ford, ed., *The Nature and Status of Ethnobotany*, Anthropological Papers No. 67 (Museum of Anthropology, University of Michigan), 1987.

Aldous Huxley discusses the meaning of art in his book *Heaven and Hell* (New York: Harper & Row, 1954).

Richard Evans Schultes pays homage to the great scientific explorers of the nineteenth century in *Where the Gods Reign: Plants and People of the Colombian Amazon*. For his comments on medicine men, see p. 152.

The quotation from Schultes's field journal is taken from Krieg's *Green Medicine*.

In addition to interviews with Richard Schultes, I have drawn from a profile of Schultes by E. J. Kahn, Jr., "Jungle Botanist," *The New Yorker*, June 1, 1992, pp. 35–58, and interviews with his students.

Schultes recalled his trips into the Amazon in Arthur F. Joy and Richard E. Schultes, "Twelve Years in a Green Heaven," *Natural History* 44, no. 3, 1955.

The phytochemistry of hallucinogens is colorfully and entertainingly described in Schultes and Hoffman, *Plants of the Gods*, and in Schultes and Hoffman, *The Botany and Chemistry of Hallucinogens* (Springfield, Ill.: Charles C. Thomas, 1980). See also Julie Ann Miller, "Botanical Divinities," *Science News* 118 (August 2, 1980): 75–77. Richard Spruce's experience with caapi and other hallucinogenic and medicinal plants is recounted in his *Notes of a Botanist in the Amazon and Andes*, Vol. 2, pp. 415–455.

The human attachment to landscape forms is discussed in Yi-Fu Tuan, *Topophilia: A Study of Environmental Perception, Attitudes and Values* (Englewood Cliffs, N.J.: Prentice-Hall, 1974). See also Tuan's book *Passing Strange and Wonderful: Aesthetics, Nature, and Culture* (Washington, D.C.: Island Press, 1993).

On the subject of *Virola* snuff, see Schultes, "A New Narcotic Snuff from the Northwest Amazon," *Botanical Museum Leaflets* (Harvard University) 16, no. 9

(July 12, 1954): 241–260; "*Virola* as an orally administered hallucinogen," *Botanical Museum Leaflets* 22, no. 6 (June 25, 1969): 229–239; "*Virola* as an Oral Hallucinogen among the Boras of Peru," *Botanical Museum Leaflets*, 25, no. 9 (November 30, 1977): 259–272; "Notes on Biodynamic Plants and Aboriginal Use in Northwestern Amazon," *Botanical Museum Leaflets* 26, no. 5 (May 30, 1978): 183; and B. Holmstedt et al., "Indole Alkaloids in Amazonian Myristicaceae: Field and Laboratory Research," *Botanical Museum Leaflets* 28, no. 3 (September 1980): 215–234. See also Schultes and Raffauf, *The Healing Forest*, and Schultes, *Where the Gods Reign* and *Plants of the Gods*.

Mark Plotkin's research on *Virola* (with coauthor Richard Schultes) is found in "*Virola:* A Promising Genus for Ethnopharmacological Investigation," *Journal of Psychoactive Drugs* 22, no. 3 (July-September 1990): 357–361. And finally, a chemical analysis of *Virola* alkaloids appears in A. Lai et al., "Phytochemical Investigation of *Virola peruviana*, A New Hallucinogenic Plant," *Journal of Pharmaceutical Sciences* 62, no. 9 (September 1973): 1561–1563.

Mark Plotkin's ethnobotanical work in Suriname is described in Donald Dale Jackson, "Searching for Medicinal Wealth in Amazonia," *Smithsonian* 19, no. 11 (February 1989): 95–103. See also Anne Fadiman, "Dr. Plotkin's Jungle Pharmacy: An Ethnobotanist Goes Native for Science," *Life*, June 1987, pp. 14–16. See also Mark J. Plotkin, "Ethnobotany, Conservation and the Future of the Tropical Forest," *IUCN/SSC Primate Specialist Group Newsletter*, no. 4 (March 1984): 49–54.

Several articles on economic botany, ethnobotany, extractive reserves, conservation, and ethnobotanical ethics appear in a special issue of the magazine *Garden* (New York Botanical Garden), November-December 1990. The authors are Michael J. Balick, Elaine Elisabetsky, Charles M. Peters, Douglas Daly, Steven R. King, and Brian M. Boom.

An account of snakebite and ritualistic healing is described by Michael Balick, "Modern Medicine and Shamanistic Ritual: A Case of Positive Synergistic Response in the Treatment of a Snakebite," *Journal of Ethnopharmacology* (Lausanne, Switzerland) 5 (1982): 181–185.

Comments by Michael Balick on Belize are drawn from interviews with the author and published reports. The latter include Samantha Franklin, "Traditional Healers Lead Scientists to Biologically Active Plants," *Oncology Times* 13, no. 11 (November 1991); Robin Eisner, "Botanists Ply Trade in Tropics, Seeking Plant-Based Medicinals," *The Scientist* 5, no. 12 (June 10, 1991): 1; Eugene Linden, "Lost Tribes, Lost Knowledge," *Time* 138, no. 12 (September 23, 1991); William K. Stevens, "Shamans and Scientists Seek Cures in Plants," *New York Times*, January 28, 1992, p. C1; Michael Balick, "The Belize Ethnobotany Project," *Fairchild Tropical Garden Bulletin* (Fairchild Tropical Gardens, Miami), April 1991, pp. 17–24.

The economic value of tropical rainforest medicinals, rainforests as a source of medicinal plants is discussed by Michael Balick, "Assessing the Economic Value of Traditional Medicines from Tropical Rain Forests," *Conservation Biology* 6, no. 1 (March 1992): 128–130. Balick's study of hits from randomly and ethnobotanically collected plants in Belize appears in D. J. Chadwick and J. Marsh, eds., *Bioactive Compounds from Plants* (Chichester, England: J. Wily and Sons, 1990), pp. 22–38. See also Constance Holden, "Saving Forests with Their Own Medicine," *Science* 256 (April 17, 1992): 312.

Chapter 5 — Biophilia

Spruce's quotation, "The largest river in the world . . ." is from *Notes of a Botanist*. Also quoted in Schultes, *Where the Gods Reign*.

For discussions of what rainforests are, and deforestation and extinction rates, see Wilson and Peter, eds., *Biodiversity*, especially chapters by Paul Ehrlich and Norman Myers, and Wilson's book *The Diversity of Life*.

On the subject of why rainforests are so biodiverse, see Eric R. Pianka, *Evolutionary Ecology* (New York: Harper & Row, 1978); Carol Kaesuk Yoon, "Rainforests Seen as Shaped by Human Hand," *New York Times*, July 27, 1993, p. C1; Joseph H. Connell, "Diversity in Tropical Rain Forest and Coral Reefs," *Science* 199 (March 24, 1978): 1302–1310; Jared Diamond, "Factors Controlling Species Diversity: Overview and Synthesis," *Annals of the Missouri Botanical Garden* 75 (1988): 117–129; John Flenley, "The Origins of Diversity in Tropical Rain Forests," *Tree* 8, no. 4 (April 1993): 119; and David Jablonski, "The Tropics as a Source of Evolutionary Novelty Through Geological Time," *Nature* 364 (July 8, 1993): 142–144. On the topic of rainforest refugia, see Paul A. Colinvaux, "The Past and Future Amazon," *Scientific American* 260, no. 5 (May 1989): 102–108.

The tenfold area/species doubling rule is fully described in Edward O. Wilson and Robert H. MacArthur's *The Theory of Island Biogeography* (Princeton, N.J.: Princeton University Press, 1967).

For discussion of human genetics and the culture, see Edward O. Wilson and Charles Lumsden, *Genes, Mind and Culture* (Cambridge, Mass.: Harvard University Press, 1981).

On the link between habitat selection, landscaping, and human origins, see Gordon H. Orians, "Habitat Selection: General Theory and Applications to Human Behavior," in Joan Lockard, ed., *The Evolution of Human Social Behavior* (New York: Elsevier, 1980), pp. 49–66. See also Tuan, *Topophilia*.

Edward O. Wilson's views on mankind's relationship with nature and biodiversity are explored in his books *Biophilia* and *On Human Nature* (Cambridge, Mass.: Harvard University Press, 1978), and in personal interviews with the author. For a profile of Edward O. Wilson, see Robert Wright, *Three Scientists and Their Gods* (New York: Harper and Row, 1988). A collection of essays on the subject of biophilia appears in Stephen R. Kellert and Edward O. Wilson, eds., *The Biophilia Hypothesis* (Washington, D.C.: Island Press, 1993).

Chapter 6 — Biodiversity Prospecting

Deforestation rates in the tropics and in the United States are taken from reports by the United Nation's Food and Agricultural Organization. See William Booth, "Tropical Forests Disappearing at Faster Rate," *Washington Post,* September 9, 1991.

Early efforts by Chico Mendes and others to establish extractive reserves are described in Alex Shoumatoff, *The World Is Burning* (Boston: Little, Brown, 1990).

"Valuation of an Amazonian Rainforest," by Charles M. Peters, Alwyn H. Gentry, and Robert O. Mendelsohn, is widely believed to have brought economics and tropical botany together in a way that pointed conservationists and biologists toward a solution to the deforestation of tropical forests. It was published in *Nature* 339 (June 29, 1989): 655–656.

Sustainable harvesting of timber by strip-cutting is described by Gary S. Hartshorn, "Natural Forest Management by the Yanesha Forestry Cooperative in Peruvian Amazonia," in A. B. Anderson, ed., *Alternatives to Deforestation: Steps Toward Sustainable Use of the Amazon Rain Forest* (New York: Columbia University Press, 1990), pp. 128–137.

Rates of discovery in drug exploration and related costs are the subject of a paper by James D. McChesney, "Biological Diversity, Chemical Diversity and the Search for New Pharmaceuticals," delivered at the symposium *Tropical Forest Medical Resources and the Conservation of Biodiversity,* January 24–25, 1992, held in New York City by the Rainforest Alliance. See also Walter V. Reid et al., eds., *Biodiversity Prospecting: Guidelines for Using Genetic and Biochemical Resources Sustainably and Equitably* (Washington, D.C.: World Resources Institute, INBio, Rainforest Alliance, and the African Centre for Technology Studies, 1993).

The renaissance in natural drug discovery is described in Varro E. Tyler, "Plant Drugs in the 21st Century," *Economic Botany* (New York Botanical Garden) 40, no. 3 (1986): 279–288.

Ardent support for tropical ethnobotany and the revival of pharmacognosy comes from The Conservation Foundation's Mark J. Plotkin, in "Conservation, Ethnobotany, and the Search for New Jungle Medicines: Pharmacognosy Comes of Age . . . Again," *Pharmacotherapy* 8, no. 5 (1988): 257–262.

For numbers on the percentage of drugs derived from natural products from the tropics, see Soejarto and Farnsworth, "Tropical Rainforests: Potential Sources of New Drugs?", supra.

Chapter 7 — From Osa to New Jersey

An account of Janzen's research into the guanacaste tree is described by Jeremy Cherfas, "The Tropical Tree That Travels by Horse," *New Scientist,* June 11, 1987, pp. 46–52. Janzen outlines his philosophy for forest restoration in Janzen, "Tropical Ecological and Biocultural Restoration," *Science* 239, no. 837 (January 15, 1988): 243–244. See also Don Lessem, "From Bugs to Boas, Dan Janzen Bags the Rich Coast's Life," *Smithsonian* 17 (December 1986): 110–116.

Reforestation techniques for tropical forests is the subject of Daniel H. Janzen, "Management of Habitat Fragments in a Tropical Dry Forest: Growth," *Annals Missouri Botanical Garden* 75 (1988): 105–116.

In addition to numerous interviews with staff at INBio and Merck & Company and two visits to INBio, I have drawn on the articles that describe their collecting arrangement, including: Laura Tangley, "Cataloging Costa Rica's Diversity," *BioScience* 40, no. 9 (October 1990): 633–636; Leslie Roberts, "Chemical Prospecting: Hope for Vanishing Ecosystems?" *Science* 256 (May 22, 1992): 1142–1143; and Diane Gershon, "If Biological Diversity Has a Price, Who Sets It and Who Should Benefit?" *Nature* 359 (October 15, 1992): 565. I have also drawn on internal documents from INBio and Merck.

Costa Rica's flora and fauna are cataloged in the compendium edited by Daniel Janzen, *Costa Rican Natural History* (Chicago and London: The University of Chicago Press, 1983). One hundred and seventy-four scientists contributed abstracts delineating the country's storehouse of wildlife, along with descriptions of climate, geology, soils, agriculture, and biotic history.

For a history of land-use and conservation in the tropics, see Roger D. Stone, *The Nature of Development* (New York: Alfred A. Knopf, 1992).

Eisner's insect work is reviewed by Diane Ackerman, "Insect Love," *The New Yorker,* August 17, 1992, pp. 34–54; Joyce and Richard Wolkomir, "Uncovering the Chemistry of Love and War," *National Wildlife* 28, no. 5 (August-

September 1990): 44–50; John Horgan, "The Man Who Loves Insects," *Scientific American* 265, no. 6 (December 1991): 660–664; and Christopher Joyce, "The Beetles, the Frogs, and the French Legionnaires," *New Scientist* 129, no. 1750 (January 5, 1991): 17.

Thomas Eisner's views on chemical prospecting and the INBio contract with Merck are described in Eisner's "Prospecting for Nature's Chemical Riches," *Issues in Science and Technology* (National Academy of Sciences), Winter, 1989–1990, pp. 31–34.

A short history of Merck's discoveries from natural products appears in a Merck magazine, *Merck World* 12, no. 5 (November 1991).

Details of the Merck contract with INBio were obtained from INBio internal documents, interviews in Costa Rica and the United States, and from news sources. See also the analysis of the value of biodiversity in general and the INBio experiment in particular in Reid et al., eds., *Biodiversity Prospecting*.

A scientific inventory of the flora of the Osa Peninsula and the forests near Golfito is described by Gary Hartshorn in Janzen, *Costa Rican Natural History*, pp. 132–136.

For details of the research into spider venom and neurotransmitters, see Kathryn Phillips, "Spider Man," *Discover*, June 1991, pp. 48–53.

Chapter 8 — Shamans, Profits, and Ethics

Details of the presentations at the January 24–25, 1992, meeting at Rockefeller University can be obtained in the proceedings, Rainforest Alliance, New York, New York.

Details of Merck's investigation of *tike-uba* appear in John W. Jacobs et al., "Characterization of the Anticoagulant Activities from a Brazilian Arrow Poison," *Thrombosis and Haemostasis* (Stuttgart) 63, no. 1 (1990): 31–35. The Indians who use it are the Urueu-Wau-Wau in the province of Rondonia, described in Loren McIntyre, "The End of Innocence," *National Geographic*, December 1988, pp. 813–817.

Articles describing Shaman Pharmaceuticals include: Deanna Hodgin, "Seeking Cures in the Jungle," *Insight*, October 7, 1991, pp. 30–31; Anon., "Rainforest Pharmaceuticals," *Natural Health*, May/June, p. 17. Three articles by Steven King are "Conservation and Tropical Medicinal Plant Research," *HerbalGram*, no. 27, 1992, pp. 28–35; "The Source of Our Cures," *Cultural*

Survival Quarterly (Cambridge, Mass.), Summer 1991, pp. 19–22; and "Among the Secoyas," *The Nature Conservancy Magazine* 41, no. 1 (January/February 1991): 6–13.

Part 2: Rainforest Rx

Chapter 9 — Blood of the Dragon

Bradley C. Bennett's research on western Amazonian plants appears in "Plants and People of the Amazonian Rainforests," *BioScience* (American Institute of Biological Sciences, Washington, D.C.) 42, no. 8 (September 1992). See also "Biological and Economic Studies to Support the Development of Extractive Reserves in Amazonian Ecuador," U.S. Agency for International Development Report, Grant No. 518-0780-G-00-0247-00, 15 May 1991–15 November 1991.

For general information about Ecuador, see Rob Rachowiecki, *Ecuador and the Galápagos Islands* (Hawthorne, Victoria, Australia: Lonely Planet Books, 1989).

Data on Ecuador's natural forest resources are taken from a report by Bruce Cabarle, "An Assessment of Biological Diversity — Ecuador" (Center for International Development and Environment of the World Resources Institute, Washington, D.C.), n.d. See also Alwyn H. Gentry, "Patterns of Neotropical Plant Species Diversity," *Evolutionary Biology* 15 (1982): 1–84; Gentry, "Phytogeographic Patterns in Northwest South America and Southern Central America as Evidence for a Choco Refugium," in Ghillean Prance, ed., *Biological Diversification in the Tropics* (New York: Columbia University Press, 1982), pp. 112–136; and, with Calaway H. Dodson, "Contribution of Non-trees to Species Richness of Tropical Rain Forest," *Biotropica* 19:149–156. The Rio Palenque mahogany is described in Cabarle, ibid, and also in Wilson's *The Diversity of Life*. Wilson quotes Norman Myers's account of the hot spots of biodiversity.

Archidona and Tena are two of the many places visited by Don George Juan and Don Antonio de Ulloa and described in *A Voyage to South America*. The colonial city of Quito and its environs are described in Book V, "Journey from Guayaquil to the City of Quito."

Ecuador's flora in the Oriente is described in David Neill, "Ecuador Forest Sector Development Project, Flora of Ecuador Subproject, Final Report," Missouri Botanical Garden, September 1991.

The story of Orellana's voyage down the Napo and the Amazon, and Carvajal's description of the Amazon warriors, are recounted in von Hagen's *South America Called Them.*

Quichua use of plants and some details of the culture's history are published in a paper by Robin J. Marles, David A. Neill, and Norman R. Farnsworth entitled "A Contribution to the Ethnopharmacology of the Lowland Quichua People of the Amazonian Ecuador," in the *Review of the Colombian Academy of Exact Physical and Natural Sciences* 16, no. 63 (1988): 111–120.

The history of the candirú or carnero fish is elucidated in gory detail by John R. Herman, M.D., in the journal *Urology* 1, no. 3 (March 1973): 265–267.

Comments on being a naturalist by Edward O. Wilson are from personal interviews in 1991 and 1992. Wilson describes the "naturalist's trance" and the organisms that are the object of such a trance in his book *Biophilia.*

For early research on sangre de drago, see a letter concerning the Euphorbiaceae from S. Morris Kupchan et al. to *Science* magazine, February 1976, pp. 571–572. These researchers found an extract, a diterpene diester, was active against tumors in rats. John A. Beutler discusses the chemistry of the plant in an unpublished paper, "Sangre de grado" (*grado* appears to be interchangeable with *drago* in the nomenclature), Chemistry Department, Northeastern University, n.d. See also Richard E. Schultes, "*Croton glabellus,*" *Botanical Museum Leaflets* (Harvard University, Cambridge, Mass.) 28, no. 1 (March 1980): 21. More recent chemical research is described in an unpublished doctoral thesis by Luc Peters, University Antwerpen, Belgium, 1992.
   P. Bernabe Cobo's comments on sangre de drago appear in *Historia del Nuevo Mundo* (Madrid: Ediciones ATLAS, 1964), p. 271.

Chapter 10 — The Vainilla Express

The activities of oil companies in Ecuador were described to the author in interviews with a company official in Quito in June 1992, and with staff members of Cultural Survival and the Missouri and New York Botanical Gardens. See also Joe Kane, "With Spears from All Sides," *The New Yorker,* September 27, 1993, pp. 54–79; and Michael Stott, "U.S. Oil Firm Seen Threatening Amazon Tribal Ways," Reuters News Service, September 6, 1993.

In addition to Spruce's *Notes of a Botanist in the Amazon and Andes,* see Alexander von Humboldt's *Aspects of Nature* for descriptions of western Amazonian flora and fauna. A popular account of the area appears in Richard Conniff, "RAP: On the Fast Track in Ecuador's Tropical Forests," *Smithsonian* 22, no. 3 (June 1991): 36–48.

The flora of Cotacachi-Cayapas are believed to be part of the southern tip of the Choco, the world's wettest and most biodiverse forests. Choco flora are described by Alwyn H. Gentry, "Species Richness and Floristic Composition of Choco Region Plant Communities," *Caldasia* 15, nos. 71–75 (October 30, 1986): 71–91.

The world record for diversity of tree species, in Iquitos, Peru, was established by Alwyn H. Gentry and published in *The Proceedings of the National Academy of Sciences* (Washington, D.C.) 85 (1988): 156–159.

The latitudinal species gradient is discussed, along with a list of publications on the subject, in George C. Stevens, "The Latitudinal Gradient in Geographical Range: How So Many Species Coexist in the Tropics," *American Naturalist* 133, no. 2, 240–256.

Of La Condamine's voyage from Esmeraldas to Quito, see Juan and Ulloa's work, *A Voyage to South America*. See also von Hagen, *South America Called Them*, Chapter 3.

The agricultural practices in and around Borbón were described to the author by Bruce Cabarle, personal communication.

A history and anthropology of the Chachi, also called the Cayapas, was written by S. A. Barrett, *Cayapa Indians of Ecuador*, July 1908, after he spent nine months living with them on the Río Cayapas. It has not been published commercially.

Chapter 11 — San Miguel

The Jívaro are the subject of an ethnography by Michael J. Harner, *The Jívaro: People of the Sacred Waterfalls* (Berkeley: University of California Press, 1972). Also see the volume edited by Harner, *Hallucinogens and Shamanism*.

Harner's ethnography of the Jivaro quotes several historical texts on Jívaro history. These include Marcos Jiménez de la Espada, *Relaciones Géograficas de Indias*, Tomo 4, *Peru* (Ministerio de Fomento, Madrid), 1897; Juan de Velasco, *Historia del Reino de Quito in la América Meridonial*, Tomo 3 and part 3 of *La Historia Moderna* (Imprenta del Gobierno por J. Campusano, Quito, 1842); and William Bollaert, "On the Idol Human Head of the Jívaro Indians of Ecuador, with a Translation of the Spanish Document Accompanying It, the History of the Jívaro and their Conspiracy against the Spaniards in 1599," *Transactions of the Ethnological Society of London*, 2:112–118.

Brad Bennett's research with the Shuar appears in Bennett, Marc Baker, and Patricia Gomez Andrade, "Ethnobotany of the Untsuri Shuar of Eastern Ecuador," *Advances in Economic Botany* (in press).

Waorani use of forest species was studied by E. Wade Davis and James A. Yost, "The Ethnobotany of the Waorani of Eastern Ecuador," *Botanical Museum Leaflets* (Harvard University) 29, no. 3 (Summer 1983): 159–217.

Darrell Posey's discussion of Kayapó usage of plants and animals appears in *Ways and Means of Strengthening Sustainable and Environmentally Sound Self-Development of Indigenous Peoples*, U.N. Doc. E/CN.4/Sub.2/1992/31/Add 1.

Morpho butterflies are the subject of a chapter in the naturalist's journal of Allen M. Young, *Sarapiqui Chronicle* (Washington, D.C.: Smithsonian Institution Press, 1991), pp. 85–153.

Von Humboldt describes the Amazonian river swimmers in *Aspects of Nature*, p. 420.

Chapter 12 — The End of the Pipeline

Medical uses including cancer treatments from temperate plants are cataloged in Foster and Duke, *Medicinal Plants*. Drugs from tropical plants are listed in "Medicine: Our Stake in the Rainforest," Rainforest Alliance, New York, New York, and other documents compiled by this environmental group.

Vincristine and vinblastine are described in Mark J. Plotkin's "Ethnobotany, Conservation and the Future of the Tropical Forest," supra.

Plants with medical uses, including anti-cancer activity, are discussed by James A. Duke in "Promising Phytomedicinals," *The Journal of Naturopathic Medicine* 2, no. 1, 48–52, and Duke, "Tropical Botanical Extractives," lecture for the symposium on rainforest conservation, Panama, June 18–21, 1991.

Nontraditional cancer treatments and the controversy over their potential merit is the subject of a report by the Office of Technology Assessment, *Unconventional Cancer Treatments* (U.S. Congress, OTA: Washington, D.C.), Government Printing Office Document H-405, September 1990.

For a discussion of *Artemisia* and malaria research, see Lisa Hooker, "Molecules for Medicine," *Johns Hopkins Magazine* 54, no. 3 (June 1992): 16–21.

Sources of drugs from the sea are described in "Sea Is the New Frontier for Developing Drugs," *New York Times*, November 10, 1992, p. C5.

The National Cancer Institute's natural products screening program is discussed in several publications, including: Erik Eckholm, "Quest for Cancer

Drugs: U.S. Devises Major New Strategy," *New York Times,* December 23, 1986, p. C1; Ann Raver, "A Botanical Hunt," *New York Newsday,* November 4, 1986, pp. 4–5.

For an account of NCI's resurgent natural products drug discovery program, see Saul A. Schepartz et al., "Summary of the Workshop on Drug Development, Biological Diversity, and Economic Growth," *Journal of the National Cancer Institute* 83, no. 18 (September 18, 1991): 1294–1298; Kari Smigel, "Scientists Find Better Ways to Find Better Drugs," *Journal of the National Cancer Institute* 83, no. 19 (October 2, 1991): 1370–1372; Dick Thompson, "Giving Up on the Mice," *Time,* September 17, 1990, p. 79.

Developing drug screens for natural products is described by Michael R. Boyd in "Status of the NCI Preclinical Antitumor Drug Discovery Screen," *Principles and Practice of Oncology* 3, no. 10 (October 1989): 1–11, and Michael R. Boyd, "The Future of New Drug Development," in J. E. Niederhuber, ed., *Current Therapy in Oncology* (Philadelphia: B. C. Decker, Inc., 1991). See also Rebecca Kolberg, "Casting a Wider Net to Catch Cancer Cures," *Journal of NIH Research* 2 (April 1990): 82–84.

Chapter 13 — The Yew

A history and biology of the yew tree has been written by Hal Hartzell, Jr., *The Yew Tree: A Thousand Whispers* (Eugene, Oreg.: Hulogos, 1991).

James Duke has studied Native American uses of the yew as well as taxol content in various species and cultivars. See Duke's *Handbook of Northeastern Indian Medicinal Plants* (Lincoln, Nebr.: Quarterman Publications, 1986), p. 156. Also James Duke, "You, Yew, and Yule: America's Most Valuable Tree," unpublished paper.

Historical information about the discovery of taxol appears in Douglas Daly, "Tree of Life," *Audubon* 94, no. 2 (March/April 1992): 76–85. See also (Anon.), "Taxol — Thirty Years in the Wings," *Washington Insight,* September 15, 1990, p. 7; Tom Reynolds, "Government Moves to Increase Supply of Taxol," *Journal of the National Cancer Institute* 83, no. 15 (August 7, 1991): 1054–1057; and Tom Reynolds, "House Subcommittee Scrutinizes Taxol Agreements," *Journal of the National Cancer Institute* 83, no. 16 (August 21, 1991): 1134–1135; Marilyn Chase, "A New Cancer Drug May Extend Lives — At Cost of Rare Trees," *Wall Street Journal,* April 9, 1991, p. A8.

Environmentalists' concerns about the Pacific yew were laid out in a letter from the Environmental Defense Fund, Washington, D.C., to U.S. Secretary of the Interior Manuel Lujan, September 19, 1990.

For taxol chemistry, see Elizabeth Pennisi, "Beyond Yew: Chemists Boost Taxol Yield," *Science News* 141, April 18, 1992, p. 244; Paul A. Wender and Thomas P. Mucciaro, "A New and Practical Approach to Synthesis of Taxol and Taxol Analogues: The Pinene Path," *Journal of the American Chemical Society*, no. 114, 1992, pp. 5878–5879; Richard Pazdur et al., "Phase I Trial of Taxotere: Five-Day Schedule," *Journal of the National Cancer Institute* 84, no. 23 (December 2, 1992): 1781–1788; and the proceedings of the "Second National Cancer Institute Workshop on Taxol and *Taxus,* September 23–24, 1992. National Cancer Institute, National Institutes of Health, Bethesda, Maryland.

Results of early clinical trials of taxol are reported by William P. McGuire III and Eric K. Rowinsky et al., "Taxol: A Unique Antineoplastic Agent with Significant Activity in Advanced Ovarian Epithelial Neoplasms," *Annals of Internal Medicine* 111, no. 4 (August 15, 1989): 273–279; and Frankie Ann Holmes, "Phase II Study of Taxol in Patients with Metastatic Breast Cancer," Proceedings of the annual meeting of the American Society for Clinical Oncology, Houston, Texas, May 19–21, 1991.

A summary of taxol results up to early 1993, by Eric K. Rowinsky, William P. McGuire III, and Ross C. Donehower, appears in William J. Hoskins et al., eds., *Principles and Practice of Gynecologic Oncology Updates* (Philadelphia: J. B. Lippincott Company, n.d.), Vol. 1, pp. 1–16.

The fungus that produces taxol was reported by Gary Strobel et al., "Taxol and Taxane Production by *Taxomyces andreanae,* an Endophytic Fungus of Pacific Yew," *Science* 260 (April 9, 1993): 214–216. See also in the same issue "Lorem Ipsum Dominae Here We Go Again," by Richard Stone.

Chapter 14 — Disappearing Cures

Details on Shaman Pharmaceutical's business plans can be found in *Prospectus: Shaman Pharmaceuticals, Inc.,* S. G. Warburg Securities, the First Boston Corporation, January 26, 1993.

The chemistry of calanolide A is described in Yoel Kashman et al., "A Novel HIV-Inhibitory Class of Loumarin Derivatives from the Tropical Rainforest Tree *Calophyllum lanigerum,*" *Journal of Medicinal Chemistry* (American Chemical Society) 35, no. 15 (1992): 2735–2743. The hunt for *Calophyllum* is described by Ron Dorfman, "Potential AIDS Drug from Malaysian Rain Forest," *In the Field* (Bulletin of the Field Museum of Natural History), November/December 1992, p. 1; and internal NCI documents. Costatolide and the fate of the *Calophylla* tree are outlined in internal NCI documents presented at the Drug Decision Network Committee meeting at the National Institutes of Health, Bethesda, Maryland, May 24, 1993.

The Samoan anti-AIDS plant is described in Kirk R. Gustafson et al., "A Non-promoting Phorbol from the Samoan Medicinal Plant *Homolanthus nutans* Inhibits Cell Killing by HIV-1," *Journal of Medicinal Chemistry* 35, no. 11 (May 29, 1992): 1978–1986. See also Tonya Whitfield, "A Botanist Fights to Save the Samoan Rain Forest," *Chronicle of Higher Education*, November 18, 1992, p. A5.

The scope of intellectual property rights vis-à-vis biodiversity is discussed by Michael Gollin, Esq., "An Intellectual Property Rights Framework for Biodiversity Prospecting," in Reid et al., eds., *Biodiversity Prospecting*, pp. 159–197. See also Josephine R. Axt, M. Lynne Corn, Margaret Lee, and David M. Ackerman, *Biotechnology, Indigenous Peoples, and Intellectual Property Rights* (Washington, D.C.: Congressional Research Service, Library of Congress), Doc. 93-478-A, April 16, 1993.

A special issue of *Cultural Survival Quarterly*, Summer 1991, is devoted to intellectual property issues.

For details on the neurotoxin homobatrachotoxin, see Natlie Angier, "Rare Bird Indeed Carries Poison in Bright Feathers," *New York Times*, October 30, 1992, p. A1.

Cultural Survival's views on NCI's letter of intent were put forward in a letter from CS attorney Janet McGowan to Gordon Cragg at NCI, June 6, 1991.

For a short description of the search for Australia's *Conospermum*, see Sue Katz Miller and Leigh Dayton, "Australia Takes Tough Line on 'HIV plant,' " *New Scientist*, July 3, 1993, p. 4.

Chapter 15 — The Flowers of *Ancistrocladus*

Korup National Park and the Thomases' work there is described in Duncan Thomas et al., *Korup Ethnobotany Survey*, a report to the World Wide Fund for Nature, Godalming, Surrey, U.K., July 1989.

The first scientific paper to describe Michellamine was Kirk P. Manfredi et al., "Novel Alkaloids from the Tropical Plant *Ancistrocladus abbreviatus* Inhibit Cell Killing by HIV-1 and HIV-2," *Journal of Medicinal Chemistry* (American Chemical Society), December 1991, pp. 3402–3405.

Chapter 16 — Time Holds Us Green

Descriptions of the organization of reserves by the Awá and Kuna appear in Jason Clay, *Indigenous Peoples and Tropical Forests*, Cultural Survival Report 27 (Cultural Survival, Cambridge, Mass.), 1988.

Equitable sharing of biodiversity profits is the subject of an essay by Darrell Posey, "Intellectual Property Rights and Just Compensation for Indigenous Knowledge," *Anthropology Today* 6, no. 4 (August 1990): 13–16.

Edward O. Wilson's statement on the folly of allowing species extinction to continue at such a high rate is quoted by Mark Plotkin in "Traditional Knowledge of Medicinal Plants — the Search for New Jungle Medicines," in Akerele, Heywood, and Synge, eds., *Conservation of Medicinal Plants*. See also Wilson's article "Is Humanity Suicidal?" *New York Times Magazine,* May 30, 1993, p. 24. His calculations of the rate of species loss appear in his book *The Diversity of Life.*

Index